Manipal Manual of
Clinical Medicine
for Postgraduate Students

Manipal Manual of
Clinical
Medicine

for Postgraduate Students

BA Shastry

Professor
Department of Medicine
Consultant Physician
Kasturba Medical College and Hospital
Manipal, Karnataka, India

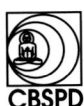

CBSPD

CBS Publishers & Distributors Pvt Ltd

New Delhi • Bengaluru • Chennai • Kochi • Kolkata • Lucknow • Mumbai
Hyderabad • Jharkhand • Nagpur • Patna • Pune • Uttarakhand

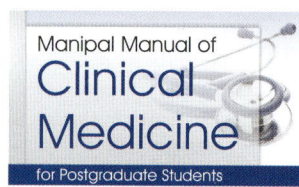

Manipal Manual of
Clinical Medicine
for Postgraduate Students

ISBN: 978-93-89688-04-7

Copyright © Author and Publisher

First Edition: 2021
Reprint: 2023

Published by Satish Kumar Jain and produced by Varun Jain for

CBS Publishers & Distributors Pvt Ltd
4819/XI Prahlad Street, 24 Ansari Road, Daryaganj, New Delhi 110 002, India
Ph: 011-23289259, 23266861

Website: www.cbspd.com
e-mail: delhi@cbspd.com

Corporate Office: 204 FIE, Industrial Area, Patparganj, Delhi 110 092, India
Ph: 011-4934 4934   Fax: 011-4934 4935   e-mail: publishing@cbspd.com; publicity@cbspd.com

Branches

- **Bengaluru:** Seema House 2975, 17th Cross, K.R. Road, Banasankari 2nd Stage, Bengaluru 560 070, Karnataka, India
  Ph: +91-80-26771678/79   Fax: +91-80-26771680   e-mail: bangalore@cbspd.com
- **Chennai:** 7, Subbaraya Street, Shenoy Nagar, Chennai 600 030, Tamil Nadu, India
  Ph: +91-44-26680620, 26681266   Fax: +91-44-42032115   e-mail: chennai@cbspd.com
- **Kochi:** 42/1325, 1326, Power House Road, Opp KSEB, Power House, Ernakulam, Kochi, 682 018, Kerala, India
  Ph: +91-484-4059061-65   Fax: +91-484-4059065   e-mail: kochi@cbspd.com
- **Kolkata:** 147, Hind Ceramics Compound, 1st Floor, Nilgunj Road, Belghoria, Kolkata 700 056, West Bengal, India
  Ph: +91-33-25633055/56   e-mail: kolkata@cbspd.com
- **Lucknow:** Basement, Khushnuma Complex, 7-Meerabai Marg (behind Jawahar Bhawan), Lucknow 226 001, UP, India
  Ph: +91-522-4000032   e-mail: tiwari.lucknow@cbspd.com
- **Mumbai:** PWD Shed, Gala no. 25/26, Ramchandra Bhatt Marg, Next to JJ Hospital Gate no. 2,
  Opp. Union Bank of India, Noorbaug, Mumbai 400 009, Maharashtra, India
  Ph: +91-22-66661880/89   e-mail: mumbai@cbspd.com

Representatives

- **Hyderabad**   0-9885175004
- **Patna**   0-9334159340
- **Jharkhand**   0-9811541605
- **Pune**   0-9923910676
- **Nagpur**   0-9421945513
- **Uttarakhand**   0-9716462459

Printed at HT Media Ltd., Greater Noida, UP, India

to

---

my wife and children

Preface

*M*anipal Manual of Clinical Medicine has been written to help the postgraduate students in internal medicine to prepare for their final examination.

Keeping in view the vastness of clinical medicine especially for postgraduates, four main topics (CNS, CVS, RS and GIT) have been covered in detail and smaller topics have been covered in brief. Standard textbooks of medicine and clinical methods and monograms have been used as references while preparing this book.

Since all the basic aspects of clinical medicine have been covered in my book *Manipal Manual of Clinical Medicine*, they are not repeated in this book. Postgraduate students and readers are requested to read *Manipal Manual of Clinical Medicine* before reading this book.

I sincerely thank my colleagues, artist and computer operators for their constant support and for the initial preparation of the manuscript and computer work.

I sincerely thank Mr SK Jain, CMD, CBS Publishers & Distributors, New Delhi, for the support given to me while preparing this book.

I welcome any suggestion and criticism by the students to improve the quality of this book.

BA Shastry

Contents

Cardiovascular System

APPROACH TO A PATIENT OF CARDIAC DISEASE

Suspect cardiac disease under the following circumstances

- History of dyspnea, chest pain and palpitation.
- Recurrent syncope (due to severe aortic stenosis, cardiac conduction defect).
- History of sudden cardiac death in the family (due to acute myocardial infarction or obstructive cardiomyopathy, prolonged QT, etc.).
- Known hypertensive, diabetes mellitus and IHD.
- Taking cardiac medications
- On anticoagulants/antiplatelet drugs.

Suspect following cardiac disease depending on the history

- Congenital heart disease
- Rheumatic heart disease
- Hypertensive heart disease
- Ischemic heart disease
- Cardiomyopathy.

Congenital heart disease (*see* under approach to congenital heart disease).

Rheumatic heart disease (*see* under valvular heart disease).

Hypertensive heart disease

Suspect

- If there is history of hypertension.
- Presence of cardiac symptoms usually after 35–40 years of age.

- Sudden onset of acute coronary syndrome/aortic dissection/cerebrovascular accident
- Sudden onset of LVF.

 Note

Early morning occipital headache, irritability, epistaxis, blurring of vision and dizziness are nonspecific symptoms of hypertension.

Suspect ischemic heart disease if there are symptoms of

1. Precordial pain—angina
2. Symptoms of cardiac disease after 4th decade
3. Presence of chest pain, palpitation, dyspnea
4. Sudden onset of LVF
5. Sudden cardiac death
6. Recurrent arrhythmias
7. Associated diabetes mellitus and hypertension, smoking and obesity.

Cardiomyopathy: *Primary*: Is a diagnosis of exclusion.

If there are symptoms of cardiac disease without evidence of HT, IHD, RHD and congenital heart disease, consider the diagnosis of cardiomyopathy.

Normal Hemodynamics of Cardiovascular System

Cardiac output: It is the amount of blood which is pumped by the heart/minute = 70 ml × 72 = around 5 L/min.

Stroke volume: It is the amount of blood which is pumped by the ventricle = 70 ml/each LV contraction.

Ejection fraction: It is the amount of ventricular blood which is pumped out by the heart out of total amount of blood which is collected in the ventricle (expressed as % or fraction). It indicates systolic function of the ventricle.

- Normal ejection fraction: 50 to 70%
- Below normal: 36 to 49%
- Low ejection fraction: Less than 35%
- Ejection fraction >70 to 75%, e.g.: Obstructive cardiomyopathy.

Preload: It is the load with which the cardiac muscle (ventricle) contracts. It is determined by the end diastolic volume which stretches ventricular muscle fiber.

After load: It is the stress/load against which the cardiac muscle has to eject blood—depends on the aortic root pressure and systemic vascular resistance.

Systolic dysfunction: Occurs due to disease of the ventricles.

Results in decrease contraction of the ventricle and decrease in the cardiac output with decreased ejection fraction.

Diastolic dysfunction: Inability of the ventricle to relax with decreased filling of the ventricle due to decrease compliance of the ventricle. Associated with increased ventricular wall resistance.

Heart failure with preserved ejection fraction: It is mainly due to diastolic dysfunction. Ejection fraction is > 50%. There is increased stiffness with decreased relaxation of the ventricle.

Pulmonary hang out interval: It is the time interval taken by the pulmonary valve to close after equalization of pressure between the right ventricle and pulmonary artery. Even after equalization of pressure blood continues to flow into the pulmonary artery till the pulmonary vascular resistance increases as it is a low resistance vessel (normal pulmonary hang out interval = 60 to 80 milliseconds).

Aortic hang out interval: Compared to pulmonary valve, aortic valve closes immediately due to high systemic vascular resistance.

Aortic hang out interval is negligible.

Important Laws of Physics in the Hemodynamics of Cardiovascular System

Frank Starling's law: Energy of contraction is proportional to the initial length of the cardiac muscle fiber.

In cardiac muscle, length of cardiac muscle fiber is proportional to the end diastolic volume of the ventricle. As the end diastolic volume is increased, force of contraction of the ventricle is increased.

Coanda effect: Fluid attaches to the nearby surface whenever the jet of flow occurs through a pipe or a vessel. Even if the surface it flows takes a curved direction, it remains attached to the surface it is flowing.

Clinical significance: In supravalvular aortic stenosis jet of aortic flow is predominantly directed to the right innominate, as a result left carotid, left radial pulse and blood pressure on the left side becomes lower than the right side.

Venturi effect: There will be reduction in the fluid pressure occurs when the fluid flows through a narrower section of a pipe.

Clinical significance: There will be decreased pressure on the atrial side of mitral and tricuspid regurgitation and ventricular side of aortic and pulmonary regurgitation. Because of sudden decrease of pressure causing injury to the endothelium, the vegetations can occur over the following sites in infective endocarditis.

- In MR—vegetations on the left atrial side
- In TR—vegetations on the right atrial side
- In AR—vegetations on the LV side

- In PR—vegetations on the RV side
- In VSD—vegetations on the RV side
- In PDA—vegetations on the pulmonary artery side.

Measurement of pressures in different cardiac chambers: Different chambers of the heart and their hemodynamic measurements.
Right ventricular pressure: 15–30 mm Hg
Right atrial pressure: 5–10 mm Hg
Left atrial pressure: 5–12 mm Hg
Left ventricular pressure:
- Systolic: 90–140 mm Hg
- Diastolic: 5–12 mm Hg

Pulmonary artery pressure: 9–20 mm Hg
Aortic root pressure
- Systole: 110–140 mm of Hg
- Diastole: 70–90 mm Hg

Pulmonary capillary wedge pressure: 4–12 mm of Hg
Pulmonary vascular resistance: <250 dynes/sec/cm^{-5}
Systemic vascular resistance: 900–1500 dynes/sec/cm^{-5}

CORONARY CIRCULATION

Normal coronary arteries
- Right coronary artery
- Left coronary artery

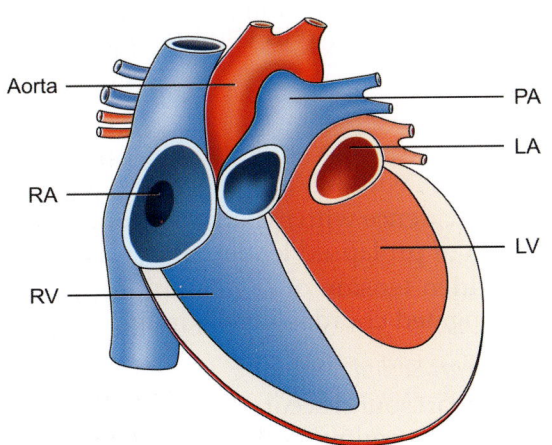

Fig. 1.1: Different chambers of heart

Right coronary artery
- *Branches*: Right marginal artery, posterior descending artery.
- *Supplies*
  - Right side of heart
  - LV inferior wall
  - Interventricular septum
  - Posterior papillary muscle
  - In 60% of persons sinus node is supplied by right coronary artery
  - In 40% of persons sinus node is supplied by left circumflex artery.

Left coronary artery
Branches
- Left anterior descending (LAD)
- Left circumflex
- LAD-branches—diagonal artery
- Left circumflex branches: Obtuse marginal artery
- Left circumflex artery: Supplies left atrium, side and base of LV
- LAD: Supplies front and bottom of LV and front of interventricular septum.

Coronary dominance: If the posterior descending artery is from right coronary artery, this is called right dominant (70%).

If the posterior descending artery is from left coronary artery, this is called left dominant (20%).

It is the AV nodal artery which is deciding the dominance.

Normal coronary blood flow: 225 ml/min.

EXAMINATION OF CARDIOVASCULAR SYSTEM

JVP (Jugular Venous Pressure)
- JVP at bed side is measured in cm of water
- "a" wave occurs just before the 1st heart sound
- In TR-V wave is prominent with rapid Y descent (rapid fall in pressure)
- In TS and cardiac tamponande Y descent can become less prominent due to obstruction to the flow of blood into the right ventricle.

Positive Abdominojugular Reflux

Apply pressure over the right hypochondrium for at least 10 seconds.

Increase in the height of the JVP for more than 3 cm which is persisting for more than 15 seconds after the release of pressure from the hand.

JVP in Pericardial Disorders

In cardiac tamponade X-descent is present with absent Y-descent.

Explanation

- Jugular venous pressure changes occur due to changes in the right atrial pressure and venous filling of the atrium.
- In patient with severe cardiac tamponade the total intracardiac volume is fixed. Venous blood can get into the right atrium only when the blood is leaving the heat.
- X-descent appears when blood is getting out from the heart during ejection of blood from the ventricle as blood is entering into the heart. There is X-descent.
- Y-descent appears when tricuspid valve is opening (ventricular filling). So blood is getting into the heart. As total cardiac volume cannot further increase in tamponade—Y-descent is lost.

Constrictive Pericarditis

- X-descent with prominent Y-descent.
- Early diastolic filling is rapid in constrictive pericarditis (due to high atrial pressure and small end systole) (LV volume). There is rapid Y-descent.

INSPECTION OF CARDIOVASCULAR SYSTEM

Shield Chest

Angle between the body of the sternum and manubrium—greater than normal.

Widely separated nipples: For example, Turner and Noonan's syndrome.

Pectus Excavatum

- Sternum displaced posteriorly

For example:
- Marfan's syndrome
- Homocystinuria
- Ehlers-Danlos syndrome
- MVP

In pectus excavatum:
- Signs of heart disease—apparent than real.
- May be associated with palpitation, tachycardia, fatigue and dyspnea.

Important Clinical Signs while Examining the Precordium

Shaking of entire precordium with each heart beat: For example, AR, MR, PDA, VSD, HOCM, complete heart block.

Biventricular hypertrophy: Can cause systolic retraction between RV and LV impulse.

Left atrial enlargement: Keep the index finger of one hand at the apex and index finger of the other hand in left parasternal region in the 3rd intercostal space. Movement and lifting of latter finger begins and ends slightly later than the first.

Right atrial enlargement: Marked pulsation at right of sternum.

Normal apex: Palpable single outward pulsation. Normal apex is less than 2 cm and is well circumscribed. Apex more than 10 cm left to mid-sternal line—consider LVH.

LVH: Persistent outward systolic pulsation of the apex with retraction of parasternal region.

Mid-systolic click

- High frequency and clicking sound—in patients with MVP.
- Coincidence with maximal systolic excursion of prolapsed leaflet.
- Sudden tension of redundant leaflet and elongated chordae results in the click.

First heart sound

- 1st heart sound occurs due to simultaneous closure of mitral and tricuspid valves.
- It is heard loudest at the apex.

Causes of loud 1st heart sound
- Mitral stenosis
- Tachycardia.

Causes of soft 1st heart sound
- Acute AR
- Rheumatic mitral regurgitation
- Bradycardia.

Causes of split 1st heart sound
- Due to delayed tricuspid component— RBBB
- VPCs

Causes of loud 1st heart with loud tricuspid component
- ASD
- Ebstein's anamoly
- In LBBB—1st heart sound is single due to delayed mitral component

2nd heart sound
- 2nd heart sound is produced by the closure of aortic and pulmonary valves.
- It marks the end of ventricular systole.
- Normally aortic valve closes earlier than the pulmonary valve causing physiological split of 2nd heart sound (normal split— 0.02 to 0.08 sec).

Physiological splitting of 2nd heart sound
- Normally aortic valve closes earlier than pulmonary valve.
- During inspiration pulmonary valve closure is further delayed causing widening of split.
- During expiration pulmonary valve closes earlier than inspiration causing narrowing of splitting of 2nd heart sound.

Wide and persistent split of 2nd heart sound
Causes
- Pulmonary embolism
- VSD
- PAPVC
- RBBB due to delayed pulmonary closure.
- Severe MR—early closure of aortic valve.

Wide and fixed split of 2nd heart sound
Cause: Septum secundum ASD

Paradoxical splitting: During expiration—both A_2 and P_2 are audible.
Causes: In severe AS and LBBB—aortic component is delayed due to delayed closure of aortic valve.

Loud aortic component of 2nd heart sound
Causes
- Systemic hypertension
- Severe AR (syphilitic AR—tambour quality of A_2).

Loud pulmonary component—Loud P_2
- P_2 can be palpated in the pulmonary area.
- It is heard with greater intensity than A_2 at the base of the heart.
- Loud P_2 can be appreciated even at the apex on auscultation.

Causes of loud P_2
- For example, all causes of pulmonary hypertension.
- ASD
- Straight back syndrome
- Idiopathic dilation of pulmonary artery.

Causes of soft A_2: Severe valvular aortic stenosis.

Causes of soft P_2
- Severe pulmonary stenosis.
- Fallot's tetralogy

Persisting splitting of 2nd heart sound (not fixed)
(split is present during expiration and inspiration)
- Due to delayed RV systole: RBBB
- Due to prolonged RV systole: ASD (fixed split)
- Pulmonary stenosis and pulmonary embolism
- Due to shorter LV systole with early closure of aortic valve: Severe MR, VSD.

3rd heart sound
- 3rd heart sound is produced—during passive left ventricular filling.
- Occurs when the blood is striking the left ventricle which is compliant.

- Physiological 3rd heart sound occurs in
  - Children
  - Athletes
  - Pregnant females.

Characteristics of 3rd heart sound
- Low-pitched sound.
- Better heard with the bell of the stethoscope.
- Left-sided 3rd heart sound is best heard at the apex (on expiration).
- Right-sided 3rd heart sound is heard in the tricuspid area (on inspiration).
- Pathological 3rd heart sound indicates systolic heart failure.
- 3rd heart sound is heard in the diastole after the 2nd heart sound. It is called proto-diastolic sound.

Table 2.1: Differences between 3rd heart sound and split S₂	
S_3	Split S_2 (A_2 and P_2)
Low-pitched sound	High-pitched sound
Better heard with the bell of the stethoscope	Better heard with the diaphragm of the stethoscope
Left-sided S3—best heard in the left lateral—position at the apex	Better heard in the pulmonary area.

4th heart sound
- 4th heart sound occurs during the presystolic phase of the ventricular filling.
- It is heard due to forceful contraction of the atrium into a noncompliant ventricle which cannot expand further.

Characteristics
- Low-pitched sound.
- Heard better with the bell of the stethoscope.
- Heard before the 1st heart sound (presystolic sound).
- Left-sided S_4—best heard in the apex.
- Right-sided S_4—best heard at 4th/5th intercostal space—left sternal border.

Conditions associated with 4th heart sound
Left-sided S_4
- Essential hypertension

- Aortic stenosis
- HOCM.

Right-sided S_4
- Pulmonary hypertension
- Pulmonary stenosis.

 Note

4th heart sound does not occur in a patient of atrial fibrillation.

Ejection clicks/sounds
- Ejection click occurs due to rapid movement of aortic or pulmonary leaflet during opening of corresponding valves.
- For example, aortic ejection click—bicuspid aortic valve.
- Pulmonary ejection click—valvular pulmonary stenosis.
- Ejection sounds: Occurs in dilated artery either due to dilatation of aorta or pulmonary artery.
- Ejection sound occurs due to vibrations of walls of dilated arteries.

DYNAMIC CARDIAC AUSCULTATION
Following physiologic maneuvers are performed during cardiac auscultation.

Purpose: To differentiate different cardiac auscultatory events and cardiac lesions.

Different Maneuvers
- Respiratory variation
- Postural changes
  - Standing
  - Squatting
- Isometric exercise
- Valsalva maneuver
- Passive leg raising
- Left lateral position
- Stooping forward position.

Respiration
- Best to assess the cardiac events during normal respiration.

- There is negative intrathoracic pressure and increase in the venous blood flow into the right heart and decreased pulmonary vascular resistance during inspiration.
- All right-sided cardiac events increase during inspiration except pulmonary ejection click.
- Severe pulmonary hypertension and right-sided cardiac failure—does not cause increase of cardiac events during inspiration.

Cardiac events which increase on inspiration
- RVS_3 and RVS_4
- Opening snap of tricuspid valve
- Normal splitting of 2nd heart sounds—widening of split occurs during inspiration.

Murmurs of right sided
TS, TR, PS and PR murmurs increase during inspiration.

Events better heard during expiration
- Heart sounds—LVS3 and LVS4. Mitral opening snap.
- Left-sided murmurs—like MS, MR, AS and AR, VSD may or may not increase on expiration but does not decrease.
- Pulmonary ejection click: Better heard during expiration.

Postural Standing
Hemodynamic consequences
- Decrease of systemic venous return
- Decrease of cardiac output

Heart sound: Decrease in the split of 2nd heart sounds.

Murmurs: All left-sided murmurs decrease.
   There is decrease in the size of LV and murmur of HOCM increase and occurrence of click and murmur of MVP earlier.

Squatting
Hemodynamic Consequences
There is increase of venous return initially.
   Increase in the peripheral vascular resistance (kinking of femoral arteries).

Murmurs: Most of the left-sided murmurs increase except—there will be decrease murmur of HOCM and delayed click and murmur of MVP (due to increased LV size and decrease of LVOT obstruction).

Isometric Exercise
Perform bilaterally with handgrip or handball and hold it for about 30 to 40 seconds.

Contraindicated in
- Acute and severe ischemic heart disease
- Severe/accelerated hypertension
- Ventricular arrhythmias.

Hemodynamic consequences
- Increase of peripheral vascular resistance
- Increase systolic and diastolic pressure
- Increase in LV size

Murmurs
- All left-sided regurgitant murmurs increase (AR, MR)
- Murmur of aortic stenosis decrease
- Murmur of HOCM decrease
- Click and murmur of MVP delayed.

VALSALVA MANEUVER
- Person is asked to breath out against closed glottis.
- Asked to blow against aneroid manometer.
- To maintain the pressure around 40 mm of HG for about 30 seconds.

Different Phases of Valsalva
Phase I: Initial straining phase for about 1–3 seconds.
Phase II: Maximum straining phase.
Phase III: Cessation of straining
Phase IV: Relaxation phase.
   Most of the hemodynamic changes occur during (phase II) valsalva maximum strain phase.

Physiological Consequences of Valsalva Maneuver
- There is increase in the intra-thoracic pressure

- Decrease of venous return
- Increase of heart rate
- Decrease in the cardiac output

Murmurs: Most of the murmurs and heart sounds decrease during valsalva strain.

Murmur of HOCM and MVP (decrease LV size)

- Increase in the intensity of HOCM murmur
- Early occurrence of click and murmur of MVP.

Left Lateral Position

Events which are better heard in left lateral position

- 1st heart sound
- LVS_3
- LVS_4

Opening snap of mitral stenosis and murmur of mitral stenosis and Austin Flint murmur—better heard during expiration and in left lateral position.

Sitting and Leaning Forward Position

Murmur of aortic and pulmonary valves are better heard (comes closer to the chest wall) in sitting and leaning forward position.

Passing Leg Raising

- Increase of venous return.
- Murmur of tricuspid valve increases except in patients with hepatic outflow obstruction and RVF.

Effect of Premature Ventricular Contraction (PVC) on Cardiac Hemodynamics

After PVC: There is complete compensatory pause with increased time for LV filling with increase in the aortic flow. As the aortic stenotic murmur depends on the aortic flow, there is increase in the intensity of aortic stenosis after VPC but murmur of MR does not change as it does not depend on LV filling.

Beat to beat variation of murmur in multiple VPCs occur with murmur of aortic stenosis.

Pharmacological Agents in Dynamic Auscultation

Amyl nitrate inhalation

- Produces vasodilation and decreases peripheral resistance.
- There is decrease of AR and MR murmur.
- There is increase in AS murmur.

Important Clinical Points while Examining the Cardiovascular System

Palmar crease xanthoma is associated with type 3 hyperlipidemia.

While examining JVP a wave precedes 1st heart sound and v wave follows after 2nd heart sound and v wave is smaller compared to a wave.

Pulsus Bisferiens is better appreciated in the brachial artery: Prosthetic valve dysfunction is indicated by change in the murmur with change of quality of murmurs.

Pulsus Paradoxus

Occurs in a patient of cardiac tamponade.

There will be decrease of blood pressure more than 10 mm of Hg during inspiration.

What is the Paradox?

In spite of decrease of blood pressure and pulse volume decrease, heart sound is still heard.

Recording of Pulsus Paradoxus

BP cuff is inflated 20 mm of Hg above systolic pressure.

Deflate the cuff 2 to 3 mm of Hg/sec till the first Korotkoff's sound is heard (during expiration and may not be heard during inspiration). Record the blood pressure.

Deflate the cuff further till the Korotkoff's sound is heard during both inspiration and expiration. Record the BP recording. If the difference between the two recordings is more than 10 mm of Hg, it is suggestive of pulsus paradoxus.

Reverse Pulsus Paradoxus

There will be inspiratory increase in the blood pressure during inspiration and decrease during expiration.

Causes

- HOCM
- Intermittent positive pressure breathing

In HOCM there will be increase of LVOT obstruction during expiration. During inspiration intra-LV pressure increases with decrease of obstruction (during inspiration there is decrease of intra-thoracic pressure and intra-pericardial pressure with increase in the LV transmural pressure with decrease LVOT obstruction).

DIFFERENT CARDIAC POSITIONS IN THE CHEST

Normal position of heart in the chest is called situs solitus.

Situs Solitus (Fig. 1.2)

- Normal heart and viscera position
- Heart position—left side in the thoracic cavity.
- Doom of the diaphragm—left lower.
- Aortic position—left side.
- Cardiac chamber—LV and LA on the left side of RA and RV
- Stomach—on the left side of the abdomen.

Situs Solitus with Dextrocardia (Fig. 1.3)

- Heart in the right thoracic cavity (apex of the heart points to the right).

- Left atrium and ventricle are on the left side of the heart (Fig. 1.3).
- Right atrium and right ventricle—placed to the right of LA and LV.
- Right doom of the diaphragm—lower than the left.
- Liver, lungs and all the viscera—normal (situs solitus).

Situs Inversus with Dextrocardia (Fig. 1.4)

All the thoracic and abdominal viscera are exactly mirror image of normal position (mirror image of situs solitus).

Visceral Position in Situs Inversus

- Heart side: Right side
- Heart chambers: Right atrium and right ventricle are positioned to the left of left atrium and left ventricle.
- Fundus of stomach: Right side
- Liver: Left side
- Right doom of the diaphragm is lower than the left side
- Descending aorta: Right side.

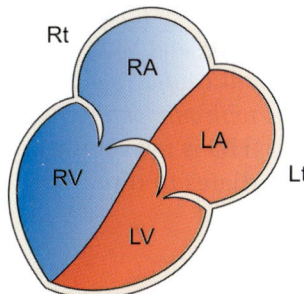

Fig. 1.3: Situs solitus with dextrocardia

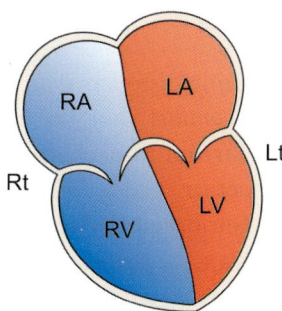

Fig. 1.2: Normal position situs solitus

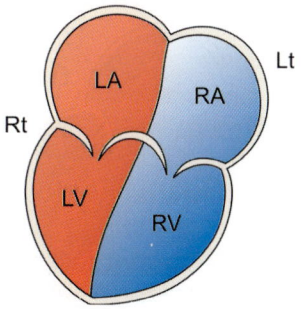

Fig. 1.4: Situs inversus with dextrocardia

Situs Inversus with Levocardia (Fig. 1.5)

- All the thoracic and abdominal viscera are placed: Mirror image of normal position except the heart.
- Heart is placed on the left side of the thoracic cavity.
- Left cupola of the diaphragm is lower than right.

Cardiac chambers: LA and LV are on right of RA and RV.

Mesocardia (Heart Midline)

- Heart is in the middle of thoracic cavity.
- All the abdominal and thoracic visceral structures are in normal position (situs solitus).

Congenital anomalies associated with cardiac malposition

Situs inversus with dextrocardia: Not associated with cardiac abnormalities.

Isolated dextrocardia: Can be associated with septal defects or pulmonary or aortic outflow obstruction.

Levocardia with situs inversus: Can be associated with complicated congenital heart disease.

Cardiac examination and symptoms of heart disease in different cardiac malpositions

Situs inversus with mirror image dextrocardia: Chest pain of IHD is felt on the anterior part of the chest radiates to ulnar border of right upper limb.

Cardiac examination

Situs inversus with mirror image dextrocardia:
- Cardiac apex—right side.

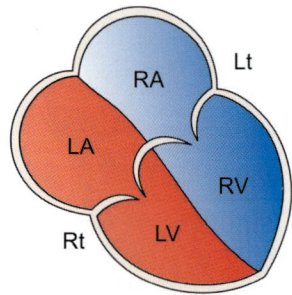

Fig. 1.5: Situs inversus with levocardia

- Cardiac dullness—percussed on the right side of the chest.
- Liver dullness—on the left side of the abdomen.
- Fundal resonance of stomach—on the right side.
- Heard sounds—1st and 2nd heart sounds are heard better on the right side.
- 2nd heart sound—splitting is better on the right 2nd intercostal space.

ECG and X-ray Chest in Situs Inversus with Dextrocardia

X-ray chest
- Fundal gas—on the right side
- Liver shadow left of the abdomen.
- Cardiac shadow—right side of the chest

ECG
- QRS—negative in lead I and aVL
- P wave negative lead I and aVL
- Prominent R wave in V1.

Dextroposition of the Heart

Position of the heart is in the right side of the chest due to noncardiac causes like right lung fibrosis or eventration of the diaphragm on the left side.

Dextroversion of the Heart

- Due to severe right-sided rotation of the heart.
- Heart is in the right side of the chest. LV lies anteriorly. Relation of the cardiac chambers is normal. LV lies to the left of RV.

CHEST PAIN

Four life-threatening disorders which cause acute chest pain or discomfort
- Acute myocardial infarction
- Aortic dissection
- Pulmonary embolism
- Pneumothorax.

Other causes of acute chest pain—cardiac causes
- Stable angina

- Unstable angina
- Acute pericarditis.

Other causes of ischemic pain—cardiac causes
- Aortic valve disease
- Mitral regurgitation
- HOCM
- Pulmonary artery hypertension.

Cardiac causes of chest pain which mimic angina but with normal coronaries due to
- MVP
- Pulmonary artery hypertension.

Causes of chest pain which can mimic angina but not of cardiac origin
- Costochondritis
- Pleuritis
- Gastroesophageal reflux, herpes zoster
- Gall bladder disease
- Cardiac neurosis

Clinical approach to the chest pain for cardiac origin

Acute myocardial infarction (MI)
- Precordial pain—typical angina pain—severe, prolonged more than 30 minutes.
- Pain is radiating to the jaw, interscapular area.
- Pain does not radiate below the umbilicus.
- If the pain radiates to the trapezius—pain is more likely to be due to pericarditis.
- Associated features like sweating, hypotension, dyspnea, syncope can be present.
- Diabetics and elderly need not have chest pain in acute myocardial infarction.

Description of symptoms favoring angina: Symptoms like heaviness of chest, feeling of breathlessness, anxiety, sweating (angina equivalents) usually favor pain of coronary artery disease.

Cardiac syndrome X
- Patient c/o angina pain with ECG changes
- Abnormal stress test.
- Normal coronary angiography
- May be microvascular disease.

There will be abnormality of coronaries like coronary spasm, and increased coronary vasoconstrictor response.

 Note

Other conditions cause chest pain which can be considered as differential diagnosis of angina are discussed in separate chapters.

Features of typical angina
- Site of pain: Retrosternal
- Type of pain: Pressing/heaviness
- Duration: 2–5 minutes

Brought on by
- Exertion
- Emotional stress

Relieved by
- Rest
- Sublingual nitroglycerin

Radiation: Tip of shoulder, jaw, left upper limb, ulnar border.

Unstable Angina
- Anginal pain which is lasting for more than 10 minutes and occurs at rest.
- New onset of angina pain with increased severity.

Aortic dissection
- Sudden onset of sharp central chest pain radiating to back: In between the shoulders.
- Patient can suddenly have a cardiovascular collapse.
- Patient is usually a hypertensive and can have aortic valve disease with aortic dilatation.
- Other conditions like Marfan's syndrome and Ehlers-Danlos syndrome may cause aortic dissection.
- There will be spreading subclinical hematoma within the wall of aorta.

Pulmonary embolism
- Sudden onset of chest pain—massive occlusion of pulmonary artery can cause substernal pain.

- Pain can occur due to infarction of the lung causing pleuritic pain or due to rapid dilatation of pulmonary artery.
- Pulmonary artery embolism can cause hemoptysis due to pulmonary infarction.
- Miniature emboli cause pulmonary infarction and pleuritic pain.
- Patient of pulmonary embolism can present with acute dyspnea.
- There will be risk factors for pulmonary embolism.

Pneumothorax
- Sudden onset of unilateral pleuritic pain.
- Sudden onset of cough and dyspnea.
- History of pulmonary tuberculosis/COPD.

> **Key Points: Regarding chest pain**
> - Consider always possible dangerous life-threatening causes whenever patient complains of chest pain especially with risk factors for IHD.
> - Gradual worsening of pain over a few minutes-may be possible acute MI/pulmonary embolism.
> - Pain of myocardial ischemia usually radiates to left upper limb but rarely it can also radiate to the right side.

PALPITATION

> **Key Points:**
> - Many episodes of palpitation are benign and self-limiting.
> - Persons with dangerous arrhythmias may not complain of palpitation.
> - History of drug intake, alcohol, smoking, caffeine is important in the evaluation of palpitation.

Approach to a Patient of Palpitation
Palpitation Type and Clinical Significance and Type of Arrhythmia
- Sustained regular or racing type—suggests SVT.
- Sustained irregular palpitation—atrial flutter/atrial fibrillation.
- Abrupt onset with fluttering feeling in the chest—atrial/ventricular tachy arrhythmias.

- With abrupt termination of palpitation—SVT.
- Feeling of sudden heart stopping with thumping sensation in the chest—atrial or ventricular premature contractions.
- Pulsatile feeling with increased heart beat may be due to aortic regurgitation, fever, anemia, thyrotoxicosis.

Relationship of Palpitation to Body Position
- Palpitation changes with body position—AV nodal tachycardia.
- Palpitation on lying left lateral position—severe aortic regurgitation.

Relationship of Palpitation to Exercise
- Exercise-induced palpitation: Physiological
- Prolonged palpitation after exercise—may indicate SVT/atrial fibrillation (? due to ↑ sympathetic stimulation).
- Palpitation: May be on awakening can occur due to obstructive sleep apnea.
- Feeling of pounding like sensation in the neck: Due to regular/irregular cannon waves due to—complete heart block/AV nodal rhythm/reentry tachycardia/supraventricular arrhythmias
- Palpitation which is related to anxiety and emotional stress: Due to panic attack/long QT syndrome/torsades de pointes/pheochromocytoma
- Palpitation which suddenly stops after
  - Pressure on the neck
  - Change of breathing
  - Valsalva
  } AV nodal re-entry tachycardia

History of syncope/presyncope/dizziness can be associated with supraventricular and ventricular arrhythmias/Stokes-Adams attack.

Enquire following history in a patient of palpitation
- Alcohol intake
- Quinalone intake
- Sympathomimetic drugs
- Diabetes, hypertension, ischemic heart disease

- Thyroid disease
- Smoking
- Caffeine intake
- Infection—especially pulmonary
- Neurological disorder.

History of polyuria—after an attack of palpitation—due to supraventricular tachycardia—release of atrial natriuretic factor.

🔑 Key Points:

- Macrolides and fluoroquinalones can cause prolonged QT syndrome with polymorphic VT.
- Family history of sudden death can be present in patients with long QT syndrome.
- Valvular heart disease can cause palpitation either due to—arrhythmia/chamber hypertrophy or compensatory tachycardia because of decreased cardiac output during exertion.

Examination of a Patient of Palpitation

Look for
- Presence of pallor
- Blood pressure
- Cannon wave in the JVP
- Evidence of RHD
  - Congenital heart disease
  - HOCM
  - MVP
- Complete heart block
- Thyroid swelling/pheochromocytoma/autonomic neuropathy.

SYNCOPE

Syncope in Cardiac Disease

Cardiac Causes of Syncope

a. *Structural heart disease*
  - Severe aortic stenosis
  - Severe mitral and pulmonary stenosis
  - Hypertrophic obstructive cardiomyopathy
  - Left atrial myxoma
  - Pericardial effusion.

b. *Due to abnormal cardiac rhythm*
  Due to decreased heart rate
  - Sick sinus syndrome

- Complete AV block
- Type II-A.V block (Mobitz type 2 block)
Due to increased heart rate
- Due to ventricular tachyarrhythmias
- Due to disorders causing cardiac arrhythmias:
  - Prolonged QT syndrome.
  - Brugada syndrome
- Arrhythmias due to myocardial ischemia
  - Acute myocardial infarction

c. *Postural syncope*: Left atrial myxoma, antihypertensive drugs, diuretic therapy.

Clinical approach to a patient of cardiac syncope:

Structural heart disease producing syncope:
- Exertional syncope—typically occurs in severe aortic stenosis
- Post-exertional syncope: Occurs in patients with obstructive cardiomyopathy.
- Syncope, dizziness can also occur in patients with severe mitral stenosis, pulmonary stenosis and severe pulmonary hypertension.
- Structural heart disease can predispose to arrhythmias causing syncope.
- Ventricular stretch can result in baroreceptor response causing bradycardia, vasodilatation and syncope (e.g. aortic stenosis).

Syncope due to arrhythmias
- Sick sinus syndrome (SA node dysfunction) can cause bradycardia-tachycardia syndrome.
- Syncope can also occur due to Mobitz type 2 block and complete heart block in whatever position of the patient.
- Prolonged pause following tachycardia is usually associated with syncope in a patient of sinus node dysfunction.
- Brugada syndrome also predisposes to ventricular arrhythmias and can cause sudden cardiac death.
- IHD can cause syncope due to arrhythmias.

- Ventricular rate (>200/minute) causes decrease diastolic ventricular filling and ventricular dysfunction causing syncope.
- Prolonged QT interval (congenital/drug induced) can cause syncope and sudden cardiac death due to ventricular arrhythmias like torsades de pointes and ventricular fibrillation. Acute myocardial infarction predisposes to cardiac arrhythmias causing syncope.
  - Acute MI can cause hypotension, peripheral circulatory failure and syncope.
  - Chronic myocardial ischemia can predispose to dangerous ventricular arrhythmias causing syncope.

Syncope in cardiac disease due to drug therapy
- Treatment of cardiac disease with drugs like anti-hypertensives and diuretics.
- Beta blockers and vasodilators can cause orthostatic hypotension and can cause postural syncope.

Clinical approach to a patient of cardiac syncope
Syncope irrespective of position of the patient
- Complete heart block.
- Mobitz type 2 block
- Sick sinus syndrome

Exertional/post-exertional syncope: Valvular AS/HOCM

Associated with palpitation: Cardiac arrhythmias.

Associated with dyspnea/chest pain:
- Valvular heart disease
- IHD

History of intake of cardiac medication and syncope: Due to postural hypotension.

Syncope on standing: Can also be due to left atrial myxoma.

Family history of sudden cardiac death:
- Cardiac arrhythmias
- HOCM
- MVP
- IHD

HYPERTENSION

Staging of Hypertension

Normal Blood Pressure (at all ages)
- Systolic less than 120 mm of Hg
- Diastolic less than 80 mm of Hg

Prehypertensive state: Systolic blood pressure: 120–139 mm of Hg or diastolic blood pressure 80–89 mm of Hg.

Stage I hypertension: Systolic blood pressure 140–159 mm of Hg or diastolic blood pressure 90–99 mm of Hg

Stage II hypertension: Systolic blood pressure ≥160 to 179 mm of Hg and diastolic blood pressure ≥100 mm to 109 mm of Hg.

Stage III hypertension: Systolic blood pressure of 180 and above and diastolic BP of 110 mm of Hg and above.

Isolated systolic hypertension
- Systolic blood pressure ≥140 mm of HG
- Diastolic blood pressure ≤90 mm of Hg.

Causes of isolated systolic hypertension
Due to increase cardiac output states:
a. Valvular heart disease: Aortic regurgitation
b. Congenital heart disease: PDA
c. Endocrine disease: Thyrotoxicosis
d. AV: Fistula
e. Febrile state

Due to increased stiffness of artery with decreased compliance: Atherosclerosis.

Clinical Approach to a Patient of Hypertension

Most of the patients of hypertension may not have any symptoms and are detected on routine clinical examination.

Some patients of hypertension can directly present with acute/chronic complications of hypertension without prior history.

Historical Aspects in a Patient of Hypertension

Nonspecific symptoms of hypertension
- Early morning occipital headache

- Dizziness
- Blurring of vision

They can also have symptoms like irritability, epistaxis and impotence.

Enquire following history in all patients of hypertension

1. If he is already on treatment.
2. Time duration of hypertension.
3. Dietary salt intake and socioeconomic history.
4. Smoking, alcohol, weight gain, lipid abnormality and diabetes mellitus.
5. *Symptoms of cardiovascular disease*: Chest pain, palpitation, dyspnea.
   Cerebrovascular disease: TIA, decreased vision and CVA.
   Peripheral vascular disease: Claudication pain in the lower limb.

Patient of hypertension can also present with acute LVF, intracerebral hemorrhage and renal insufficiency.

Examination of a Patient of Hypertension

General Physical Examination

- Height, weight, BMI.
- Features of secondary hypertension (*see* under secondary hypertension).

Proper BP recording

- Two times—office recordings—in basal conditions
- If white coat hypertension is suspected or sudden episodes of hypertension or autonomic neuropathy: 24 hours monitoring of blood pressure is required.
- BP recording should also be done in:
  - Supine and standing position.
  - Both arms
  - Also lower limb

Cardiovascular System Examination

Peripheral cardiovascular system

Pulse: *For rate, rhythm*

- Tachycardia may occur due to atrial fibrillation, common in patients of hypertension.

Volume of the pulse: High volume pulse—in patients of isolated systolic hypertension.

Condition of vessel wall: Thickening of vessel wall—arteriosclerosis.

Peripheral pulse: For peripheral vascular disease.

Ophthalmic fundus for hypertensive retinopathy and carotid and aortic bruit for occlusive vascular disease.

Precordial Examination

- For evidence of LVH: Hearing apex
- Left-sided S4: Due to less compliant left ventricle
- Loud A2: Due to forcible closure of aortic valve
- Ejection systolic murmur: Across aortic valve
- Evidence of CCF.

Acute Complications of Hypertension

Cerebrovascular

- Ischemic/hemorrhagic stroke
- Hypertensive encephalopathy
- Subarachnoid hemorrhage
- TIA
- Posterior reversible ischemic encephalopathy syndrome (PRES).

Cardiovascular

- Acute pulmonary edema
- Acute myocardial infarction
- Acute aortic dissection

Renal: Acute renal failure.

PRES (Posterior Reversible Ischemic Encephalopathy Syndrome)

- Acute onset of neurological disturbance
- Headache, visual disturbance, altered sensorium and seizures
- Imaging studies demonstrate posterior cerebral involvement (especially occipital cortex)
- Abnormalities are reversible

Chronic Complication of Hypertension

- Chronic cerebrovascular disease
- Left ventricular hypertrophy and LV dysfunction.
- Aortic valve disease.
- Chronic renal failure.
- Peripheral vascular disease
- Hypertensive retinopathy

Routine Laboratory Testing in a Patient of Hypertension

- Urine routine examination
- Serum-urea and creatinine
- Hb% and packed cell volume
- Serum electrolytes (sodium, potassium)
- TSH and calcium
- Fasting lipid profile and blood sugar.

APPROACH TO A PATIENT OF SECONDARY HYPERTENSION

Suspect Secondary Hypertension under following Circumstances

- Young hypertensives (less than 25 years of age) and persons developing hypertension more than 55 years of age.
- Uncontrollable hypertension.
- Accelerated/malignant hypertension.

History in a Patient of Suspected Secondary Hypertension

Symptoms of renal disease: Puffiness of face and pedal edema and decreased urine output.

Symptoms of endocrine disease:

- Like thyroid disease, Cushing's syndrome, acromegaly.
- Palpitation, sweating, tremor and episodes of hypertension: Pheochromocytoma.

Other causes of episodic hypertension: Porphyria, Guillain-Barré syndrome.

Wait gain and fatigue: Cushing's syndrome.

Fatigue and proximal muscle weakness: Primary aldosteronism.

Lower extremity fatigue: Coarctation of aorta.

Intake of medications—like corticosteroids, NSAIDs, nasal decongestants, cyclosporine, estrogen preparations.

Snoring while sleeping, disturbed sleep and daytime sleepiness: Sleep apnea with hypertension.

Pregnancy status: Pregnancy-induced hypertension.

Examination of a Patient of Secondary Hypertension

General Examination

- Severe pallor—chronic renal parenchymal disease.
- Evidence of polycythemia—polycystic kidney, pheochromocytoma
- Puffiness of face and pedal edema—parenchymal renal disease.
- Neck swelling—thyroid disease
- Fine tremors ⎱ Thyrotoxicosis
- Eye signs ⎰

Plethoric face, moon face, buffalo hump, abdominal striae: Cushing's syndrome. Enlarged extremities with prognathism: Acromegaly.

Pulse and Blood Pressure

Radiofemoral delay: Coarctation of aorta.

BP recording

- Observe for degree of hypertension, stage of hypertension
- Upper limb BP is more compared to lower limb—coarctation of aorta.

Postural recording of blood pressure

- Decrease of systolic BP on standing (without medication/autonomic neuropathy)—possible pheochromocytoma.
- Increase of diastolic pressure on standing—possible essential hypertension.

Systemic Examination

- Cardiovascular system for evidence of hypertensive heart disease.
- Ophthalmic examination—corkscrew arteries: Coarctation of aorta.

- Bilateral mass palpable in the abdomen: Polycystic kidney.
- Auscultate for renal artery bruit.
- Sudden raise of blood pressure—on massaging the abdomen—possible pheochromocytoma.
- For evidence of complications of hypertension.

Secondary Hypertension

Causes

Renal parenchymal disease

- Acute glomerulonephritis
- Chronic glomerulonephritis
- Chronic pyelonephritis
- Polycystic disease of kidney
- Renal tumors especially renin producing

Renovascular

- Renal artery stenosis
- Fibromuscular dysplasia
- Atherosclerosis.

Endocrine Disease

- Acromegaly
- Hypothyroidism—diastolic hypertension
- Thyrotoxicosis—systolic hypertension
- Hyperparathyroidisam
- Primary aldosteronism
- Cushing's syndrome
- Pheochromocytoma
- Adrenal enzyme deficiency.

Vascular causes: Coarctation of aorta, vasculitis syndrome.

Drug induced

- Intake of corticosteroids, large dose of estrogen.
- NSAIDs.
- Nasal decongestants
- Cyclosporin

Pregnancy-induced hypertension

Neurological: Increased intracranial pressure, porphyria, Guillain-Barré syndrome.

Investigation of a Patient of Secondary Hypertension

- Routine investigations—already discussed under hypertension
- Urine—RBCs, casts, protein: Parenchymal renal disease.
- Serum electrolytes—potassium low:
  - Conn's syndrome
  - Cushing's syndrome
  - Adrenal enzyme defect.
- 24 hours urinary VMA and catecholamines—pheochromocytoma.
- 24 hours urinary cortisol and serum cortisol levels.
- Serum calcium, thyroid function tests.
- Renal artery Doppler/angiogram for renal artery stenosis.
- Echocardiogram/ECG for evidence of coarctation of aorta/hypertensive heart disease.
- Sleep study—to rule out obstructive sleep apnea syndrome.
- MRI brain—for pituitary pathology and intracranial lesions.
- Ultrasound abdomen/CT scan for kidney size, cysts, adrenal pathology.

Pseudohypertension and Osler's Sign

Pseudohypertension occurs due to thickening of arterial walls and occurs in conditions like—Monckeberg's sclerosis of arteries. Manual recording of blood pressure is overestimated even though intra-arterial recording of blood pressure is normal.

Osler's Sign

Normally when the blood pressure cuff is inflated above systolic pressure both the radial pulse and the artery are not palpable. In patients with positive Osler's sign radial pulse is absent but vessel is still palpable when the BP cuff is inflated above the systolic pressure. This occurs in a patient of pseudohypertension.

Monogenic Hypertension

Several inherited defects in the synthesis of adrenal steroid results in hypertension and hypokalemia due to synthesis of increased levels of mineralocorticoids.

Characteristic Features of Monogenic Hypertension

- Early onset of hypertension
- Severe refractory hypertension
- Family history of childhood hypertension
- History of consanguinity between parents.

Examples of Monogenic Hypertension

- Glucocorticoid remediable aldosteronism.
- 17-alpha hydroxylase deficiency
- 11-beta hydroxylase deficiency
- Administration of steroid decreases over-production of aldosterone, causes lowering of blood pressure and there will be correction of hyperkalemia.
- In apparent mineralocorticoid excess administration of spironolactone and glucocorticoids may be required.

Peripheral Arterial Disease

Risk Factors

- Diabetes mellitus
- Hypertension
- Hyperlipidemia
- Hyperhomocysteinemia
- Smoking

Causes of Peripheral Arterial Disease

- Atherosclerosis
- Trauma
- Thromboembolic occlusion
- Vasculitis
- Fibromuscular dysplasia

Clinical Approach to a Patient of Peripheral Vascular Disease

Symptoms: Peripheral vascular disease is more likely to involve lower limb than upper limb.

🔑 Key Points:

- Lower limb arteries are more likely to be occluded compared to upper limb.
- Atherosclerotic vascular occlusion: Usually presents at 6th/7th decade of life.
- Characteristic presenting features of peripheral vascular disease is claudication.

Site of obstruction of peripheral artery depending on the site of claudication:

- Claudication of calf—femoral/popliteal occlusion.
- Claudication of proximal lower limb—buttocks, hip, thigh: Iliac/aortic occlusion.
- Vascular claudication: Usually occurs during exercise.
- If rest pain occurs—indicates severe obstruction to the artery—associated with signs of ischemia like cold extremities, pallor and paresthesia.
- Symptoms of ischemia is more likely to occur when the limb is kept horizontal and less when the blood flow increases during dependent position.

Examination of a Patient of Peripheral Vascular Disease

Rule out: Diabetes mellitus, hypertension.

Pulse: Examination of peripheral arteries like radial, carotid, dorsalis pedis artery.

Signs of peripheral vascular disease
- Pallor of the limb
- Feeble pulse or pulse absent
- Decrease of temperature
- Bluish discoloration of the limb
- *Other features*: Lack of hair, skin becomes shiny and atrophy of muscles.
- If severe obstruction—ulcer and gangrene and edema of limbs.
- *Due to ischemia*: Neuropathic manifestations can occur.
- Auscultate for arterial bruit over the major arteries.

Ankle brachial index
- Record the blood pressure in the legs and arms.

- Normally ankle blood pressure is slightly higher the upper limb.
- Recording of ankle BP.

Apply the Sphygmomanometer cuff above the ankle and auscultate over the posterior tibial or dorsalis pedis artery for the BP recording. Doppler recording can also be done.

$Normal$: $\dfrac{\text{Ankle blood pressure}}{\text{Brachial blood pressure}}$ ratio is more than 1

Peripheral vascular disease

$= \dfrac{\text{Ankle blood pressure}}{\text{Brachial blood pressure}}$ ratio is more than 1

If the ratio <0.5—severe ischemia of the limb.

THORACIC OUTLET OBSTRUCTION

Compression of Artery/Vein at the Thoracic Outlet

Causes

- Cervical rib
- Scaleneus anticus muscle
- Rarely by pectorals minor or by clavicular compression
- Can press over the subclavian artery, vein or brachial plexus
- Can produce ischemia to the upper limb and gangrene of the limb.

On Examination

- It may be normal examination of the limb.
- Distal pulse in the upper limb:
  - May be absent.
  - Associated with digital cyanosis and edema of the limb.

Adson's Test

To detect the compression of subclavian artery.

Test

Position of the patient: Upright position of the patient and abduct, extend and externally rotate the affected limb.

Respiration: Patient takes deep inspiration.

Position of head and neck: Neck extended and head rotated to the affected side.

Interpretation: There is decrease or disappearance of volume of radial pulse on the affected side.

ISCHAEMIC HEART DISEASE

Important Clinical Aspects

Typical Angina Pain (Refer before)

Factors which does not favor angina:
- Tenderness over the chest.
- Stabbing or sharp pain over the left infra-mammary area.
- Localisation of pain to single anatomical area.
- Dull aching precordial pain.

Factors which indirectly indicate angina pain
- Family history of IHD
- Presence of peripheral vascular disease
- Presence of carotid bruit
- History of TIA/CVA.

Nocturnal angina—angina occurring at night

Mechanisms: Development of tachyarrhythmias at night
- Return of splanchnic blood and from lower extremities to the left heart.
- Increase in the intrathoracic volume with increase of myocardial oxygen demand.
- Decrease of respiratory center drive with decrease oxygenation.

Patients with syphilitic aortic regurgitation can have nocturnal angina.

Angina Equivalents

- Presence of discomfort of the chest which is interpreted as fatigue, breathlessness instead of typical angina.
- Suspect IHD/angina in an elderly diabetic with above symptoms and search for other evidences like TAO, cerebrovascular disease.

Note

Women patients with angina can have normal epicardial coronary arteries—on angiogram—will be having microvascular disease—coronary syndrome 'X'.

Suspect acute myocardial infarction in a patient of angina under the following circumstances:
- Duration of pain—more than 30 minutes
- Tachycardia
- Hypotension.

Examination of A Patient of Ischemic Heart Disease

Look for risk factors
- Hypertension
- Diabetes mellitus
- Hyperlipidemia
- *Smoking*: Nicotine staining of fingertips.

Look for
- Waist/hip ratio
- Body mass index
- Xanthelasma
- Xanthoma
- Extra ear lobe crease.

Other important clinical findings
- Look for peripheral vascular disease.
- Abdominal aortic aneurysm.
- Carotid bruit.
- Blood pressure comparison between upper and lower limbs—ankle bronchial index.
- Fundus—for arteriosclerotic changes.
- Other signs like anemia, thyroid disease.
- Pulse—for thickening of vessel wall.
- Ankle brachial index—for evidence of peripheral vascular disease.

Cardiac Examination
- Look for cardiomegaly with hyperdynamic apex.
- Dyskinetic segment (suggestive of ventricular aneurysm).
- Left-sided 3rd and 4th heart sound.

- Apical systolic murmur—due to papillary muscle dysfunction.
- Signs of cardiac failure.

During an Attack of Angina
- Patient can have left-sided 3rd or 4th heart sound
- Dyskinetic segment
- Transient MR
- LVF

HEART FAILURE

Symptoms of Heart Failure

Left heart failure symptoms
- Dyspnea, orthopnea and PND
- Hemoptysis.

Right heart failure symptoms
- Anorexia
- Nausea
- Right hypochondrial pain
- Swelling of feet and decreased urine output

Symptoms due to decreased cerebral perfusion in heart failure
- Confusion
- Disorientation

Other symptoms of heart failure
- Fatigability
- Cachexia

Chronic right heart failure can also result in
- Jaundice
- Abdominal distension due to ascites

Mechanisms of Dyspnea in Heart Failure

Interstitial/intra-alveolar fluid collection causing stretch of J receptors resulting in rapid shallow breathing.

Other Factors Contributory for Dyspnea in Heart Failure
- Compliance of the lung is decreased.
- Airway resistance is increased.
- Fatigue of muscles of respiration including diaphragm.

Orthopnea: Dyspnea in recumbent position.

Mechanism: Lying down position—from splanchnic circulation fluid is shifted to pulmonary circulation with increase in the pulmonary venous congestion.

 Note

In chronic left heart failure, due to increase in the lymphatics draining the fluid in the lungs— crepitations may be absent during auscultation.

Pleural Effusion in Heart Failure

- Due to increased hydrostatic pressure in the capillaries of pleura—fluid accumulates in the pleural cavity due to transudation of fluid.
- Biventricular failure produces pleural effusion.
- Cardiac failure producing unilateral pleural effusion is predominantly right sided.
- If unilateral effusion and if there is associated fever and pleuritic pain—requires analysis of pleural fluid in a patient of cardiac failure.

Cardiac Examination in a Patient of CCF

- Cardiomegaly with LVH and RVH
- Heart sounds: Tachycardia
  - Left-sided S_3 and S_4
- *Murmurs*: Mitral and tricuspid regurgitant murmurs.

Abdomen

- Congestive hepatomegaly, splenomegaly
- Ascites and ANASRCA.

Respiratory system: Pleural effusion, bilateral basal crepitations.

Mechanisms of cardiac cachexia

- Due to hepatic and IVC congestion: Loss of appetite and impaired absorption.
- ↓ Blood flow to the muscles and cellular hypoxia.
- Dyspnea causing increased basal metabolic rate.

- Increased cytokine release like TNF causing increased metabolic turnover.

Factors which Precipitate Acute Worsening of Heart Failure in a Chronic Cardiac Disease

- Acute myocardial infarction.
- *Arrhythmias*: Atrial fibrillation
- *Infection*
  - Infective endocarditis
  - Pulmonary infection.
- Increased fluid intake
- Stopping of treatment and intake of drugs like diuretics.
- Drugs which can precipitate/worsen heart failure—NSAIDs, corticosteroids, beta blockers.

Paroxysmal Nocturnal Dyspnea (PND): Manifestation of Left Heart Failure

After sleeping for 1 to 3 hours patient complains of dyspnea and cough (wheeze may be associated).

Mechanisms

- Shift of fluid to pulmonary capillaries.
- Compression of airways by the bronchial arteries due to increased pressure in them.
- Increase in the airway resistance.

Cheyne-Stokes respiration: Can occur in left heart failure.

Due to decreased cardiac output and altered sensitivity of respiratory center.

Anorexia, nausea and pain in the right hypochondrium and jaundice (in right heart failure) can occur due to: Congestion of bowel wall and liver and stretching of liver capsule.

Ascites, pedal edema in heart failure: Ascites, swelling of feet and decreased urine output: Occurs due to decreased renal blood flow, retention of salt and water due to altered hemodynamic mechanisms.

Clinical Signs

Pulse

- Sinus tachycardia

- Low volume pulse
- Pulsus alternans in left heart failure

Blood pressure: Systolic blood pressure is lower than normal

Extremities cool ⎫ due to peripheral
Peripheral cyanosis ⎭ vasoconstriction

Signs of right heart failure
- Raised JVP
- Tender enlarged liver, pedal edema and ascites.

Signs of left heart failure
- Low volume pulse/pulsus alternans
- Left-sided S_3
- Central cyanosis
- Bilateral basal crepitations
- Cheyne-Stokes respiration

Other conditions/factors which can cause worsening of heart failure
- Increased of blood pressure
- Progressive anemia
- Thyrotoxicosis
- Pregnancy
- Alcohol
- Progressive worsening of heart disease like IHD, valvular disease.

Conditions which results in sudden worsening of heart failure
- Atrial fibrillation
- Infective endocarditis
- Systemic infections—especially pulmonary infection
- Stopping of diuretics/fluid overload.

PULMONARY HYPERTENSION

Normal pulmonary artery pressure: 12–16 mm of Hg

Pulmonary hypertension: Pulmonary artery pressure is more than 25 mm Hg.

Classification
- Primary
- Secondary

Primary or idiopathic pulmonary artery hypertension—no secondary cause made out—diagnosis of exclusion.

Secondary Causes
- Left heart disease.
- Congenital left to right intracardiac shunts.
- Chronic lung disease and hypoxia.
- Thromboembolic pulmonary hypertension.
- Chronic hemolytic anemias
- Myeloproliferative disorders.
- Sarcoidosis.

What is Primary Pulmonary Hypertension?

Pulmonary artery pressure is high without any apparent cause.

Different Mechanisms of Development of Pulmonary Hypertension

Left-sided heart disease: Mitral stenosis and left heart disease with persistently elevated left atrial and pulmonary venous pressure will lead on to pathological changes in the pulmonary arteries resulting in increased pulmonary vascular resistance. There will be an additional factor like changes in the vascular muscle tone with defective vascular relaxation. Backward transmission of pressure: From pulmonary veins to pulmonary arteries also play a role in the genesis of pulmonary hypertension in patients with left heart disease.

Pulmonary hypertension in intracardiac shunt lesion: Increased pulmonary blood flow with high pressure will lead on to changes in the pulmonary vascular structure and function resulting in pulmonary hypertension.

Pulmonary hypertension in COPD and hypoxic conditions: COPD and chronic hypoxic conditions predominantly will result in pulmonary vasoconstriction leading to increased pulmonary vascular resistance.

Other factors like changes in the vascular structure and function, polycythemia will also contribute for pulmonary hypertension.

Pulmonary hypertension in chronic pulmonary thromboembolism: Chronic pulmonary thromboembolism will result in obliteration of the pulmonary vascular bed leading on to increased pulmonary vascular resistance and pulmonary hypertension.

Other conditions which are considered responsible for the development of pulmonary hypertension

1. Collagen vascular disease.
2. Drugs: Phenfluramine and anorexiants
3. Portal hypertension

Idiopathic (Primary) Pulmonary Hypertension

- More common in females.
- Can be familial with autosomal dominant inheritance.
- There is mutation in the genetic coding for bone morphogenetic protein receptor (BMPR II) leading to different cellular response.
- Progressive disease leading on to RVH and right-sided cardiac failure.
- Leads on to significant changes in the pulmonary vasculature.

Pathophysiology of Pulmonary Hypertension

- There is increase in the pulmonary vascular resistance.
- Increase pulmonary vascular resistance leads to increase in the pulmonary artery pressure.
- Increase in the pulmonary vascular resistance leads to:
  - RVH
  - Prominent 'a' wave in the JVP
  - Opening of the patient foramen ovale
  - Right-sided cardiac failure.

Clinical Features

Symptoms

- Easy fatigability
- Dizziness and syncope
- Exercise intolerance and dyspnea

- Chest pain (RV ischemia/pulmonary artery dilatation).

Less common symptoms

- Hoarseness of voice (pulmonary artery dilatation causing pressure on the left recurrent laryngeal nerve).
- Hemoptysis.

Severity of Pulmonary Hypertension

Mild: Pulmonary artery pressure: 25–40 mm of Hg

Moderate: Pulmonary artery pressure: 41–55 mm of Hg

Severe: Pulmonary artery pressure:> 55 mm of Hg

Primary Pulmonary Hypertension

Pathology

- Endothelial cell proliferation.
- Plexiform lesions of arterioles
- Muscularisation of arterioles
- Smooth muscle proliferation with thickening of media.
- Fibrotic changes of arterioles
- Vessels show inflammatory changes.
- Small arterioles will be occluded by thrombi.

Signs of pulmonary hypertension: *See* under cor pulmonale.

COR PULMONALE
(Pulmonary Heart Disease)

Features

- Right ventricular hypertrophy or dilatation.
- Right-sided cardiac failure may or may not be present.
- Presence of pulmonary artery hypertension.
- Presence of respiratory disease/disease of pulmonary vasculature or abnormal respiratory mechanism.
- There is no left-sided cardiac disease with normal pulmonary capillary wedge pressure.

- Right ventricular hypertrophy occurs in patients with chronic cor pulmonale.
- Right ventricular dilatation occurs in patients with acute cor pulmonale, e.g. acute massive pulmonary embolism.

Causes

Lung parenchymal disease
- Chronic obstructive pulmonary disease.
- Bronchiectasis.
- Cystic fibrosis.
- Interstitial lung disease.
- Pneumoconiosis.

Pulmonary vascular disease
- Acute pulmonary embolism (acute cor pulmonale)
- Chronic pulmonary embolism
- Veno-occlusive disease of the lungs.
- Chronic pulmonary vascular disease.

Conditions causing chronic hypoxia
- Chronic obstructive pulmonary disease.
- Obesity hypoventilation syndrome.
- Neuromuscular dysfunction.
- High altitudes.
- Diseases of the chest wall.

Clinical manifestations
- Symptoms of primary disorder causing cor pulmonale.
- Symptoms of dyspnea, orthopnea.
- Symptoms of abdominal pain and anasarca (due to cardiac failure).

Clinical signs
Signs of pulmonary hypertension
- Prominent 'a' wave in the JVP
- Left parasternal heave—due to RVH
- P_2 palpable
- P_2 loud (narrow splitting of 2nd heart sound—except in a patient of acute pulmonary embolism)
- ESM pulmonary area
- Early diastolic murmur of PR (Graham Steell murmur)
- TR murmur.

Signs of congestive cardiac failure—in late stages
- JVP increased
- Enlarged tender liver
- Pedal edema
- Central cyanosis occurs either due to chronic lung disease or due to opening of patent foramen ovale
- *ECG*: P pulmonale, RVH, right axis deviation.
- *Chest X-ray*
  - Enlarged main pulmonary artery
  - RVH
  - Evidence of chronic lung disease

CLINICAL ASPECTS OF RHEUMATIC FEVER

Organism: Any strain of streptococcus can cause rheumatic fever.

Common strains responsible for rheumatic fever: Serotypes: 1, 3, 5, 6, 14, etc.

Rheumatic fever is more likely to be associated with HLA class II alleles DR7 and DR4.

Immune response: Cross-reacting antibodies attacking valvular endothelium allowing the entry of primed CD4 cells leading onto subsequent T cell-mediated inflammation.

Pathogenesis

- Autoantibodies against cardiac endothelium.
- There is cross-reaction between streptococcus M protein and cardiac myosin.
- There is also cross-reaction between autoantibodies and neuronal cell surface gangliosides and dopamine receptors.
- There is a genetic susceptibility with more incidence with HLA class II antigens.

Clinical Features

- 50% may not give classical history of rheumatic fever except for pharyngitis
- Usual latent period between streptococcal infection and acute rheumatic fever is 3 weeks.

- In India and other tropical regions mitral stenosis can occur as early as 5 years of age: Juvenile mitral stenosis.
- Chorea and low grade arthritis can occur after 6 months after acute streptococcal pharyngitis.

Carditis
- Acute/chronic pancarditis
- Common valve involved: Mitral valve
- Can cause acute MR and Carey Coombs murmur
- Pericarditis and CCF can occur in acute rheumatic fever.

Joint involvement
- Asymmetrical polyarthritis
- Migratory joint pain can migrate even over a period of hours.
- Occasionally only arthralgia/aseptic mono-arthritis can be a feature. Pain is usually for 2 weeks, pain more than 4 weeks—consider alternate diagnosis.

  Joint involvement that persists more than 1–2 days after starting salicylates is unlikely to be acute rheumatic fever.

Chorea
- Can occur alone after a prolonged latent period.
- More common in females.
- It may be generalized or may be restricted to one side of the body (hemichorea). Disappears during sleep.
- Chorea usually resolves completely within 6 weeks.
- Risk of carditis is higher in patient with rheumatic chorea.

Skin manifestations
Erythema marginatum: Can appear and disappear in front of the examiner (evanescent)/central clearing with spreading lesions usually associated with carditis.
Usual sites: Trunk, limbs not on the face.

Subcutaneous nodules
- Commonly associated with carditis

- Rheumatic nodules over the olecranon indicate severe carditis
- Appear 2–3 weeks after the onset of the disease and lasts for only 2–3 weeks.

Fever—high grade common
Endemic area of rheumatic fever: There can be only arthralgia/monoarthritis.

Diagnosis criteria: Verify Manipal Manual of Clinical Medicine.

Treatment
- Salicylates
- Glucocorticoid: Prednisolone 1–2 mg/kg for 3 weeks for carditis can be given for severe disorder/refractory to other treatment.
- Penicillin prophylaxis is given once in 2–3 weeks, if the risk is high but with person with normal compliance once in 4 weeks is adequate.

Jaccoud's Arthritis
- Occurs due to repeated attacks of inflammation in rheumatic fever.
- Results in hand deformities
- Deformities are reducible/correctable
- There is non-erosive arthritis and no joint/bone destruction
- May be due to laxity of ligaments/soft tissue inflammation.
- It can also occur in a patient of SLE

Post-streptococcal reactive arthritis
- Symmetrical small joint involvement.
- Latent period between arthritis and streptococcal infection: 1 week
- Non-group A beta hemolytic streptococcus can cause.
- Less response to salicylates.
- Carditis: Absent.

APPROACH TO A PATIENT OF VALVULAR HEART DISEASE
- Rheumatic fever is the most common cause of valvular heart disease.
- Mitral and aortic valves are mainly affected.

- Occasionally pulmonary and tricuspid valve can be affected.
- Rheumatic fever causes pancarditis.

Suspect rheumatic heart disease under following circumstances

- Symptoms of cardiac disease usually around 3rd or 4th decade of life onwards. Rheumatic fever usually occurs in between the age of 5–15 years and symptomatic chronic valvular heart disease develops after 10–15 years.
- Isolated mitral stenosis: Usually rheumatic
- Multivalvular disease: Usually rheumatic
- If there is previous history suggestive of rheumatic fever. Only in 50% of patients with rheumatic valvular disease give previous history of rheumatic fever. In another half of patients it would have been subclinical.
- If the patient is on Inj Benzathine Penicillin prophylaxis (against streptococcal infection).

Suspect mitral stenosis under following circumstances

- History of exertional dyspnea, PND, palpitation in the 2nd or 3rd decade of life (person develops symptoms of pulmonary venous congestion due to early raise in the left atrial pressure). Usually manifests after about 10 years after an attack of acute rheumatic carditis. In juvenile mitral stenosis symptoms of mitral stenosis develops as early as 2 years after an attack of rheumatic fever.
- Presentation like embolic CVA may also be a manifestation of mitral stenosis due to the development of atrial fibrillation.
- Infective endocarditis is usually not a manifestation of severe mitral stenosis because of the low pressure jet across the mitral valve.
- Isolated mitral stenosis alone without regurgitation can occur in female patients.
- Suspect mechanical prosthetic valve or atrial fibrillation if the patients is on anticoagulation.

Suspect mitral regurgitation under following circumstances

- Prolonged history of palpitation (due to volume overload of LV)
- History of easy fatigability (due to low cardiac output)
- Development of dyspnea due to pulmonary venous congestion occurs much later compared to mitral stenosis (it is predominantly volume overload of the left atrium compared to pressure overload in mitral stenosis)
- Manifests much later 10–20 years after an attack of rheumatic fever.
- Isolated rheumatic MR is not very common (occasionally in males isolated rheumatic MR can occur) and rule out always other causes of MR like MVP/papillary muscle dysfunction in such cases.
- Infective endocarditis is common in patients with MR due to rapid jet of flow across the mitral valve.

Suspect aortic stenosis under following circumstances

- History of exertional syncope and chest pain.
- Palpitation due to left ventricular hypertrophy
- Dyspnea and PND occur much later as development of pulmonary venous congestion occurs much later as LV has got enormous capacity to enlarge/hypertrophy without raising the pressure.
- Patient can have sudden cardiac death due to severe stenosis or due to ventricular arrhythmias.
- Infective endocarditis is not a usual manifestation of severe aortic stenosis.
- Manifests 15–20 years after an attack of rheumatic fever.

Suspect aortic regurgitation under following circumstances

- Prolonged history of palpitation (volume overload of LV) for 15–20 years.

- Later on development of chest pain and dyspnea.
- Person can make out the heart beat especially on lying to left lateral side and can feel the throbbing sensation throughout the body.
- Nocturnal angina may be a manifestation of syphilitic AR.
- Occasionally aortic dissection can occur in patients with Marfan's syndrome.
- Isolated AR is not a common feature of rheumatic heart disease.
- Endocarditis may be a common complication of AR.

 Note

Rheumatic aortic valve disease manifests much later (15–20 years) compared to mitral valve disease but deteriorates faster once the symptoms appear.

APPROACH TO A PATIENT OF VALVULAR HEART DISEASE

 Note

Main 4 valvular heart disease involving mitral and aortic valves are discussed in this chapter.

- Common valves involved—mitral and aortic valves.
- Incidence of isolated mitral stenosis—around 25%.
- Incidence of combined mitral stenosis and regurgitation—around 40%. Mostly multivalvular involvement. Pulmonary valve-less common to be involved.

Symptoms of Rheumatic Valvular Heart Disease

Mitral stenosis
- Dyspnea, PND, orthopnea
- Palpitation
- Can present as embolic CVA

Mitral regurgitation
- Easy fatigability
- Palpitation
- Later dyspnea, chest pain.

Aortic stenosis
- Palpitation
- Syncope—exertional, chest pain, later dyspnea, PND
- Can cause sudden cardiac death.

Aortic regurgitation
- Palpitation
- Chest pain
- Later dyspnea, PND

 Note

Syphilitic AR can present as nocturnal angina.

Other historical points in valvular heart disease
- Previous history of migratory arthritis—suggestive of attack of rheumatic fever.
- Previous history of taking benzathine penicillin (penidure) prophylaxis against streptococcal infection (rheumatic fever).
- History of taking anticoagulation—possible atrial fibrillation and possible mechanical valve replacement.

Less common symptoms in valvular heart disease
- Hemoptysis—in mitral stenosis
- Recurrent bronchitis (winter bronchitis) in mitral stenosis
- Hoarseness of voice due to LA enlargement in mitral stenosis/mitral regurgitation.

GENERAL EXAMINATION IN VALVULAR HEART DISEASE

Build and nourishment
- Mitral stenosis—usually normal. Can have mitral facies.
- Mitral regurgitation—usually normal.
- Aortic stenosis—usually normal
- Aortic regurgitation—may have features of Marfan's syndrome.

Chronic valvular heart disease with CCF
- Presence of icterus—due to hepatic congestion.
- Presence of abdominal distention due to ascites—due to CCF/cardiac cirrhosis.
- Cachexia—due to cardiac cachexia.

Note

Observe always for evidence of goiter and features of hypo and hyperthyroidism in all patients of cardiac disease.

Radial pulse in valvular heart disease
- Mitral stenosis—usually normal.
  - Low volume—if severe mitral stenosis
- Mitral regurgitation—normal
  - Severe MR: High volume (minicollapsing): High volume but collapsing nature need not be present as the diastolic pressure is not very low.
- Aortic stenosis—severe AS—low volume and slow raising (parvus et tardus).
- AR severe—typical collapsing pulse—Corrigan's pulse.

Blood pressure in valvular heart disease
- Mitral stenosis—usually normal.
- MR (severe)—high systolic pressure.
- AS (severe)—lower systolic pressure.
- AR (severe)—high systolic and low diastolic pressure—wide pulse pressure—can have Hill's sign.

JVP in valvular heart disease
- Mitral stenosis. Normal, if severe—prominent 'a' wave due to pulmonary hypertension.
- MR: Normal. If severe, prominent 'a' wave due to pulmonary hypertension.
- AS: Normal. If severe, 'a' wave prominent due to pulmonary hypertension.

 Note

Patients of severe aortic stenosis can have prominent 'a' wave without pulmonary hypertension. This is due to Bernheim effect, causing decrease compliance of RV with forceful RA contraction.

- AR (severe)—prominent 'a' wave in pulmonary hypertension.
- TS—prominent 'a' wave (due to higher RA pressure)
- TR—prominent 'v' wave.

Carotid pulse in valvular heart disease
- MS: Normal
- MR: Normal
- Severe AS—slow upstroke of carotid. Apico-carotid delay and carotid thrill.
- In HOCM—jerky carotid upstroke.
- AR-dancing carotids—Corrigan's sign
- Severe AR—pulsus bisferiens.
- If AS with AR, with AR dominant, pulsus bisferiens.

Cardiac apex in valvular heart disease
- *Mitral stenosis*
  - Tapping apex
  - Palpable first sound
  - Diastolic thrill
- *Mitral regurgitation*
  - Hyperdynamic apex
  - Systolic thrill
  - Palpable S_3
- *AS:*
  - Heaving apex
  - Palpable S_4
- *AR:* Hyperdynamic apex

Precordium in valvular heart disease
- MS—left parasternal heaving due to RVH (due to pulmonary hypertension).
- MR—left parasternal pulsation due to RVH/giant left atrium.
- Aortic stenosis—systolic thrill in the aortic area.
- AR—pulsatile precordium (due to LV volume overload)
- Diastolic thrill—aortic area.

Heart sounds in valvular heart disease
- *Mitral stenosis*
  - Loud 1st heart sound
  - Opening snap
  - Severe MS—no S3
  - Loud P2
- *Mitral regurgitation*
  - 1st heart sound—muffled—if rheumatic.
  - Normal 1st heart sound in MR—MVP MR/ischemic MR

- 2nd heart sound—widely split—due to early closure of aortic component (due to less aortic flow).
- *Aortic stenosis*
  - 1st sound: Normal.
  - Ejection click: If bicuspid valve
  - 2nd sound: A2 muffled
  - If severe AS—paradoxical split of S2
  - S4 at the apex.
- *AR*
  - 1st sound may be normal/muffled
  - S3—at the apex
  - A2 loud
- *AR*—can have aortic ejection sound due to sudden dilatation of aorta.
- *Syphilitic AR*—Tambour quality of 2nd heart sound.

Murmur in valvular heart disease
- *MS*: Typical MDM at the apex.
- *MR*
  - Pansystolic murmur at the apex.
  - Can have MDM at the apex as a flow murmur—severe MR
- *AS*
  - Ejection systolic murmur at the aortic area conducted to carotids.
  - If HOCM—murmur not conducted to carotids
  - If sclerotic valve—Gallaverdin phenomenon.
- *AR*—early diastolic murmur in the aortic area.
- Rheumatic AR—murmur better heard in the left sternal border.
- Syphilitic/Marfan's syndrome—AR—murmur better heard in the right sternal border. Austin Flint murmur at the mitral area.

ECG in valvular heart disease
MS
- "P" mitrale
- LA—enlargement
- Features of AF.

MR
- "P" mitrale
- LV volume overload

AS
- LA enlargement
- LV pressure overload

AR
- LV volume overload
- LA—enlargement.

Chest X-ray in left-sided valvular heart disease
- Cardiomegaly (massive in MR and AR)
- Straightening of left heart border (mitralisation).
- Lifting up of left main bronchus.
- Splaying of carina
- Double atrial shadow: If severe MR with left atrial enlargement.
- Hilar congestion/bat wing appeerence
- Kerley B lines
- Prominent upper lobe veins.

Other chest X-ray evidences
- Calcification of mitral/aortic valve
- Evidence of pulmonary hypertension
  - Dilated right descending pulmonary artery.
  - Peripheral pruning of vessels.

> **Note**
>
> *Look for following signs—depending on the history and clinical signs in a patient of valvular disease*
> 1. *Peripheral signs of severe AR*
> 2. *Signs of rheumatic activity*
> 3. *Signs of infective endocarditis*
> 4. *Signs of atrial fibrillation*
> 5. *Signs of pulmonary hypertension*
> 6. *Signs of CCF.*

Complications of valvular heart disease
- *Due to valve abnormality*
  - Infective endocarditis
  - Valve calcification
  - Left heart failure
  - Pulmonary hypertension
  - Right heart failure
  - Hemoptysis

- *Due to LA enlargement*
  - Presence of a thrombus
  - Ortener's syndrome.
- *Due to arrhythmias*
  - AF—precipitation of CCF
  - AF—systemic embolisation
  - Ventricular arrhythmias—sudden death.

MITRAL STENOSIS

- Normal mitral valve orifice—surface area 4–6 cm^2.
- Mild mitral stenosis—valve orifice <2 cm^2.
- Moderate mitral stenosis—valve orifice: 1 to 1.5 cm^2
- Severe mitral stenosis—valve orifice: <1 cm^2

Common causes of mitral stenosis

- R: Rheumatic heart disease
- C: Congenital
- C: Calcified valve.

Other causes

- SLE
- Rheumatoid arthritis

Conditions which mimic mitral stenosis

- Left atrial myxoma
- Cor triatrium

Pathology of Rheumatic Mitral Stenosis

Mitral valve narrowing occurs due to

- Cusps are thickened and rigid.
- Commissures are fused
- Chordae tendineae become fused and shortened.
- *Added factors:* Calcification of the valve along with mechanical and hemodynamic trauma.

Thrombus Formation in Mitral Stenosis

- Usual site of thrombus—left atrial appendage with dilated left atrium.
- Thrombus formation occurs with atrial fibrillation and can occur over the calcified valve.

Pathophysiology of Mitral Stenosis

- Narrowing of mitral valve leads to decrease of left atrial blood flow to the left ventricle.

- There will be increased left atrial pressure with increased pulmonary venous pressure.
- Further increase in the pulmonary venous pressure causes pulmonary venous congestion and decrease pulmonary compliance.
- Any increase in the heart rate causes further increase in the pulmonary venous pressure and pulmonary edema.

Consequences of mitral stenosis

- Severe mitral stenosis—leads to decrease in cardiac output.
- Severe mitral stenosis—leads to increase in left atrial pressure which is transmitted to pulmonary artery. Changes in the pulmonary vascular bed becoming obliterated.
- There may be pulmonary vasoconstriction. There will be pulmonary venous congestion developing interstitial edema.
- Increase in the pulmonary artery pressure leads to pulmonary HT, RVH and pressure is reflected onto JVP with prominent 'a' wave.

Left Atrial Changes in Mitral Stenosis

- Dilatation of the atrium
- Fibrosis of the atrial wall and atrial musculature becomes disorganised.

Mitral facies

- Pinkish and purplish patches over the cheek.
- It is due to the combination of low cardiac output with systemic vasoconstriction.

Hemoptysis in mitral stenosis occurs due to

- Sudden raise in pulmonary venous pressure with rupture of bronchial veins called pulmonary apoplexy.
- Pink frothy sputum in acute pulmonary edema.
- Recurrent pulmonary infection and winter bronchitis.
- Pulmonary embolism and infarction.

Mechanisms of pulmonary hypertension in mitral stenosis

1. Increased LA pressure which is transmitted backwards to pulmonary circulation.

2. Reactive pulmonary HT: This occurs due to vasoconstriction of pulmonary arterioles due to increased left atrial and pulmonary venous pressure.
3. There will be edema involving small pulmonary vessels.
4. Anatomical changes in the pulmonary vascular system … obliterating the arterial system.

Physical Findings

- Tapping apex
- Diastolic thrill at the apex
- Loud 1st heart sound
- Opening snap
- Typical MDM at the apex
- Signs of pulmonary hypertension
- Signs of CCF.

Severity of mitral stenosis depending on the 2nd heart sound and opening snap interval

- *Mild mitral stenosis*: Interval is around 0.08 seconds.
- *Moderate mitral stenosis*: Interval is around 0.06 seconds.
- *Severe mitral stenosis*: Interval is less than 0.04 seconds.

Table 1.1: Differentiating points between 2nd heart sound associated with opening snap and 2nd heart sound associated with 3rd heart sound	
2nd heart sound associated with S3	2nd heart sound associated with opening snap
Associated lesions	
MR/TR	MS/TS
Pulmonary hypertension	
Mild	Severe
Area heard	
Only apex	Medial to apex and/or all over the precordium
First heart sound	
Muffled	Loud
On standing	
Does not change	Increases the interval

Table 1.2: Differentiating points between 2nd sound associated with opening snap (A2–OS) and split 2nd heart sound (A2 and P2)	
Split 2nd sound (A2–P2)	A2 with OS
Area of auscultation	
Pulmonary area	Medial to the apex/all over the precordium
On standing	
Narrows the splitting	Widens the gap between A2 and OS
On inspiration	
Widens the splitting	Narrows the A2–OS gap

Differential diagnosis of mitral stenosis

Left atrial myxoma

- Features—systemic symptoms
- Tumor plop sound
- MDM—varying with position.

Flow MDM at the apex: Due to MR, AR, PDA, VSD.

Complications: See under Approach to Valvular Heart Disease

ECG

- 'P' mitrale
- RVH
- RA enlargement.

Chest X-ray in mitral stenosis

- Cardiac size—minimal cardiomegaly
- Prominent pulmonary artery
- Straightening of left upper border (due to enlarged pulmonary artery and enlarged left atrium).
- Widening of carina of bronchi
- Lifting up of left main bronchus
- Kerley B lines
- Hilar congestion due to pulmonary edema
- Calcified valve.

Kerley B lines

Type of lines: 1 to 2 CMs perpendicular lines.

Site: At costophrenic angles perpendicular to pleura.

Significance: Indicate increased left atrial and pulmonary venous pressure >20 mm of Hg

Due to: Dilatation and thickening of lymphatics and interlobular septae.

Kerley A lines: Lines running from periphery to hilum (same significance as above lines).

Significance of prominent upper lobe veins in mitral stenosis

Location of veins: Dilated upper lobe veins.

Predisposing condition: Chronic left heart failure.

Pathogenesis: In patients of chronic left heart failure, there will be accumulation of fluid in the interstitium and venules are compressed predominantly in the lower zones compared to upper zones (in upright position). There will be increased vascular resistance in the lower zones diverting the blood to upper lobe veins resulting in dilatation of upper lobe veins (veins diameter becomes >3 mm).

Risk of endocarditis in mitral stenosis

- Less infective endocarditis risk due to no jet of blood flow across the valve.
- Occurs in early stage of mitral stenosis before the valve becomes calcified.

Indications for surgery in mitral stenosis

For balloon mitral valvotomy: Isolated mitral stenosis with valve orifice size less than 1 cm² and NYHA class II, III, IV.

Contraindications:
- Calcified valve.
- Presence of a thrombus in the left atrium

Open mitral valvotomy

- If balloon mitral valvotomy is not possible or unsuccessful.
- Restenosis after balloon valvotomy.

Open mitral valvotomy can remove

- Left atrial thrombus
- Deposits of calcium.
- It can also perform opening of commissures.
- Removal of subvalvular fusion.

Mitral valve replacement

- In patients with MS and severe MR.
- Significant deformed valve.

 Note

Occurrence of atrial fibrillation in mitral stenosis depends on the severity of mitral stenosis and advanced age. Long standing atrial fibrillation can cause atrophy of atrial muscle and atrial enlargement.

MITRAL STENOSIS

Important Clinical Points

- Mitral stenosis (MS) can be associated with AF and embolic CVA: May be the first presenting manifestation of MS.
- Fish mouth appearance of mitral valve in rheumatic MS occurs due to chronic rheumatic process.
- Severe MS is indicated by MV orifice surface area 1–1.5 cm² and very severe MS—surface area is <1 cm².
- Kerley B lines in the chest X-ray occur when LA pressure >20 mmHg.
- Surgery—mitral valvotomy—by balloon—in symptomatic patients—NYHA I to IV and mitral valve orifice less than 1 cm.²
- Mitral valve replacement; in patients with MS + significant MR/valve distorted by previous procedure.

MITRAL REGURGITATION (MR)

Causes of MR

MR due to mitral leaflet abnormality

- Rheumatic heart disease—causes—chordae abnormality—shortening and fusion of chordae.
- Cuspal abnormality in RHD: Rigidity, deformity and shortening of cusps.

Disorders which cause valvular abnormality causing MR

- SLE
- Trauma
- Infective endocarditis
- Acute rheumatic fever

MR due to chordae tendinae abnormality

- Infective endocarditis.
- Rupture of posterior leaflet
- Rheumatic fever.

MR due to papillary muscle dysfunction: Ischemia and acute MI causing posterior mitral leaflet involvement (posterior papillary muscles are more vulnerable to ischemia as it has got single blood supply).

MR due to abnormality of mitral annulus: Causes dilatation of mitral annulus causing MR (any cause of LV enlargement).

MR due to prolapse of the leaflet: MVP with MR.

Pathophysiology of MR

Chronic MR

- There will be steady increase in the volume of left ventricle with decreased function of left ventricle.
- In chronic MR—cardiac output is reduced with slow development of LV dysfunction and increase in the left atrial pressure with increase in the pulmonary venous pressure.
- Massive LA enlargement predisposes to atrial fibrillation.
- Chronic MR predisposes to endocarditis.

Acute MR

Causes

- Acute MI/acute infective endocarditis.
- Rapid increase in the left atrial pressure and pulmonary venous pressure leads to rapid left heart failure.

Clinical Features of MR

Symptoms

Acute MR: Presents with acute pulmonary edema.

Chronic MR

- Mild to moderate MR—asymptomatic for a long period of time
- Chronic rheumatic MR—may be asymptomatic up to 15–20 years after the attack of rheumatic fever.
- Chronic severe MR—causes decrease in the cardiac output causing fatigue.
- There will be symptoms of dyspnea, PND and orthopnea due to pulmonary venous congestion.

- Irregular palpitation occurs due to AF.
- Symptoms like hemoptysis, CVA and embolism are less common compared to mitral stenosis.
- Long standing MR can result in pulmonary hypertension and right heart failure.
- Infective endocarditis may be a presenting feature of chronic MR.

Signs

- Radial pulse—high volume pulse
- Cardiac apex—out and down and hyper-dynamic
- Massive enlarged LA–pulsation in the left parastenral area.
- Systolic thrill at the apex.

Heart sounds

- 1st heart sound—rheumatic MR—soft
- MR with normal 1st heart sound—MVP and papillary muscle dysfunction.
- 2nd heart sound in severe MR—widely split—A2 occurs early—early aortic closure—due to less aortic flow.
- Left-sided 3rd heart sound—S3 in severe MR due to rapid filling of LV—rules out significant associated mitral stenosis.

Murmur

- Rheumatic—pan systolic—due to constant pressure gradient between LA and LV.
- MR with late systolic murmur—MVP and papillary muscle dysfunction
- MR in HOCM—papillary muscle is displaced anteriorly and there will be systolic anterior motion of anterior mitral leaflet.
- Cooing/seagull murmur of MR—chordae tendinae rupture.
- Musical quality of murmur—due to flail leaflet.
- MDM at mitral valve in MR—due to increase flow across mitral valve during diastole (functional narrowing of mitral valve) in severe MR.

Important clinical points

- Mitral annular calcification occurs in elderly hypertensives and diabetes mellitus and can cause MR.

- Endocardial cushion defect can cause congenital MR.
- Fibrosis of papillary muscle occurs in chronic IHD causing MR.
- Chronic LV enlargement further aggravates mitral regurgitation.

Complications of MR
- *Acute MR*: Acute pulmonary edema.
- *Chronic MR*
  - Pulmonary artery hypertension.
  - Atrial fibrillation
  - Ortner's syndrome
  - Infective endocarditis
- *ECG changes in MR*
  - Marked left atrial enlargement
  - LV enlargement
  - RVH
- *Chest X-ray in MR*
  - Massive cardiomegaly.
  - Left atrial and ventricular enlargement.
- *Acute MR*
  Causes—IHD
  - Ischemia of papillary muscle
  - Infective endocarditis
  - Dysfunction of prosthetic valve.

Table 1.3: Differences between acute MR and chronic MR

	Acute MR	Chronic MR
Apical impulse	Hyperkinetic	Heaving
Thrill	Absent	Present
JVP	Large 'a' wave	Normal/prominent 'a' wave
Murmur	At base	At the apex
	Soft	Harsh
	Not pan systolic	Pan systolic

Mitral regurgitation
Indication for surgery (valve replacement):
- Symptomatic patients.
- Recent onset atrial fibrillation.
- Pulmonary hypertension with PA pressure >50 mm of Hg
- *LV dysfunction*: LV ejection fraction <60%.

MITRAL REGURGITATION
Clinical Points
- Calcified valve (can occur due to HT, DM) and dilated cardiomyopathy can cause MR.
- Congenital AV canal defect can cause MR.
- Angina can be associated with transient MR. Because of the single blood supply to the posteromedial leaflet, it can get damaged in acute myocardial infarction producing mitral regurgitation.

Auscultatory events in MR
- S3 in severe MR—there is sudden tensing of chordate, papillary muscle and leaflets.
- Seagull type of murmur can occur due to chordae tendinae rupture.
  Musical types of murmur of MR—can occur due to flail valve leaflet.

AORTIC STENOSIS (AS)
Causes
- Congenital
  - Bicuspid aortic valve
- Sclerotic aortic valve
- Rheumatic heart disease.

Normal aortic valve orifice: 3–4 cm^2
Mild aortic stenosis: 1.5 to 2 cm
Moderate aortic stenosis: 1 to 1.5 cm
Aortic valve orifice less than <0.75 cm^2 suggests severe obstruction.

Pathophysiology
- Aortic stenosis produces systolic pressure gradient between left ventricle and aorta.
- Aortic stenosis will lead onto LV hypertrophy and dilatation with decrease in the stroke volume.
- There will be left ventricular systolic dysfunction and diastolic dysfunction.
- There will be myocardial fibrosis.
- There will be decreasing stroke volume with increased left side pressure increase

with ultimate result of pulmonary hypertension.

- There may be associated coronary artery disease.

Consequences and Effects of LVH

- There will be increased oxygen demand and increased oxygen consumption.
- There will be decrease in the coronary blood flow and associated subendocardial ischemia.

Clinical Features

Symptoms: May be asymptomatic for a prolonged duration.

Common symptoms

- Palpitation
- Chest pain
- Exertional syncope.

Later dyspnea, PND and orthopnea

Clinical signs: If aortic stenosis is associated with mitral stenosis, findings of aortic stenosis will decrease.

Signs: Low volume, slow raising pulse.

- Carotid thrill.
- If atrial fibrillation is present—suspect associated mitral stenosis.
- JVP prominent 'a' wave—due to septal hypertrophy causing bulging of interatrial septum causing right ventricular dysfunction.
- Apex: Heaving due to LVH.
- Thrill: Systolic thrill in the aortic area.
- *Auscultation*: Ejection click—bicuspid aortic valve without calcification.
- A2—soft (due to severe AS/calcified or immobile valve)
- Paradoxical splitting of 2nd heart sound in severe aortic stenosis.
- S4—at the apex due to LVH
- S3—at the apex due to LVF
- ESM at the aortic area conducted to the carotids. Low pitched, diamond-shaped murmur.

- If severe aortic stenosis—late peaking of the murmur—kite shaped.
- If sclerotic aortic valve—Gallavardin phenomenon.
- Paradoxical splitting occurs due to prolonged LV ejection and delayed closure of aortic valve.

Complications of Aortic Stenosis

- Left-sided cardiac failure.
- Pulmonary hypertension and right heart failure.
- Cardiac syncope
- Conduction abnormalities due to associated calcification of conduction tissue.
- Ventricular arrhythmias.
- Endocarditis—risk: More with bicuspid aortic valve.

ECG: LVH with pressure overload

Chest X-ray: LVH

- Dilatation of aorta (post-stenotic)
- Calcified aortic valve.
- Later enlargement of RV, RA and pulmonary artery.

Indications for Surgery (Valve Replacement)

- Symptomatic patients with aortic valve area less than 1 cm^2.
- LV ejection fraction less than 50%.
- Requires coronary angiogram and CABG for associated coronary artery disease
- Balloon aortic valvuloplasty
- Usually not performed in AS: Because there is high chance of restenosis and more complications of the procedure.

AORTIC STENOSIS

Clinical Points

- AS: May be a manifestation of chronic atherosclerotic process.
- Aortic sclerosis may occur in elderly without significant stenosis.
- Rheumatic inflammation, bicuspid valve and degeneration of aortic valve can result in AS.

- Bicuspid aortic valve is the most common form of congenital heart disease and can be silent throughout life.
- Aortic valve surface area of <1 cm^2 is suggestive of severe AS.
- Presence of mitral stenosis in a patient of aortic stenosis predisposes the patient for AF and MS can mask the clinical signs of AS.
- Double apex in a patient of AS may be due to LVS4.
- If aortic pressure gradient >60 mm of Hg and aortic valve area of <1 cm^2 and LV ejection fraction <50% is indication for surgery in aortic stenosis.
- Patient who is undergoing CABG with symptomatic AS requires valve replacement.

AORTIC REGURGITATION (AR)

Clinical Aspects of AR

Common Presenting Symptoms

- Palpitation
- Chest pain
- Dyspnea, PND, orthopnea.

Nocturnal Angina in AR

- Common in patients with syphilitic AR
- Associated with coronary osteitis.
- Due to decrease heart rate and low diastolic blood pressure during sleeping—causing decrease coronary filling.
- May not respond to nitrates.
- Patients of AR can become conscious of their heart beating especially on lying in left lateral position.

Causes of AR

- *Due to valvular dysfunction*
  - Rheumatic
  - Bicuspid valve with AR
- *Due to dilatation of aortic root*
  - Syphilis
  - Marfan's syndrome
  - Ankylosing spondylitis.

Consequences of AR

- Dilatation and hypertrophy of left ventricle.
- Dilatation of aortic valve ring and also mitral valve ring due to LV dilatation.
- Chronic AR leads to thickening of LV and LV dysfunction.
- Due to LVH there will be increased oxygen demand of left ventricle
- Due to decreased diastolic pressure there will be decreased filling of coronary and LV ischemia.

Clinical Feature: Chronic AR

- May be asymptomatic for a long time.
- Can have palpitation, chest pain and dyspnea.

Signs

- Signs of wide pulse pressure.
- S1 may be soft
- Ejection sound of aorta due to sudden distention of aorta.
- A2 loud in syphilitic AR (tambour quality sound)
  EDM at the aortic area.
  Perforated or everted aortic cusp—cooing dove murmur.
  Severe AR—early diastolic murmur is lengthier.
  Austin Flint—MDM at the apex.
  ESM across the aortic valve conducted to carotids.

ECG: LV diastolic/volume overload.

- Left axis deviation
- LV conduction defect.

Chest X-ray

- Massive cardiomegaly
- Aneurysmal dilatation of aorta
- If severe left atrial enlargement—suspect mitral valve disease.
- If associated AS is present—calcification of aortic valve.
- Linear calcification of aorta occurs in patients with syphilitic AR.

Acute AR

Causes

- Infective endocarditis
- Trauma to the chest
- Aortic dissection.

Clinical Differences between Acute AR/Chronic AR

Acute AR		Chronic AR
Pulse rate	Increase	Normal
Pulse pressure	Near normal	Wide
LV impulse	Normal	Hyperdynamic
EDM of AR	Shorter	Longer duration
Peripheral signs	Absent	Present

Complications of AR

- LV dysfunction and LV failure
- Pulmonary hypertension
- Infective endocarditis
- Ventricular arrhythmias
- Aortic aneurysm—ascending aorta

Indications for Surgery in AR

- Severe symptomatic patients
- LV ejection fraction less than 50%
- LV end diastolic dimension more than 65 mm
- LV end systolic dimension of >50 mm

Aortic Regurgitation

Clinical Points

- Combined lesion of AS with AR—usually occurs due to either rheumatic/congenital cause.
- Rheumatic AR is invariably associated with mitral valve involvement.
- In severe isolated AR—consider phase IV of Korotkoff's sounds as diastolic pressure
- In severe AR—because the diastolic pressure of LV increases—arterial diastolic pressure can increase as aortic root pressure cannot be below the LV pressure.
- Severe AR can be associated with diastolic thrill.

- In a patient of severe AR—there can be associated ESM in the aortic area due to increased flow which can be associated with systolic thrill but does not indicate aortic stenosis.
- In severe AR—2nd heart sound can be soft and can be associated with low pitched MDM—Austin Flint murmur at the apex.
- EDM of AR is usually high pitched and can become musical due to eversion of cusps.

TRICUSPID STENOSIS

Causes

- Rheumatic heart disease
- Congenital
- Infective endocarditis
- Carcinoid syndrome

Clinical Features

Symptoms

- Fatigue due to decreased cardiac output
- Symptoms due to systemic venous congestion:
  - Swelling of feet
  - Abdominal distention
  - Right hypochondrial pain
- Rheumatic tricuspid stenosis can be associated with mitral stenosis.
- Associated tricuspid stenosis will decrease pulmonary blood flow and decrease the symptoms of mitral stenosis.

Signs

- JVP prominent 'a' wave
- Pedal edema
- Ascites
- 1st heart sound split
- 2nd heart sound—single due to decrease blood flow across pulmonary valve.
- Presence of tricuspid opening snap.
- Mid-diastolic murmur at the tricuspid valve which increases on inspiration
- Pulsatile liver—pre-systolic pulsation

Conditions which mimic tricuspid stenosis
a. Constrictive pericarditis.
b. Restrictive cardiomyopathy.
c. Right atrial myxoma.

Chest X-ray
- Cardiomegaly
- Right atrial enlargement.

ECG
- Right atrial enlargement
- Atrial flutter and fibrillation.

TRICUSPID REGURGITATION

Causes
- Severe pulmonary hypertension.
- Infective endocarditis.
- Ebstein's anomaly

Rarer causes
- Carcinoid syndrome
- Rheumatic fever

Clinical features
- Can be detected on routine examination without symptoms
- Can have the following features
  - Swelling of feet
  - Abdominal distension
  - Prominent neck veins
  - Decreased urine output
  - Symptoms of primary cardiac disease causing pulmonary hypertension.

Signs
JVP is showing prominent 'v' wave.
- If severe pulmonary hypertension—prominent 'a' wave in the JVP
- Pulsatile liver—systolic pulsations.
- Ascites present.
- Pansystolic murmur increasing on inspiration (de Carvallo's sign)—in the tricuspid area.
- There will be signs of pulmonary hypertension.

ECG: Right atrial enlargement.
- RVH

- Evidences of associated other cardiac disease.

Chest X-ray
- Right atrial enlargement
- RVH

PULMONARY STENOSIS

Causes
- Congenital
- Rarely rheumatic/carcinoid syndrome
  For details—*see* under congenital pulmonary stenosis.

PULMONARY REGURGITATION

Causes
- Pulmonary hypertension.
- Infective endocarditis.
- RHD
- Connective tissue disease
- Carcinoid syndrome

Clinical features
- Easy fatigue
- Dizziness/syncope
- Chest pain palpitation
- Symptoms of right ventricular failure.
- Symptoms of basic heart disease.
- Signs of pulmonary hypertension
- Early diastolic murmur—Graham Steell murmur

ACUTE PERICARDITIS

Acute inflammation of the pericardium.

Causes of acute pericarditis
Infectious disorders
- Viral
  - HIV virus
  - Coxsackie virus
  - Herpes virus.
- Bacterial
  - Pyogenic organisms
  - Tuberculosis.
- Systemic causes
  - Rheumatic fever

- SLE
- Rheumatoid arthritis
- Scleroderma

Metabolic: Uremia

Cardiac disease: Acute myocardial infarction.

Other causes
- Radiation
- Malignancy
- Trauma

Clinical features: Chest pain—characteristic of pericarditis.

Pain of pericarditis
- Type—severe catching type of pain
- Site—retrosternal—predominantly left side of precordium

Pain is referred to
- Arm
- Neck
- Shoulder
- Trapezius (pain of acute MI—not referred to trapezius)
- Pain is aggravated by lying in supine position
- Relieved by sitting and leaning forward.
- Pericarditis is usually associated with pleuritis.

Other symptoms of pericarditis
- Palpitation
- Fever
- Cough
- Can be associated with symptoms of systemic disease.
- Pericarditis can involve the myocardium due to involvement of epicardial arteries.

Clinical features
- Fever
- Tachycardia
- Pericardial rub.

Characteristic of pericardial rub

Scratchy sound

Site of the rub
- Left lower sternal border
- Firmly apply the diaphragm of the stethoscope.

Better heard on
- Inspiration
- Upright and leaning forward

Components of pericardial rub
- Systolic
- Presystolic
- Early diastolic
- Pericardial rub is heard throughout the respiratory cycle and does not stop with stopping of breathing.
- Pleural rub is not heard on stopping of breathing.
- Other features of systemic disease can be present.

Different inflammatory exudates in pericarditis
- Caseating pericarditis: Tuberculosis
- Suppurative/pyogenic: Pyogenic organisms
- Serous pericarditis: SLE, rheumatoid arthritis
- Fibrous/serofibrinous: Acute MI, uremia, radiation.
- Hemorrhagic: Malignancy, tuberculosis, uremia, bleeding disorders

Chronic Pericarditis

Causes
- Tuberculosis
- Pyogenic pericarditis
- Radiation.

ECG changes of acute pericarditis
- ST segment elevation with concavity upwards (in standard leads and leads V2–V6)
- PR—segment depression (atrial involvement)
- T wave inversion
- Normal QRS.

DD of ECG changes of acute pericarditis
- Acute MI
- Early repolarisation syndrome.

ECG changes in acute myocardial infarction
- Changes occur within hours
- ST segment elevated with convexity upwards

- Leads involved: Depends on site of myo-cardial involvement.
- Reciprocal changes: Prominent T inversion. There can be loss of R wave amplitude.

Early repolarisation syndrome:
- Benign condition
- ST segment elevated and T wave tall—present in left precordial leads.

 Note

ST/T ratio is higher in pericarditis than in early repolarisation syndrome (ratio is less than 0.25).

Complication of pericarditis: Pericardial effusion and result in chronic constrictive pericarditis.

PERICARDIAL EFFUSION

Normal fluid content of pericardial cavity: Around 50 ml

Pericardial effusion: There will be increased accumulation of fluid in the pericardial cavity which may be abnormal in character. Clinical effect depends on the rate of accumulation of pericardial fluid. If there is rapid accumulation of fluid even 80–100 ml of fluid can interfere with ventricular filling, whereas slow accumulation of even 2000 ml may be well tolerated.

Causes of pericardial effusion: Same as acute pericarditis.
Other causes:
- Hypothyroidism
- Post-cardiac surgery

Clinical features:
Chest pain of pericarditis:
- Occasionally palpitation and syncope.
- Rarely—respiratory symptoms like cough and dyspnea.

Signs:
- Tachycardia
- Increased cardiac dullness
- Cardiac apex: Not palpable
- Pericardial rub

- Muffled heart sounds
- Can have features of cardiac tamponade.
- **Ewart's sign**—dullness to percussion and presence of bronchial breathing in the left lower part of scapula due to compression of the lung (bronchus) by pericardial fluid.

Pericardial tamponade: Due to rapid accumulation of fluid in the pericardial cavity resulting in decreased ventricular filling causing hemodynamic disturbance.

Causes
- Same as acute pericarditis/pericardial effusion.
- Slow development of fluid can result in dyspnea/orthopnea.

Clinical features: Occur due to defective ventricular filling and decreased cardiac output.

Signs
- Tachycardia
- Tachypnea
- Pulsus paradoxus
- Raised JVP
- Kussmaul's sign
- Ewart's sign

Beck's triad
- JVP↑
- Decreased heart sound
- Hypotension

JVP in tamponade: JVP↑ (*see* under JVP)

Low pressure tamponade: Milder form of tamponade. Intra-pericardial pressure is raised. Central venous pressure is normal or minimally raised. It occurs in patients with severe hypotension.

ECG in pericardial effusion
- Low voltage QRS
  - <0.5 mV in limb leads.
  - <1 mV in precordial leads.
- Electrical alternans:
- Beat to beat variation in direction and amplitude of QRS—due to swinging of heart in pericardial fluid.

Chest X-ray in pericardial effusion
- Massive cardiomegaly
- Water bottle appearance—narrow pedicle with cardiomegaly.
- No pulmonary plethora or venous congestion.
- Difficult to delineate different cardiac chambers.

CONSTRICTIVE PERICARDITIS

Pathophysiology
- Constrictive pericarditis occurs due to fibrosis and thickening of pericardium.
- It can also result from pericardial effusion. Heart will be enclosed in a thick sac.
- There will be chronic scarring, fibrosis, and calcification of pericardium.
- Ultimately there will be defective filling of the ventricles.

Hemodynamic Effects of Pericardial Constriction
- There will be decreased filling of ventricles.
- Stroke volume is reduced.
- There will be increased pressure in the atrium, pulmonary and systemic circulation
- Myocardial function can be affected later by fibrosis process extending into the myocardium.

Clinical Features
- Fatigue
- Swelling of feet
- Distension of abdomen
- Right hypochondrial pain
- Cachexia.

Signs
- Cachexia
- Ascites
- Edema
- Pleural effusion
- Jaundice
- Enlarged liver

Cardiac Examination
- Pulsus paradoxus
- JVP: Prominent X and Y descent (*see* under JVP)
- Square root sign (there is early raise of diastolic pressure of RV with early filling and then the pressure contour reaches a plateau—not a clinical sign)
- Kussmaul's sign
- Apex: Not made out and can have cardiac apical retraction (Broadbent's sign)
- Heart sounds—muffled

Pericardial Knock (in Constrictive Pericarditis)
- Occurs in early diastole and is due to sudden stoppage of ventricular filling
- Heard all over the precordium
- High-pitched sound increases with inspiration

Table 1.4: Differences between restrictive cardiomyopathy and constrictive pericarditis

Constrictive pericarditis	Restrictive cardiomyopathy
Past history of pericarditis and pericardial effusion	H/o systemic disease like amyloidosis
Cardiac apex—not felt	Cardiac apex—well made out
High-pitched pericardial knock	Low-pitched S3
Murmur not heard	Murmur of TR/MR

Table 1.5: Differences between pericardial effusion and constrictive pericarditis

	Pericardial effusion	Constrictive pericarditis
Kussmaul's sign	Negative	Positive
Pulsus paradoxus	Present	Present/absent
Y descent	Absent	Prominent
Square root sign	Negative	Positive

Other causes of Kussmaul's sign
- Right ventricular infarction

- Restrictive cardiomyopathy
- Pulmonary embolism

JVP in constrictive pericarditis
- JVP is raised
- Prominent X and Y descent.

Square root sign
- This is the ventricular pressure tracing in constrictive pericarditis. There is initial dip and then plateau of pressure.
- There is initial decrease of ventricular pressure after systole and there is abnormal rapid filling during early diastole which suddenly stops due to non-distensibility of the pericardium—dip and plateau form—**square root sign**.

ECG
- Low voltage of QRS
- Diffuse T wave inversion
- Atrial fibrillation

Chest X-ray
- Minimally enlarged heart
- Pericardial calcification

ATRIAL FIBRILLATION

Common form of arrhythmia associated with increased heart rate.

In atrial fibrillation there will be irregular activation of atria with irregular ventricular response depending on the AV nodal conduction. Usual ventricular rate in atrial fibrillation is >200/minute.

Genesis of Atrial Fibrillation

Increased automaticity of the atrial musculature with micro reentry mechanism. Dilated and fibrosed atrium is more likely to initiate automaticity.

Usual site of initiation of automaticity: At the atrial entry site of pulmonary veins containing atrialised musculature.

Change in the autonomic tone, increased automaticity and re-entry mechanisms play the role in precipitating AF.

Types of Atrial Fibrillation

Intermittent/paroxysmal AF: Sudden onset of AF—starts abruptly and stops on its own. Usually within 24 hours.

Persistent: Usually continues for a week and stops on its own/with treatment.

Permanent AF: Cannot be reversed.

Causes of Atrial Fibrillation

Common
- IHD
- Mitral stenosis and mitral regurgitation
- Hypertension
- Thyrotoxicosis

Less common
- COPD
- Pneumonia
- Pericardial disorders
- ASD
- Lone atrial fibrillation.

Effects of Atrial Fibrillation
- Loss of atrial contractility (loss of atrial booster pump).
- Increased ventricular rate interfering with filling of the ventricles.
- Risk of systemic embolisation.
- Tachycardia cardiomyopathy

Clinical Features
- May be asymptomatic.
- May complain of fatigue/irregular palpitation
- Can precipitate cardiac failure and can precipitate anginal chest (pain and syncope)
- Increased ventricular rate interferes with ventricular filling and loss of atrial contraction leads to pulmonary venous congestion.
- Stagnation of blood at the atrial appendage leads to formation of left atrial thrombus with systemic embolisation.

Signs
- Irregularly irregular pulse.
- Pulse apex deficit >10/minute.
- Absence of a wave in JVP.
- Varying intensity of 1st heart sound.
- Presystolic accentuation of MDM of mitral stenosis disappears.
- There may be other evidence of RHD, congenital heart disease, thyrotoxicosis, etc.

Table 1.6: Differences between multiple VPCs and AF

	Multiple VPCs	*AF*
JVP	a wave present	'a' wave absent
Pulse	Apex deficit—less than 10	More than 10
Exercise	Reduces or disappearance of VPCs of AF	No change or increase

Embolisation in AF
- Because of the loss of atrial contractility thrombus formation occurs in the atrium—usual site is left atrial appendage.
- Dislodgement of thrombus can occur causing systemic embolisation, e.g. CVA.
- Systemic embolisation is more likely to occur during intermittent AF.
- In patients with intermittent AF clot formation will occur during an attack of AF and when the AF terminates, there will be normal contraction of the atrium with dislodgement of thrombus.

Risk factors for CVA in atrial fibrillation
- More likely to occur in patients with dilated left atrium.
- Presence of CCF
- Previous embolisation
- With associated risk factors like diabetes mellitus, hypertension

Irregular ventricular response and irregularly irregular pulse in AF
- Ventricular response is irregular in atrial fibrillation due to the varying refractory period of AV node and concealed conduction through the AV node.
- If the ventricular response is rapid (due to significant number of atrial impulses conducted across the AV node) ventricular filling becomes inadequate to produce sufficient force of contraction and the pulse is feeble and may not be felt (pulse apex deficit). If the ventricular response is slower with less impulses from atria being conducted through AV node—causing increased ventricular filling with increased force of contraction, the pulse being conducted to the periphery with feeling of pulse in the periphery.

Slow atrial fibrillation
- Atrial fibrillation with bradycardia
- Usually AF is associated with ventricular rate of around 200/min due to the AV node preventing the atrial impulses reaching the ventricle even though the atrial rate is very high.
- In some patients with AF—ventricular rate can be very low (around 60–70/min)—suspect following disorders
- Sinus node dysfunction
- AV nodal disease and AV block
- Drugs like digoxin/verapamil/beta blockers.

Role of digoxin in AF
Digoxin decreases the ventricular rate by:
1. Increases the refractory period of AV node.
2. Decreases the refractory period of atria, thereby more atrial impulses reach the AV node resulting in greater degree of concealed conduction through the AV node causing decreased heart rate.

INFECTIVE ENDOCARDITIS

Organisms Causing Endocarditis

- *Streptococcus viridans*—can affect damaged valves.
- Normal valve can be affected by
  - *Staphylococcus aureus*
  - Pneumococcus

In IV drug abusers

Normal valve can be affected by

- Usual organisms: Gram negative organisms, *Staphylococcus aureus* and fungi
- Usual valve affected: Tricuspid valve
- Because of septic embolisation to lungs from tricuspid valve endocarditis—can cause—pneumonia and lung abscess.

Prosthetic Valve Endocarditis

- Occurs within 60 days of replacement of valve.
- *Common organisms*:
  - *Staphylococcus aureus*
  - Coagulase-negative Staphylococcus
- Common source of infection in prosthetic valve endocarditis:
  - Urinary catheter
  - Intra-venous/intra-arterial lines.
  - Endotracheal tube
  - May be pacemaker.
- Early prosthetic valve endocarditis: within 60 days of valve replacement
- Late prosthetic valve endocarditis— within 1 year of valve replacement.

Infective Organisms in Endocarditis

Streptococcus viridans

- Common cause of endocarditis
- Usually causes subacute endocarditis.

Beta-hemolytic Streptococci: Common in older age group and IV drug addicts can cause acute endocarditis.

Streptococcus pneumoniae

- Can cause acute endocarditis
- Endocarditis can occur together with pneumonia and meningitis

Streptococcus gallolyticus (bovis)

- Usual source is gastrointestinal tract
- Rule out GIT pathology and carcinoma colon.

Staphylococcus aureus

- Causes acute severe endocarditis with severe systemic toxicity

- Can infect native/prosthetic valve with significant valve damage
- In IV drug abusers it can cause tricuspid valve endocarditis.

Coagulase negative staphylococcus: Commonly infects prosthetic valve and causes subacute endocarditis.

HACEK organisms: Gram-negative bacilli colonizing the URT occasionally causes endocarditis.

Enterococcus: Usual source is from genito-urinary tract and common in elderly.

Fungi: Rarely can infect prosthetic valve and common with IV lines.

Culture negative endocarditis

- May be due to partial antibiotic treatment
- Rare organisms like Brucella, Coxiella and Legionella can cause culture negative endocarditis
- Observation of the blood culture for minimum of 2 weeks may be required for the above organisms
- Conditions which predispose to infective endocarditis:
  - High velocity of flow with jet with lesions with a pressure gradient.
  - Jet of blood on the valve leaflet causing damage to the endothelium.
  - Jet lesions cause deposition of platelets, fibrin material and leads to deposition of bacteria.

Cardiac lesions predisposing to endocarditis

- Valvular diseases
- Mitral regurgitation (may be MVP with MVR)
- Aortic regurgitation
- Bicuspid aortic valve

Congenital lesions

- VSD
- PDA
- Fallot's tetralogy—RV outlet obstruction

Effects of intracardiac infection

Can cause damage to the valve

- Like abscess of the valve ring
- Valvular damage

- Infection of the pericardium: Pyoperi-cardium.
- Infection of the myocardium: Myocardial abscess.
- Damage to the conductive tissues:
  - Conduction abnormality
  - Scar formation

Embolization in endocarditis
- Left-sided endocarditis—systemic emboli-zation
- Right-sided endocarditis—pulmonary embolization, infection, abscess formation.

Septic embolization
- More common with staphylococcal endo-carditis
- Can embolise to brain and kidney
- Septic embolization causes splinter hemorr-hage and Janeway lesions
- Immune complex deposition and vascu-litis causes
  - Osler's nodes
  - Roth's spots
  - Acute glomerulonephritis
- Large vegetations in endocarditis can be caused by: Fungi and *Staphylococcus aureus*.

Mycotic aneurysm in endocarditis
- In left-sided endocarditis—embolization to cerebral vessels.
- Embolization into branches of arteries of circle of Willis.
- *Causes*: Weakening of vessel with aneu-rysm—formation which can rupture.

Usual sites of vegetation in endocarditis
- Leaflets of valves.
- Chordae tendinae
- Endocardium

Composition of vegetations: Vegetations contain platelets, fibrin, WBCs, RBCs and microorganisms.

Predisposing conditions for endocarditis
- Oropharyngeal, genitourinary, gastro-intestinal procedures.

- Tooth extraction and periodontal surgeries.
- IV line, IV drug abusers, intra-cardiac devices.

 Note

Routine brushing of teeth and chewing can result in bacteremia.

Systemic conditions predisposing to endocarditis
- Diabetes mellitus
- Internal malignancy
- Immune suppressive therapy
- CRF
- Hemodialysis

Pathogenesis of lesions in endocarditis: Lesions occur due to infection of intra-cardiac struc-tures.

Peripheral manifestations of infective endocar-ditis
Petechial hemorrhages
- Usual sites
  - Conjunctiva
  - Oral cavity
  - Upper and lower limbs
- Splinter hemorrhage—streaky hemorrhage beneath the nail.
- Janeway lesions: Macular lesions over the palms and soles, hemorrhagic painless: Due to septic embolization. Common in Staphylococcal endocarditis
- Osler's nodes: Nodular lesions
  - Site—pads of fingers and toes, painful and erythematous
  - Due to—vasculitis with immune comp-lex depression
- Roth's spots—pale centered hemorrhagic spot in the retina
  - Due to—vasculitis with immune comp-lex deposition.

 Note

Roth spots can also occur in SLE, leukemia.

- Infective endocarditis can also cause glo-merulonephritis due to immune complex deposition.

Blood culture in infective endocarditis: 3 sets of blood cultures to be drawn 1 hour apart to demonstrate continuous bacteremia.

 Note

Large doses of intravenous antibiotics are required in the treatment of endocarditis because higher concentration of drugs in the blood is required for the treatment of valve lesions as the valves do not have separate blood supply and only depend on the circulating blood.

Complications of Infective Endocarditis

Cardiac

- Valvular damage resulting in acute AR/MR
- Conduction defects
- Valve abscess
- Congestive cardiac failure
- Prosthetic valve dysfunction

Systemic

- Systemic embolization
- Mycotic aneurysm rupture
- Immune complex deposition and glomerulo-nephritis
- Sepsis syndrome

APPROACH TO A PATIENT OF CONGENITAL HEART DISEASE

Symptoms of Congenital Heart Disease

ASD

- Usually asymptomatic till 5th decade of life
- Easy fatigability
- Palpitation
- Recurrent LRTI

VSD

- Can be asymptomatic
- Can become symptomatic at 2nd to 3rd decade of life.
- Retarded growth
- Exertional dyspnea
- Recurrent LRTI
- Can present with CCF
- Can present with infective endocarditis.

PDA

- May be detected on routine examination
- Failure to thrive in a child
- Can present with CCF.

Congenital PS

- May be asymptomatic
- Dizziness
- Chest pain
- Exercise intolerance.

Congenital AS

- Fatigue
- Palpitation
- Syncope
- Angina
- Dyspnea

Coarctation of aorta

- Fatigability of lower limbs
- Can present as epistaxis
- Cardiac failure, endocarditis
- Intracranial bleed.

Ebstein's anomaly

- Exercise intolerance and dyspnea
- Central cyanosis
- Swelling of feet
- Sudden cardiac death.

Fallot's tetralogy

- Retarded growth and development
- Hypoxic spells
- Squatting episodes
- Central cyanosis.

General examination in congenital heart disease.

Marfan's syndrome

- Look for high-arched palate
- High-arched palate:
  - Height of the palate will be >2 SD above normal height from floor of the oral cavity.

Lens dislocation in Marfan's syndrome

- Partial dislocation
- Usually bilateral
- Causes tremulousness of iris—iridodonesis
- Direction of dislocation: Superior and temporal

Homocystinuria

Features

- Intellectual abnormality
- Marfanoid features
- Ectopia lentis (lens dislocation is in the inferior nasal direction)
- Thromboembolism/vascular occlusion.

 Note

Marfan's syndrome is not associated with intellectual abnormality and lens dislocation is in the superior and temporal direction.

ASD: Gracile built

- Evidence of Holt-Oram's syndrome
- Rarely trisomy 18.

VSD: Evidence of

- Down's syndrome
- Rubella syndrome
- Fetal alcohol syndrome
- Trisomy 18
- Trisomy 13.

PDA

- Features of trisomy 18
- Rocker bottom feet

Congenital PS: Features of Rubella/William's syndrome

Valvular PS

- Face: Round and bloated
- Cheek—colored

Congenital AS: Supravalvular AS—features of William's syndrome.

Coarctation of aorta

- Features of Turner's syndrome
- Noonan's syndrome
- Well-developed upper extremities
- Less developed lower extremities

Ebstein's anomaly: Central cyanosis

Fallot's tetralogy

- Cachexia and weight loss
- Central cyanosis.

Pulse in Congenital Heart Disease

ASD

- Usually normal
- Occasionally low volume

VSD

- Small VSD—normal
- Large VSD—high volume pulse
  PDA—high volume and collapsing

Congenital PS: Normal or low volume—if associated with right side cardiac failure.

Congenital AS

- Valvular—low volume. Slow raising
- Supravalvular—left upper limb pulse feeble.

Coarctation of aorta

- Radiofemoral delay
- If left subclavian is involved—left upper limb pulse—feeble

Ebstein's anomaly: Normal

Fallot's tetralogy: Normal/high volume if severe AR or large collaterals.

Blood Pressure Recording in Congenital Heart Disease

ASD: Normal

VSD: Normal

PDA: High systolic and low diastolic with wide pulse pressure

Valvular PS: Normal

Valvular AS: Low systolic pressure

Supravalvular AS: Left upper limb blood pressure is lower by 10–15 mm of Hg

Coarctation of aorta: Lower limb blood pressure is lower than upper limb blood pressure by 10–15 mm of Hg

Ebstein's anomaly: Normal

Fallot's tetralogy: Normal.

JVP in the Congenital Heart Disease

ASD: Equal amplitude of 'a' and 'v' waves

VSD: Initially normal

Prominent 'a' wave if pulmonary artery hypertension

PDA: Normal

Cong PS: Prominent 'a' wave due to RVH
Coarctation of aorta: Normal
Ebstein's anomaly: Usually normal
Fallot's tetralogy: Normal

Cardiac Apex in Congenital Heart Disease

ASD: May be formed by right ventricle.
VSD: LV apex—hyperdynamic
PDA: LV apex—hyperdynamic
Congenital PS—normal/RV apex
Congenital AS-LV apex—heaving
Coarctation—LV apex—heaving
Ebstein's anomaly: Normal
Fallot's tetralogy: Normal

Heart Sounds in Congenital Heart Disease

ASD
- 1st heart sound—loud (due to loud tricuspid component)
- 2nd heart sound—wide and fixed split (septum secundum ASD).

VSD
- 1st heart sound normal
- 2nd heart sound—wide and varying split (due to early closure of aortic valve)

PDA
- 1st heart sound normal
- 2nd heart sound widely split due to prolonged RV ejection

Congenital PS
- Presence of pulmonary ejection click
- 2nd heart sound—severe stenosis—P_2 not audible
- 2nd heart sound—wide split due to delayed P_2 (delayed RV ejection)
- Right-sided S4.

Congenital AS
- Ejection click—in valvular or bicuspid valve.
- Mild AS: A2 not delayed
- 2nd heart sound is not split.
- Severe AS—paradoxical split of 2nd heart sound.

- Left-sided S4
- Supravalvular AS—normal heart sounds
- Coarctaion of aorta—A2 loud
  Ejection click—bicuspid valve.
  LVH—left-sided S4

Ebstein's anomaly
- 1st heart sound split
- 2nd heart sound widely split
- Right-sided 3rd and 4th heart sound

Fallot's tetralogy
- 1st heart sound—normal
- 2nd heart sound P_2 absent, A_2 loud.

Murmurs in Congenital Heart Disease

ASD
- Ejection systolic murmur: Pulmonary area.
- MDM—across the tricuspid valve.

VSD
- Pansystolic murmur—left 3rd/4th intercostal space—sternal border
- MDM—across the mitral valve.

PDA
- Continuous murmur—left 1st IC space
- MDM—across the mitral valve.

Congenital PS
- Ejection systolic murmur: Pulmonary area
- Pansystolic murmur of TR.

Congenital AS
- Ejection systolic murmur—aortic area—right 2nd space.
- Supravalvular AS—ESM—right first intercostal space conducted to right carotid.

Coarctation of aorta
- ESM—at aortic area—due to bicuspid aortic valve.
- Systolic murmur at 4th or 5th thoracic spine—at the site of coarctation.
- Suprasternal systolic murmur—due to collaterals

Ebstein's anomaly: Pansystolic murmurs—tricuspid area due to TR.

Fallot's tetralogy
- ESM left 2nd or 3rd intercostals space
- Due to infundibular pulmonary stenosis.

ECG in Congenital Heart Disease

ASD
- Right atrial enlargement
- Sputum secundum ASD—rsr' pattern in lead V_1
- Supraventricular arrhythmias
- Septum primum ASD
  - QRS left axis deviation
  - V1-rsr' pattern, severe MR-LA enlargement

VSD
- Left atrial enlargement
- LV volume overload
- RVH
- Katz-Wachtel phenomenon

PDA
- LA enlargement
- LV enlargement.

Congenital PS
- Giant P wave
- Right axis deviation in V1 and V2
- V1—tall R wave with T inversion in V1

Congenital AS: LVH with ST and T changes.

Coarctation of aorta: LVH with strain

Ebstein's anomaly
- Himalayan P wave
- RBBB
- All types of supraventricular arrhythmias, Brugada syndrome.

Fallot's tetralogy
- P wave left axis deviation
- QRS—tall R wave in V1
- Lead V2—rs pattern (sudden change in pattern)
- T—not inverted in precordial leads.

Chest X-ray in Congenital Heart Disease

ASD
- Pulmonary plethora
- RA and RV enlargement
- Dilated pulmonary artery
- Hilar dance
- Jug handle appearance

VSD
- Cardiomegaly
- Pulmonary plethora
- RV and LV enlargement
- Pulmonary artery enlargement

PDA
- Pulmonary plethora
- Enlarged LA and LV
- Separated convexity between aorta and pulmonary artery on the left cardiac border—due to the ductus

Congenital PS
- Poststenotic dilatation of pulmonary artery.
- RA and RV enlargement.

Congenital AS
- Cardiomegaly—LVH
- Calcified bicuspid aortic valve.

Coarctation of aorta
- LVH
- RIB notching
- Dilatation of aorta with figure of 3 appearance.

Ebstein's anomaly: Box-like heart
Fallot's tetralogy: Boot-shaped heart.

ORTHODEOXIA

Deoxygenation of blood occurring when the person changes his position from lying down to upright position. It is associated with platypnea (dyspnea in the upright position).

Mechanisms of Orthodeoxia

- There is increasing shunting of blood from right to left on assuming upright position. Pressure in the right atrium is normal.
- It can also occur with significant shunting (A-V) in the lungs with intrapulmonary lesions or with significant ventilation perfusion mismatching.

1st Mechanism

On standing upright: There will be stretch in the interatrial communication. This allows the blood from the IVC to go through the interatrial defect into the left atrium. This becomes more significant in the presence of Eustachian valve.

Interatrial communications with orthodeoxia
- Patient foramen ovale
- ASD
- Penetrated atrial septal aneurysm.
- Cirrhosis of liver and hepatopulmonary syndrome.
  Respiratory: Pulmonary AV fistula

In cirrhotics and in patients with pulmonary A-V fistula on standing, there will be shunting of blood into the lung bases with dilated pre-capillaries with ventilation perfusion mismatch and with hypoxia.

STRAIGHT BACK SYNDROME

Straight back syndrome occurs due to:
- Loss of thoracic spine curvature.
- Anteroposterior diameter of the chest becomes narrower and heart is compressed by the narrow chest.

Clinical Findings

- Exaggerated left parasternal movement.
- Wide splitting of the 2nd heart sound (not fixed split).
- Ejection systolic murmur in the pulmonary area.
- Ejection systolic murmur may be mistaken for ASD or pulmonary stenosis.

Radiological diagnosis: By chest X-ray.
- Measure the anteroposterior diameter of the chest (measured from front of the vertebra to the back of the sternum).
- Measure the transverse diameter of the chest—from just above the right doom of the diaphragm inside of the ribs.
- AP diameter is less than 1/3 of transverse diameter is diagnostic of straight back syndrome.

VENOUS HUM IN NECK

Site of venous hum in the neck
- Right side (can be heard bilaterally) more common on the right side due to straighter right internal jugular and innominate vein
- Supraclavicular fossa
- Lateral to the sternomastoid or in between two heads of sternomastoid
- Position of the patient: Patient in sitting position. Head and neck—turned to opposite side—partial compression of the jugular vein by the transverse process of the Atlas.
- Better heard on—inspiration
- Decreases by—compression of the jugular vein at the upper part of the neck.
- Venous hum occurs due to: Increased velocity of flow in hyperdynamic circulation.

MITRAL VALVE PROLAPSE (MVP)

Prolapse of the Posterior Leaflet of the Mitral Valve into the Left Atrium

Other Physiological/Musculoskeletal Abnormalities in MVP
- Symptoms of anxiety
- Migraine headache
- Straight back syndrome
- Autonomic dysfunction and increased sympathetic activity.

Pathology in Primary MVP
- Abnormality in collagen metabolism
- Myxomatous proliferation of valve.

Key Points:
- MVP can be associated with other collagen/connective tissue disorders
- MVP can occur as a consequence of rheumatic heart disease.
- Tricuspid valve prolapse can rarely occur.

Clinical Features

Symptoms
- May be asymptomatic throughout life.
- Can present with chest pain, palpitation, dizziness and autonomic dysfunction.

Chest pain of MVP: Can have angina like pain but may not be exertional.

MVP can cause
- Increase tension on the papillary muscle and coronary spasm.
- It can also cause wall motion abnormality of the left ventricle.
- Palpitation in MVP—due to supraventricular arrhythmias.

Clinical signs
- Non-ejection click—mid to late systolic click in the mitral area.
- Mid or late systolic murmur.

Mechanism of mid-systolic click: Occurs in the mid-systole after S1—due to prolapse of the leaflet (usually posterior mitral leaflet with tension on chordae tendinae).

Murmur of MVP: Due to regurgitation of blood into left atrium due to the prolapse of the mitral leaflet.

Click and murmur of MVP on standing: Decrease return of blood to LV → decrease LV cavity size leads to increase propensity of the valve leaflet to prolapse into left atrium. Click and murmur occurs earlier and intensifies on standing.

Arrhythmias in MVP
- Tachycardia like SVT—common in patients with MVP.
- There is increased associations between AV nodal bypass tract and prolonged QT interval inpatients with MVP.

Other arrhythmias
- Ectopic beats—atrial and ventricular.
- Ventricular arrhythmias.
- SA node dysfunction

Sudden death in MVP
- Sudden death is common in patients with MVP with
  - Severe MR
  - Ventricular arrhythmias
  - Prolonged QT interval.
- Sudden death occurs with prolonged asystole and complex arrhythmias.

Endocarditis in MVP: Increased incidence of infective endocarditis—if associated with severe MR in a patient of MVP.

Embolization in a patient of MVP: Platelet aggregation can occur over the damaged endothelium of the valve and can cause embolization.

ECG changes in MVP: Non-specific ST/T changes in inferior leads and anterolateral leads.

Conditions associated with MVP
- Primary
- Secondarily associated with
  - Straight back syndrome
  - Marfan's syndrome
  - Ehlers-Danlos syndrome
- Rarely MVP may be a manifestation of rheumatic heart disease.

ATRIAL SEPTAL DEFECT (ASD)

Types of ASD

Most common type: Ostium secundum type.
Other types
- Septum primum
- Sinus venosus type
- SVC and IVC type
- Coronary sinus type

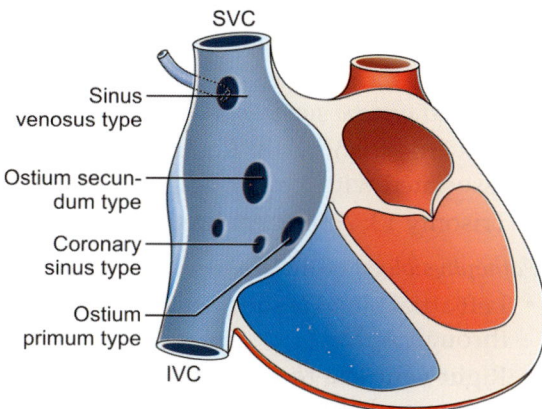

Fig. 1.6: Different types of ASD

Different Types of ASD

Septum secundum type: Due to either septum secundum growth defect or defect in septum primum.

Septum primum type: Due to atrioventricular septal defect (AV canal defect).

Sinus venosus type of defect

SVC type: Defect occurs at as SVC enters into the right atrium.

IVC type: Defect occurs at as IVC enters into the right atrium.

Coronary sinus type: At the opening of coronary sinus in the wall of left atrium.

Associated cardiac abnormalities with ASD

- Mitral valve prolapse
- Partial anomalous pulmonary venous connection
- Pulmonary artery dilatation of aneurismal type.
- Mitral regurgitation: LV cavity may become deformed and abnormal cusp movement and chordae tendineae abnormality can occur.

Associated skeletal abnormalities with ASD

Holt-Oram syndrome: Associated with ostium secundum ASD.

Skeletal abnormalties in Holt-Oram syndrome

- Presence of extraphalanx
- Hypoplasia of radius
- Thumb may be hypoplastic or absent.
- Metacarpal bones may be hypoplastic or absent.

Associated genetic syndromes with ASD

- Edwards trisomy 18: Rocker bottom feet associated with VSD, PDA
- Trisomy 13: ASD, cleft lips, palate.

Pathophysiology of ASD

- Left atrial blood is shunted to right atrium through ASD.
- Right ventricle receives blood from right atrium and also from left atrium through the shunt.

- Right ventricular compliance increases and becomes thinner after birth and there will be volume overload of right ventricle and LV becomes less volume overloaded.

Right ventricle in ASD

- Thin and compliant RV receives large volume of blood and empties into low resistance pulmonary artery without raise in pulmonary artery pressure.
- If patient develops systemic hypertension, RHD and develops LV dysfunction, more amount of blood is shunted to right side with the development of RV failure. Development of atrial arrhythmias may also contribute for RV failure.

Left ventricular function in ASD: Interventricular septum can be displaced to the left due to increase in the right ventricular volume and can cause LV dysfunction and systemic hypertension and IHD can cause further LV dysfunction. Coronary reserve can decrease due to RVH.

 Note

PAPVC can mimic ASD. Pulmonary artery dilatation can occur in ASD and pulmonary artery can become thrombosed in ASD.

Clinical Features

Symptoms: Septum secundum ASD

- Most of the patients of ASD are asymptomatic till 4th decade of life.
- Pregnancy is well tolerated.

Palpitation: Common symptom of ASD—palpitation occurs due to supraventricular arrhythmias (paroxysmal supraventricular arrhythmias, atrial flutter and fibrillation).

Breathlessness

- Not a common symptom of ASD
- Breathlessness occurs due to decrease compliance of lungs due to volume overload.
- Decrease lung compliance can also cause orthopnea.
- Platypnea can also occur due to orthodeoxia.

- *Other symptoms*
  - Recurrent lower respiratory tract infection.
  - Easy fatigability.

🔑 Key Points:

- Patient with patent foramen ovale (PFO) can present as TIA due to paradoxical embolization and can have orthodeoxia.
- Patients with aneurysm of atrial septum can develop platelet and fibrin embolization into the brain.
- Adult ASD patients can have associated IHD and hypertension and aortic valve disease and can have increased left to right shunt.

Signs of ASD

- Build and nourishment: Build can be adequate but significant low body weight can be a feature.
- Skeletal features—already discussed.

Pulse: Usually normal or due to decreased LV output can have decrease volume of pulse.

JVP: Equal amplitude of a and v waves due to communication between right and left atrium.

- Pulmonary hypertension can have prominent a wave.

Precordium

Pulsatile precordium with left parasternal lift—due to RV volume overload.

Apex: May be occupied by RV (with rotation of the apex).

Dilated pulmonary artery: Can cause prominent pulmonary artery pulsation.

Systolic thrill: Pulmonary area—either due to large ASD or associated with pulmonary stenosis.

Auscultation

- 1st heart sound—loud due to loud tricuspid component
- 2nd heart sound
  - P2 loud
  - 2nd heart sound—wide and fixed split.

Murmurs: Ejection systolic murmur in the pulmonary area which increases on inspiration.

Mid-diastolic murmur across the tricuspid area due to increased flow across the tricuspid valve.

Mechanism of Auscultatory Events in ASD

Loud tricuspid component of 1st heart sound: Large amount of blood flow at the tricuspid valve during diastole—keeping the tricuspid leaflet low into the right ventricular cavity. During RV systole the tricuspid leaflets forcibly close with moving for a larger distance causing a loud tricuspid component.

P2 loud
- Without pulmonary hypertension
- Due to dilated pulmonary artery closer to the chest wall.

Wide and fixed split of 2nd heart sound
- Typical sign of septum secundum ASD.
- Better heard on standing.

Wide splitting of 2nd heart sound
Due to
1. Large amount of blood passing through the pulmonary valve.
2. During inspiration—pulmonary artery capacitance is increased with decrease of pulmonary vascular resistance.

   Above factors cause delay of pulmonary valve closure due to delay of pulmonary hang out interval.

Fixity of 2nd heart sound split
- Equal amount of blood is passing through pulmonary valve during inspiration and expiration.
- During inspiration right atrium receives blood from IVC and SVC and less from LA through the shunt.
- During expiration more blood is coming from the shunt and less from IVC and SVC—as a result equal amount of blood passes through pulmonary valve causing P2 with fixed duration.

- Above hemodynamic changes also results in equal amount of blood filling the LV during both phases of respiration resulting in A2 with fixed duration.

 Note

PAPVC with intact interatrial septum can have wide but persistent split (but not fixed) of second heart sound.

Persistent split: Split is wider during inspiration and narrow during expiration but still audible not in septum secundum ASD.

ESM in pulmonary area: Due to the ejection of large volume of blood across the pulmonary valve into the dilated pulmonary artery.

MDM at the tricuspid valve
- Due to increased diastolic flow across the tricuspid valve.
- Other causes of wide split with varying 2nd heart sound: PAPVC, RVF and pulmonary embolism.

ASD with variable split: Sinus venosus type.

Chest X-ray in ASD
- Pulmonary plethora
- Enlargement of right atrium
- Pulmonary artery is dilated
- Enlargement of right ventricle

Jug handle appearance in chest X-ray in ASD.
Features
- Handle of the jug: Dilated right descending pulmonary artery with left-dilated pulmonary artery.
- Right border—dilated right atrium
- Left border—dilated RV
  (Jug handle appearance in the chest X-ray can also occur in primary pulmonary hypertension)

Hilar dance seen in ASD
On fluoroscopy—due to increased blood flow causing vigorous pulmonary artery pulsation.

ECG abnormalities in ASD
- RA enlargement—peaked P wave
- First degree heart block—prolonged PR interval

- P wave axis—if left axis—sinus…venosus type of ASD.
- Supraventricular arrhythmias—atrial ectopics, SVT, atrial flutter and fibrillation.

Septum secundum ASD: QRS-rsr' pattern due to enlargement and thickening of outflow tract of RV.
- If the patient develops pulmonary hypertension rsr' becomes rsR'.

Changes due to development of pulmonary hypertension in ASD
- 2nd heart sound—split becomes narrow but remain fixed.
- ESM across the pulmonary valve becomes shorter.
- MDM flow murmur across the tricuspid valve disappears.
- P_2 becomes louder.

LUTEMBACHER'S SYNDROME

Combination of congenital ASD with rheumatic mitral stenosis is called Lutembacher's syndrome.

Hemodynamic Consequences

Depends on the severity of either mitral stenosis or ASD.

If the mitral stenosis is severe with smaller ASD
- Symptoms of mitral stenosis dominate.
- Associated mitral stenosis can increase the shunt across the ASD.
- Incidence of atrial fibrillation is more in patients with mitral stenosis with ASD.
- More chance of developing early pulmonary hypertension.

If ASD is larger and less severe mitral stenosis: There is decrease of flow across mitral valve with decrease of mid-diastolic murmur of mitral stenosis with increased intensity of ejection systolic murmur across the pulmonary valve.

Scimitar Syndrome

(Otherwise called: Pulmonary venous syndrome).

Components

- Hypoplasia of right lung.
- Total or partial pulmonary venous connection.
- Hypoplastic right pulmonary artery.
- There will be anomalous right pulmonary vein—which is curved—drains into IVC.
- Curved pulmonary vein gives the appearance of a curved sword in the chest X-ray (scimitar = curved sword).
- Curved or crescent like shadow (in the chest X-ray) in the right lower lung field due to curved venous channel.

OSTIUM PRIMUM ASD

Also called endocardial cushion defect/AV canal defect

Where is the defect?

Defect is at the level of mitral and tricuspid valve in the atrial septum.

What is the defect?

Defect in the endocardial cushion.

What is endocardial cushion?

Portion of the heart which meets the atrial and ventricular septum and mitral and tricuspid valve.

What abnormality does ostium primum defect cause?

It can cause the following consequences:
- Abnormality of mitral or tricuspid valve
- Cleft mitral valve
- Single AV canal
- Shunt between RA and LA.

It causes communication between two atria causing left to right shunt
- It can result in mitral regurgitation
- Rarely LV blood may be shunted to RA.

In whom it can be associated with?

It can be associated with Down's syndrome.

What are the clinical features?

- If small defect—mild MR, no LV to RA shunting—asymptomatic.
- If large defect—severe MR—CCF at early age.
- Can have dyspnea, feeding difficulty and failure to thrive.

What are the clinical signs?

If shunt is significant—child can have:
- Tachycardia
- Tachypnea
- Precordial bulge
- Harrison's sulcus.

Precordium

Isolated defect or partial AV canal defect with mild MR
- Findings of ASD—prominent RV impulse
- ESM—at pulmonary area
- 2nd heart sound wide split may not be fixed
- Murmur of mitral regurgitation

If severe: LV enlargement and LA enlargement.

What complications patient can develop?

- If significant left to right shunt: Development of pulmonary hypertension.
- If severe defect: Severe MR and CCF.

What are the ECG changes

- QRS left axis deviation
- PR prolonged first degree heart block
- V1-rsr' pattern
- RA enlargement
- If severe MR—LA enlargement.

Chest X-ray

- Like ostium secundum ASD
- If severe MR—left heart enlargement.

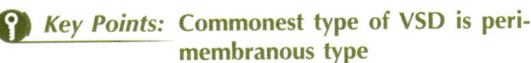
VENTRICULAR SEPTAL DEFECT

Key Points: Commonest type of VSD is peri-membranous type

- Muscular type of VSD can close at early part of life.
- Most of the VSD who have tendency to close—close by first year of life or at least by 8 years of age.

Associated Genetic Abnormalities with VSD

VSD can be a part of
- Down's syndrome
- Trisomy 18
- Trisomy 13
- Rubella syndrome/fetal alcohol syndrome

Different types of VSD (Figs 1.7–1.9)

Above crista supraventricularis: Supracristal

Below crista supraventricularis:
- Membranous
- Muscular

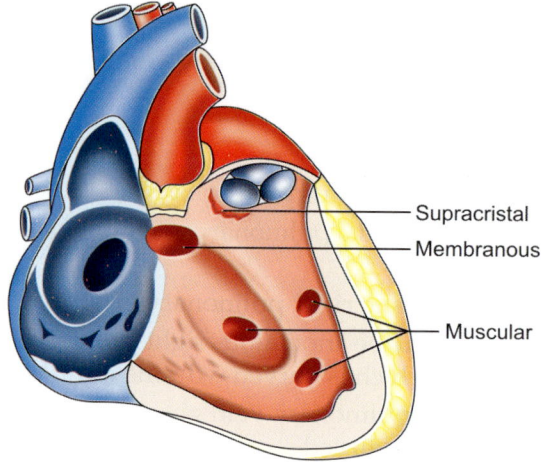

Fig. 1.9: Classification of VSD depending on the location

Membranous: Interventricular
Muscular
- Defect in the inlet septum
- Defect in the trabecular septum
- Defect in the infundibular septum

Different mechanisms of VSD closure
- Due to septal aneurysm formation.
- Aortic or tricuspid valve prolapse.
- Sinus of valsalva intrusion.

Different types of VSD—depending on the morphology
- VSD—can be single or multiple
- Sieve-like defect
- Swiss cheese defect

Physiologic consequences on the severity of VSD
1. *Maladie de Roger: Small restrictive type of defect*:
   - No significant shunt
   - Normal pulmonary artery pressure
   - Can have dangerous ventricular arrhythmias
2. *Restrictive type*: Minimal shunt across the defect. Pulmonary vascular resistance and pressure, RV pressure—normal.
3. *No restriction to blood flow or shunt*: Significant shunting of blood from LV to RV. Pulmonary artery pressure and RV pressure becomes very high. Eisenmenger's reaction can occur with reversal of shunt.

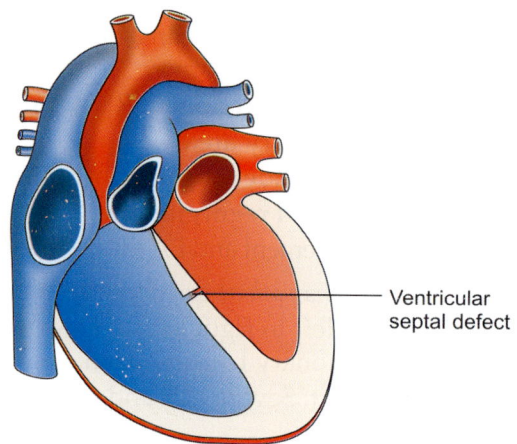

Fig. 1.7: Ventricular septal defect

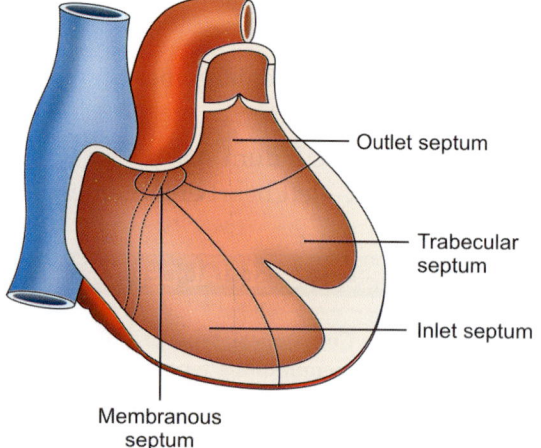

Fig. 1.8 Different parts of interventricular septum

Clinical Features of VSD

- Patient can be asymptomatic and can be detected on routine clinical examination.
- On routine examination thrill and murmur may be detectable.
- *May also present with*:
  - Retarded growth
  - Recurrent LRTI
  - Exertional dyspnea
  - Atrial fibrillation or infective endocarditis.

On examination

- Exercise-induced cyanosis
- Decreased body weight
- Delayed growth

Pulse: Small VSD: Normal

- Large VSD increased LV volume overload—high volume pulse

JVP: Normal

- If pulmonary hypertension—prominent a wave and v wave (due to TR)
- Precordium: Precordial bulge
- LV apex—due to LV volume overload
- Systolic thrill—at left 3rd and 4th intercostal space at left sternal border
- Supracristal VSD: Systolic thrill at left 2nd/first intercostal space—left sternal border.

Auscultation

- First heart sound—normal
- Second heart sound—widely split (early A2—due to early closure of aortic valve)
- *Murmur*: Pansystolic murmur heard at the left 3rd/4th intercostal space, at left sternal border—increases on expiration.
- Supracristal VSD: Pansystolic murmur heard at the 1st/2nd intercostal space—left sternal border.
- Small closing VSD can have early systolic murmur.
- Flow murmur in VSD: Due to increased diastolic flow at the mitral valve produces MDM.

Supracristal VSD

- Crista supraventricularis is a muscular ridge located between tricuspid and pulmonary valve at the junction of RV anterior wall and interventricular septum.
- Rare, located above crista supraventricularis
- Related to aortic valve
- There will be prolapse of aortic valve
- Can have associated AR
- Thrill and murmur in the 1st/2nd left intercostal space.

Pulmonary hypertension in VSD: Develops early in nonrestrictive type of VSD.

Clinical effects of pulmonary hypertension in VSD

- There will be reversal of shunt with development of central cyanosis and clubbing.
- Decrease of pansystolic murmur
- MDM across mitral valve disappears
- Signs of pulmonary hypertension.

ECG changes in VSD

- Left atrial enlargement and RVH
- Left ventricular volume overload
- Katz-Wachtel phenomenon: Large biphasic QRS in leads V2–V5 of at least 50 mm voltage (combined tall R and deep S wave) representing biventricular hypertrophy
- Ventricular arrhythmias
- *Chest X-ray in VSD*
  - Cardiomegaly
  - Pulmonary plethora
  - RV and LV enlargement
  - Pulmonary enlargement.

Gerbode defect

- A true communication between LV and right atrium.
- Blood reaches right atrium from LV through a small area of the membranous septum.
- The communication is above the tricuspid valve

PATENT DUCTUS ARTERIOSUS (PDA)

⚙ Key Points:

- Ductus arteriosus closes by 2nd week of life after birth due to increased arterial oxygen tension.
- It is less likely that ductus closes spontaneously—if it persists for more than 3 months after birth.

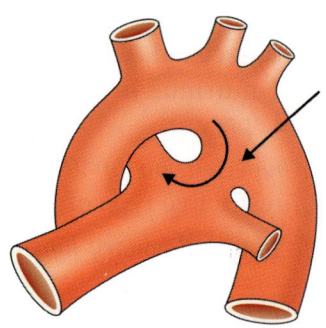

Fig. 1.10

PATENT DUCTUS ARTERIOSUS

(Shunt between aorta pulmonary artery)

Physiological Consequences of PDA

- PDA acts like a left to right shunt between aorta and pulmonary artery.
- Higher pressure zone of aorta: Aortic pressure is transmitted to pulmonary artery.
- There will be volume overload of right ventricle with development of pulmonary hypertension.

Risk Factors for Development of PDA

- 1st trimester: Rubella in the mother
- ?NSAIDs intake during pregnancy
- Born in high attitudes

Genetic syndromes associated: Trisomy 18.

Clinical Features

⚙ Key Points:

- PDA is more common in female sex.
- May be detected to have murmur at examination of a neonate.
- Failure to thrive in a child
- Can present with CCF in infancy.

General Physical Examination

Features of trisomy 18: Rocker bottom feet.

Differential Cyanosis and Clubbing

Cyanosis and clubbing of lower extremities and not the upper extremities (oxygen saturation is more in right upper limb than the lower limb)—occurs in patients with PDA with pulmonary hypertension with reversal of shunt due to shunting of unoxygenated blood to the lower limb distal to left subclavian artery.

Differential cyanosis occurs due to oxygenated blood entering into the descending aorta from the pulmonary circulation through PDA.

Reverse Differential Cyanosis

Oxygen saturation in the right hand is less than the foot.

Condition Causing

Transposition of great arteries (TGA) with PDA and pulmonary hypertension with shunt reversal.

Clinical Signs of PDA

- Pulse—high volume and collapsing pulse.
- JVP—initially normal and later prominent a wave due to pulmonary hypertension.

Precordium

- Presence of precordial bulge.
- Can have pectus carinatum and Harrison's sulcus.
- *Apex*: LV type—due to volume overload of left ventricle.
- Thrill—felt in the left infraclavicular area and left 1st intercostal space—continuous thrill.

Auscultation

- 2nd heart sound: Normal *or* widely split—due to prolonged RV ejection.
- Murmur: Continuous murmur
- Peaks late in systole

- Passes through the 2nd heart sound—enveloping it decreasing during diastole.
- Continuous murmur—when the murmur passes through the 2nd heart sound enveloping it. 2nd heart sound may not be audible.
- Classical machinery murmur (train in tunnel/Gibson's): Occurs in moderately restrictive ductus.
- Flow murmur in PDA: Due to increased diastolic flow across the mitral valve producing mid-diastolic murmur.

Development of Pulmonary Hypertension in PDA

- There will be left parasternal heave.
- Palpable pulmonary artery pulsation.
- P2 loud.
- Only systolic component of continuous murmur is heard.
- Other signs of pulmonary hypertension will be present.

Complications of PDA

- Development of pulmonary hypertension, reversal of shunt and CCF.
- Infective end arteritis (occurs at pulmonary end of the ductus—narrower with jet of blood flow)
- Rarely rupture or dissection of ductus.

Chest X-ray

- Enlarged LA and LV.
- Pulmonary plethora
- Occurrence of separate—convexity between aorta and pulmonary artery on the left cardiac border.

ECG

- Left atrial enlargement
- LV enlargement—volume overload
- If pulmonary hypertension—prominent R wave in V_1.

COARCTATION OF AORTA

Literal meaning of coarctus = contracted.

Different Types of Coarctation of Aorta

Common: Postsubclavian.

Other types: Presubclavian

- Abdominal—above or below renal artery
- May involve renal artery.

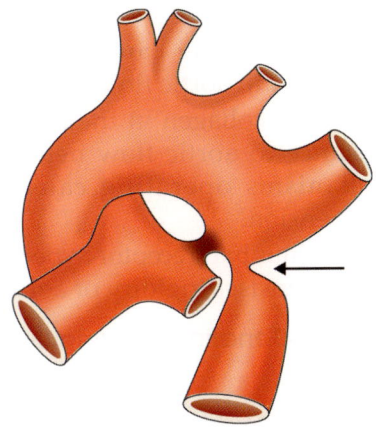

Fig. 1.11: Postductal (postsubclavian) coarctation

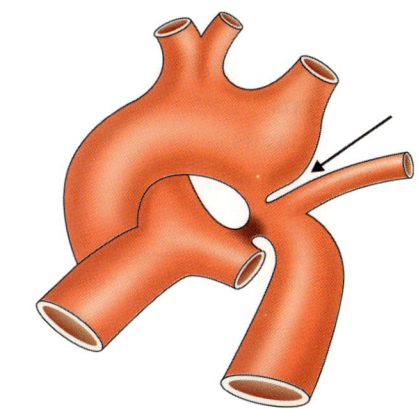

Fig. 1.12: Preductal (presubclavian) coarctation

Associated Cardiovascular Anomalies with Coarctation

Cardiac

- VSD, PDA
- Bicuspid aortic valve (normal, stenotic or regurgitant).

Vascular

- Circle of Willis aneurysm.
- Abnormalities of retinal arteries—become U-shaped

- Coronaries—premature coronary artery disease due to hypertension and abnormality of coronary arteries.

Development of Hypertension in Coarctation

Mechanisms

- Aortic narrowing causing mechanical obstruction to aortic flow.
- Increase of collagen in the aorta causing resistance to aortic flow neurohumoral mechanisms operating causing renal hypertension.
- Carotid sinus baroreceptor hypersensitivity due to increased rigidity of aorta.

Associated Genetic Abnormalities with Coarctation

Turner's Syndrome (xo)

Features

- Short statured female
- Webbing of neck
- Broad chest with widely placed nipple
- Cubitus valgus
- Pigmentary navus
- Low posterior hairline.

 Note

Webbed neck is more commonly associated with coarctation.

Noonan's Syndrome

- Can be associated with coarctation
- Features of Turner's syndrome with normal genotypes.

Coronary arteries in coarctation

- Due to hypertension—appearance of premature coronary artery disease.
- Coronary arteries themselves may be abnormal.

Different sites of coarctation depending on the site of attachment of ligamentum arteriosum

Typical site: Near the aortic attachment of lligamentum arteriosum (distal to left subclavian).

Other sites

- Preductal
- Juxtaductal
- Postductal.

Infective endocarditis in coarctation

- At bicuspid valve
- At the site of coarctation.

CVA Risk in Coarctation

- Due to rupture of circle of Willis aneurysm.
- Rupture of mycotic aneurysm with endocarditis
- Due to hypertension.

Development of collaterals in coarctation

Collaterals will be found around the scapula (Suzman's sign) around left and right sternal border and upper abdominal wall.

Retinal arteries in coarctation

- Hypertensive retinopathy is absent
- Arterial become U or cork screw shaped and tortuous.

Mitral valve in coarctation

- Parachute mitral valve
- Thickened mitral valve.

Aneurysm risk in coarctation

- Aortic aneurysms distal to coarctation and dissecting aortic aneurysm can occur.
- Aneurysm of vessels of circle of Willis.
- Intercostal artery aneurysm.

Pseudocoarctation

- No actual narrowing of aorta.
- Kinking or buckling of aorta at the site of attachment of ligamentum arteriosum.
- *Features*: No pressure gradient across the kinking of aorta.
- Not associated with hypertension and no development of collaterals.

Pregnancy with coarctation

- Toxemia of pregnancy is less common in patients with coarctation of aorta.
- There is increased risk of endocarditis.

Clinical features of coarctation of aorta
- Age of presentation—2nd to 3rd decade.
- May present as—fatigability of lower extremities.
- Epistaxis.

Other ways of presentations
- Dyspnea due to cardiac failure
- Infective endocarditis
- Intracranial bleed
- Rarely aortic dissection.

Occasionally patient may complain of
- Neck pulsations.
- Lower limb claudication due to abdominal coarctation

Clinical examination
- Build and nourishment:
- Upper extremities and chest well developed
- Lower extremities: Less well developed.
- If left subclavian is involved: Less well developed left upper limb.

Peripheral pulse
- Radiofemoral delay: Femoral pulse will be having delayed peak.
- Prominent suprasternal and neck pulsations.
- If left subclavian artery is involved—left radial artery—feeble.
- *Blood pressure*: Lower limb blood pressure is less than upper limb blood pressure.
- Left subclavian involvement—left upper limb blood pressure is less than the right upper limb by 10–15 mm of Hg

Precordium
- Heaving apex due to LVH.
- Thrill—systolic thrill in the aortic area—due to bicuspid aortic valve with stenosis.

Auscultation
- Heart sounds: Loud A2
- Aortic ejection click due to bicuspid aortic valve.
- LVH—left-sided S4.

Murmur in a patient of coarctation
1. Bicuspid aortic valve with aortic stenosis—ESM—at aortic area.
2. At the site of coarctation: Systolic murmurs at 4th or 5th thoracic spine.
- Due to collaterals: Systolic murmurs at the suprasternal notch and over brachiocephalic arteries.

Murmurs in abdominal coarctation: Systolic murmurs can be heard in the epigastrium and over the thoraco lumbar spine.

ECG changes in coarctation: LVH with strain pattern.

X-ray in coarctation
- LVH
- Rib notching
- Dilatation of aorta

Figure of 3 appearance
Combination of:
- Dilated left subclavian artery.
- Narrowing at the site of coarctation
- Dilated descending aorta
- Barium swallow will show mirror image of 3 due to compression of oesophagus by the vessels.

Rib Notching
- Notching/scalloping of ribs
- Site involved—3rd to 8th ribs—inferior part of posterior aspect of ribs
- Due to dilated tortuous posterior intercostal arteries.
- Posterior intercostal arteries run in the grooves of ribs
- Anterior intercostal arteries do not run in the grooves of ribs.
- Rib notches—may be single or multiple.
- DD for rib notching: Neurofibromas.

Complications of coarctation
- Development of hypertension and its complications.
- CCF
- Premature coronary artery disease

- Endocarditis
- Intracranial bleed—aneurysm rupture
- Dissection of aorta.

FALLOT'S TETRALOGY

It is a cyanotic congenital heart disease.

Components of Fallot's Tetralogy

- Infundibular pulmonary stenosis
- VSD—nonrestrictive
- RVH.
- Overriding of aorta on the interventricular septum.

Clinical Presentations

- Child can present with growth retardation, difficulty in gaining weight and delayed development.
- Child can present with cyanotic, hypoxic spells.

 Note

Fallot's tetralogy is the commonest cyanotic heart disease after 4 years of age.

- Patients with Fallot's tetralogy without intervention less likely to survive more than 10–15 years.

Typical Cyanotic Spell of Fallot's Tetralogy

Infant/child becomes suddenly cyanotic and can have syncope, convulsions and sudden death.

Clinical description of cyanotic spell

- Sudden activities in the child after the child had prolonged sleep or rest. Child suddenly becomes cyanosed.
- Factors/activity which can bring out cyanotic spells: Feeding of the child or when the child is crying.

Pathogenesis of cyanotic spells: When the child becomes active—develops tachycardia. Tachycardia causes increased shunting of blood to the left heart and to the systemic circulation with unoxygenated blood.

Contributing cardiac factors in bringing out cyanotic spells

- Spasm of the infundibulum of pulmonary artery leads to more shunting of unoxygenated blood to the left heart.
- Increase of venous return and increased shunting of unoxygenated blood to left heart due to activity.
- Arrhythmias like supraventricular tachycardia.
- Oversensitive respiratory center, hypoxia, acidosis and hypercarbia.

Squatting Episodes in Fallot's Tetralogy

Child tries to assume position of squatting to prevent hypoxia.

Consequences of squatting

1. Squatting leads to → increase in the peripheral vascular resistance → increase in the aortic resistance.

    Increase in the aortic resistance: More blood is going into pulmonary circulation from right heart and getting oxygenated.

2. Due to squatting less of unoxygenated blood return to the heart from lower extremities.

    Child tries to assume squatting position after exercise.

Other positions which can be advantageous to the child to prevent hypoxia

- Crossing of the child's legs while standing.
- Mother holding the child with flexion of infant's legs which are flexed over the child's abdomen.

Collateral Circulation in Fallot's Tetralogy

In a patient's of Fallot's tetralogy collateral circulation develops to perfuse the lungs.

Collaterals arise from

1. Bronchial artery to pulmonary artery
2. Aorta to the hilum of lungs
3. Can arise from internal mammary artery.

Note

Aortic cusp can herniate in a patient of Fallot's tetralogy and can result in AR.

Fallot's tetralogy can be associated with right-sided aortic arch.

Examination of a Patient of Fallot's Tetralogy

Associated conditions
- Maternal rubella
- Down's syndrome

General physical examination
- Appearance: Weight loss and cachexia.
- Central cyanosis, clubbing and hypertrophic osteoarthropathy.

Pulse
- Usually normal
- High volume pulse—if severe AR or development of large collaterals

JVP
- Normal in spite of RVH because RV is shunting blood through the aorta and VSD.
- Prominent a wave in the JVP—if there is development of systemic hypertension/development of aortic stenosis.

Examination of Precordium
- Precordium is silent
- No RV pulsation—as RV is capable of emptying into aorta and LV through the VSD without raising pressure.
- Pulsations can be present in the left 4th or 5th intercostal space because of infundibular stenosis.

 Note

There can be right sternoclavicular joint pulsation due to right-sided aortic arch in Fallot's tetralogy.

Thrill: Systolic thrill in the left 3rd space due to pulmonary infundibular stenosis (rare).

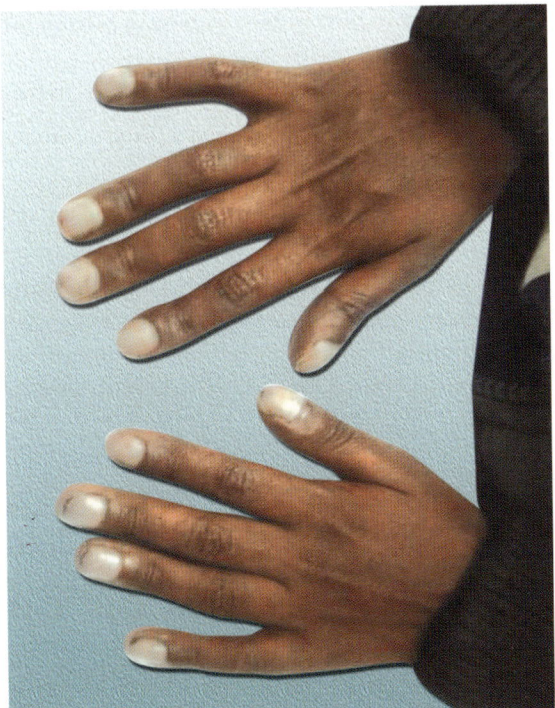

Fig. 1.13: Cyanosis and clubbing

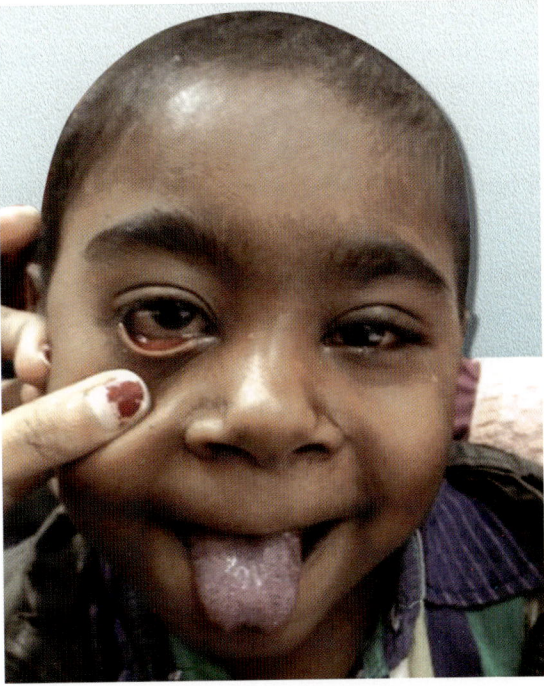

Fig. 1.14: Suffused conjunctiva due to polycythemia and central cyanosis in Fallot's tetralogy

Auscultation

- Heart sounds—1st heart sound—normal
- 2nd heart sound—P2 soft or absent (due to decreased pulmonary blood flow)
- A2 can be loud (due to anterior dilated aorta: Peacock sound)
- No pulmonary ejection click (it is infundibular pulmonary stenosis and not valvular stenosis).

Murmurs

- Ejection systolic murmur: Left 2nd or 3rd intercostal space at left sternal border.
- Murmur is due to infundibular pulmonary stenosis.
- Murmur of VSD—not heard—due to large VSD.

 Note

As the severity of infundibular stenosis increases, ESM decreases as more blood is shunted through the over-riding aorta.

Triology of Fallot's

Combination of ASD with PS with RVH and shunt—right to left.

Pentalogy of Fallot's

Combination of Fallot's tetralogy with ASD.

Pink Fallot's Tetralogy

- Mild right ventricular outflow obstruction.
- Shunt from right to left is not significant.
- No development of cyanosis.

Fallot's like physiology

- Combination of large VSD with severe PS with right to left shunt
- Conditions which are having Fallot's like physiology:
  - Tetralogy of Fallot
  - Transposition of great vessels with VSD with PS
  - Tricuspid atresia with VSD with PS.

ECG changes in Fallot's tetralogy

- No P wave enlargement
- P wave axis—left QRS—V1—tall R wave, V2-rs pattern, no T wave inversion in right precordial leads.

   If tall R wave is present in V2 with T wave inversion in leads V1 and V2—consider pulmonary stenosis with intact interventricular septum.

Chest X-ray changes

- Pulmonary oligemia—vasculature is decreased in the pulmonary circulation.
- Concave pulmonary artery segment.
- No cardiomegaly.
- Aortic arch may be right-sided.
- Boot-shaped heart in the chest X-ray due to combination of: RVH, concavity in the region of pulmonary artery, horizontal interventricular septum, small left ventricle forming the apex becoming straight.

Occurrence of Collaterals in Fallot's Tetralogy

- Bronchial collaterals—murmur—anterior chest wall on both sides.
- Murmur can also be heard over infra-clavicular area.

Occurrence of Right Heart Failure in Fallot's Tetralogy

Rare occurrence. Can occur if there is development of systemic hypertension and severe aortic stenosis, severe anemia and infective endocarditis.

 Note

Recurrent hypoxic spell in a child can give rise to CNS damage and mental retardation.

   Risk of cerebral embolization and brain abscess is more in patients with Fallot's tetralogy. There is high risk of cortical venous thrombosis in a patient of Fallot's tetralogy.

   Pulmonary valve and aortic valve endocarditis can occur in Fallot's tetralogy.

Pregnancy in Patient of Fallot's Tetralogy

- Not well tolerated
- Increase incidence of fetal wastage.
- Maturity disturbance in neonatal patient.

PARTIAL ANOMALOUS PULMONARY VENOUS CONNECTION (PAPVC)

- Pulmonary veins drain into right atrium instead of left atrium.
- Very common to have single pulmonary vein to drain into right atrium. Rarely all pulmonary veins from one lung to drain into right atrium.
- Patients with PAPVC can have associated ASD which may be of sinus venosus type or septum secundum type.
- There can be PAPVC with intact interatrial septum.
- PAPVC from right lung is more common than the left lung.
- Total anomalous pulmonary venous connection—all the pulmonary veins or most of the pulmonary veins enter right heart.
- Scimitar syndrome—discussed under ASD.

Physiological Consequences of PAPVC

- More blood is entering into the right heart from pulmonary veins.
- Right heart receives more blood and develops right atrial and right ventricular dilatation.
- If associated with ASD—further shunting of blood from left atrium to right atrium.

Consequence of PAPVC

- Development of pulmonary hypertension.
- Right-sided cardiac failure.
- Increased risk of arrhythmias.

Clinical Features

Person can be asymptomatic and may be accidentally detected.

Can present with

- Breathlessness—excess of blood into right heart and lungs.

- Palpitation due to recurrent supraventricular arrhythmias.

Edema

- Due to right-sided cardiac failure.
- Can also develop recurrent chest infection.

Signs

- May not have typical clinical signs
- Left parasternal pulsations—if right ventricular enlargement
- Pulmonary artery pulsation due to pulmonary artery dilatation.

Auscultation: 2nd heart sound—widely split but not fixed (PAPVC with intact interatrial septum).

CONGENITAL PULMONARY STENOSIS

Types of Pulmonary Stenosis

Different levels of stenosis

- Valvular
- Subvalvular
- Supravalvular

Supravalvular

- Pulmonary artery stenosis
- Main trunk or branch stenosis

Pulmonary artery stenosis: May be a part of rubella syndrome.

Consequences of Pulmonary Valvular Stenosis

- Severe pulmonary valvular stenosis causes severe right ventricular pressure raise with RVH and right ventricular failure.
- Because of RVH there will be associated dysfunction of the left ventricle.
- Due to increasing right side pressure (RV and RA) there will be shunting of blood through foramen ovale with appearance of central cyanosis.

Clinical Features of Pulmonary Valvular Stenosis

History

- Patient may be asymptomatic even with severe stenosis.

- Newborn may be detected to have systolic murmur.
- History of first trimester maternal rubella in patients with pulmonary artery branch stenosis.
- Mild to moderate stenosis—usual to survive for adult life.
- Can present with dizziness, chest pain of RV ischemia.
- Hemoptysis can occur due to dilated pulmonary artery aneurysm.
- Usual cause of death is right ventricular failure.
- Rarely can present as infective endocarditis.

Physical Appearance

- Can have features of associated following syndromes:
  - Rubella syndrome
  - William's syndrome
  - Noonan's syndrome

Facial features of pulmonary stenosis with doom-shaped valve

- Face—round bloated
- Cheeks—colored

Pulse: Normal or low volume if associated with right ventricular failure.

JVP: Giant 'a' wave and if associated with TR—prominent v wave.

Precordium

Valvular PS

- Left parasternal heave due to RVH
- Systolic thrill—left 2nd intercostal space radiating above and to left.

Auscultation

- Pulmonary ejection click due to rapid upward movement of pulmonary valve leaflets.
- Characteristics of pulmonary ejection click
  - Heard in the pulmonary area
  - Better heard on expiration.
  - Suggests valvular stenosis with mobile leaflets.

Relationship of pulmonary ejection click with respiration

On inspiration

- There is increased force of contraction of right atrium which is transmitted to right ventricle. This is transmitted to under surface of pulmonary valve. This makes the pulmonary valve to move upwards making the valve to move less during RV contraction with less prominent click.
- During expiration—converse of the above hemodynamics occurs with ejection click becoming more prominent.
- First heart sound and pulmonary ejection click interval varies inversly with the severity of pulmonary stenosis. As the severity increases the interval decreases.

Heart sounds

2nd heart sound

- More severe pulmonary stenosis due to prolonged RV ejection, P2 is delayed with wide splitting of 2nd heart sound. P2 may not be audible.
- There will be associated right-sided S4.

Murmur

Site: Left 2nd intercostal space.

Site of murmur in subinfundibular stenosis: 3rd and 4th left intercostal space—left sternal border.

Type of murmur: Ejection systolic murmur.

Radiation: Left and upwards.

Severe stenosis: Late peaking of murmur becoming kite shaped.

Other associated murmurs: TR murmur.

Murmur associated with pulmonary branch stenosis: Depends on the site of stenosis. Usually anteriorly at right and left sternal borders/axilla/back.

ECG in pulmonary stenosis

- Prominent P wave—dilated right atrium
- Positive R wave in lead V1 due to RVH

Chest X-ray in pulmonary stenosis

- Increase in the RA and RV size

- Decrease in the pulmonary vascularity
- Poststenotic dilatation of the pulmonary artery.

CONGENITAL AORTIC STENOSIS

Types of Congenital AS

- Valvular
- Subvalvular
- Supravalvular

Valvular

- Single cusp
- Bicuspid valve
- Tricuspid valve
- Single cusp—valve can become stenotic.
- Bicuspid valve—can become stenotic or regurgitant.
- Tricuspid valve—cusps can be unequal and can become stenotic.

Supravalvular aortic stenosis

- Less common
- Narrowing of aorta, above the aortic sinuses = Hourglass constriction
- Leaflets of the aortic valve may become thickened or may be dysplastic.

Coronaries in supravalvular aortic stenosis

- Obstruction to the coronary flow can occur
- High LV pressure is transmitted to coronaries with thickening of coronary arteries.

Consequences of congenital aortic valve stenosis

- Left ventricular hypertrophy
- Ischemia of endocardium
- Mitral regurgitation due to papillary muscle dysfunction.
- Pulmonary hypertension with right-sided cardiac failure.

Bicuspid Aortic Valve

- Common congenital cardiac abnormality.
- May remain asymptomatic throughout life.
- Autosomal dominant genetic disorder.
- Bicuspid valve can become sclerosed/calcified and stenotic

- Can develop AR
- Prone to infective endocarditis.

 Note

Increased level of cholesterol increases the risk of calcification of bicuspid aortic valve.

Coarctation of aorta can be associated with bicuspid aortic valve.

Clinical Features

Congenital AS

- May be asymptomatic or neonate may be detected to have murmur.
- Growth can be affected in neonates.

Can present with

- Exertional dyspnea
- Chest pain
- Palpitation
- Syncope
- Fever
- Exertional dyspnea due to LV dysfunction
- Chest pain in young—consider congenital AS
- *Palpitation due to LVH*: Due to ventricular arrhythmias especially with associated coronary artery disease.
- *Syncope*: Exertional syncope: During exertion:
  - Due to—low fixed cardiac output with increased muscular blood flow.

Syncope occurs also due to

- On exercise—increase in the LV stretch leads to activation of baroreceptors. As a result there is bradycardia, vasodilatation and hypotension with syncope.
- *Fever*: Can occur due to endocarditis.

Clinical Signs of Congenital Valvular Aortic Stenosis

Pulse: Low volume, slow raising.

JVP: Prominent 'a' wave due to LVH causes decreased distensibility of right ventricle. This leads to increased force of contraction of right atrium causing prominent a wave without pulmonary hypertension.

Precordium
- Apex: Heaving due to LVH
- Thrill: Systolic thrill in the right 2nd space and left 3rd space.
- Thrill is also felt over the carotids. Pulsation due to LA enlargement.

Auscultation
- Ejection click in valvular, and with bicuspid valve.
- Click occurs due to: Sudden upward movement of stenotic valve which is mobile and not calcified.
- *Murmur*: Ejection systolic murmur in the right 2nd space which is conducted to carotids.
- 2nd heart sounds in congenital AS:
  - If mild AS: A2 is not delayed and 2nd heart sound is split.
  - If severe AS: 2nd heart sound may become single or paradoxically split—due to delayed aortic component—due to prolonged aortic ejection.
- Fourth heart sound: S4 occurs in congenital AS due to increased left atrial force of contraction (against less compliant LV) causing presystolic distention of left ventricle:
- Left heart failure can cause left-sided 3rd heart sound.

Supravalvular AS

- Associated with William's syndrome.
- Can be associated with retarded growth
- Pulse—left subclavian, brachial and radial artery will be feeble.
- Right arm blood pressure is more than the left arm by 10–15 mm of Hg.
- Cause of difference of pulse volume in supravalvular AS
- There is narrowing of aorta above the aortic sinuses and high velocity jet of blood flow will be directed towards the right wall of the aorta and innominate artery (coanda effect) causing volume of the right radial pulse more than the left.

- *Coanda effect*: There is affinity of the jet of flow to adhere to the wall nearby.

Precordium
- LV type of apex
- Thrill—below the right clavicle and over the right carotid.
- No ejection click
- A2 normal
- ESM—right 1st intercostal space conducted to right carotid

ECG in congenital AS: LVH with ST, T changes.

Chest X-ray: Cardiomegaly. Calcified bicuspid aortic valve.

William's syndrome
Features
- Face-chin: Small
- Mouth: Large
- Nose: Upturned, blunt
- Eyes: Wide placed
- Lips: Patulous
- Brow: Broad prominent, supraorbital ridges
- Teeth maloccluded.

Associated other abnormalities
- Short stature
- Vascular abnormality
- Renal abnormality
- Mental retardation
- Associated metabolic abnormality—hypercalcemia
- Associated cardiac abnormality—supravalvular AS
- Pulmonary artery branch stenosis.

EBSTEIN'S ANOMALY

Cyanotic Congenital Heart Disease

Anatomical Abnormalities

Tricuspid leaflets—septal and posterior leaflets are downwardly displaced into the right ventricle.

Right atrium is large with atrialisation of part of right ventricle (between atrioventricular ring and orifice of the tricuspid valve).

Tricuspid valve and right ventricle may be dysplastic and tricuspid valve anterior leaflet can be larger.

There will be 3 components of the right side of the heart

1. Proper right atrium
2. Thin inlet portion of the right ventricle which is functionally part of right atrium
3. Small outlet portion of RV—functional right ventricle.

Associated anomalies coexisting with Ebstein's anomaly

- Patent foramen ovale
- Ostium secundum ASD.

Hemodynamic Consequences in Ebstein's Anomaly

- There is tricuspid valve abnormality with tricuspid regurgitation.
- This atrialised portion of right ventricle may not contribute to the atrial function.
- Because of the associated accessory pathways there will be supraventricular tachycardia with hemodynamic consequences.
- There will be gross enlargement of right atrium which can accommodate regurgitant volume/blood from TR.
- In adult patients RV pressure rises with resultant increase in RA pressure with shunting of blood from right to left through patent foramen ovale.

LV Function in Ebstein's Anomaly

- LV function is affected due to interventricular septum which is displaced to the left.
- Alteration in the shape of LV cavity.
- There will be increase in the LV free wall fibrous tissue.

Clinical Features

Progressive fatigue and dyspnea

- Due to decreased cardiac output and decrease in the left ventricular ejection.

- Central cyanosis occurs as a result of shunting of blood from right atrium to left atrium.
- Swelling of feet and ascites due to severe TR.

Sudden cardiac death and palpitation: Due to sudden cardiac arrhythmias

- Development of PSVT with or without bypass tract.
- Fatal ventricular arrhythmias.

Ebstein's anomaly can occasionally present with TIA, CVA or brain abscess due to paradoxical embolization through patent foramen ovale.

Signs

- Central cyanosis and clubbing
- JVP—initially normal
- Can have prominent c wave due to anterior tricuspid leaflet mobility
- In spite of TR V wave is not prominent because of large RA which can accommodate large amount of blood and thin atrialised RV is not capable of generating pressure.
- Radial pulse: Normal
- Precordium: Normal
- Dullness of about 1–2 cm outside the right sternal border due to enlarged right atrium (from 4th to 6th rib).

Auscultation

- 1st heart sound—widely split—due to delayed anterior tricuspid leaflet closure—due to large size of the anterior leaflet of tricuspid valve taking time to close (RBBB may also contribute).
- Tricuspid component is also loud.
- 2nd heart sound: Widely split due to delayed pulmonary component due to RBBB.
- There will be right-sided 3rd and 4th heart sounds.

Murmur

- Tricuspid regurgitation murmur in the tricuspid area.

- Murmur may not increase with inspiration because RV is hypokinetic and cannot increase its stroke volume and regurgitation.

ECG Abnormalities

- RA enlargement: Himalayan P wave
- Prolonged PR interval
- Complete heart block
- RBBB.

Arrhythmias: Supraventricular tachycardia
- Atrial flutter and fibrillation
- Brugada syndrome
- Type B: WPW syndrome

Chest X-ray

Cardiomegaly
- Markedly enlarged right atrium
- Pulmonary vasculature decreased.

Heart: Box like:
- Due to increased right heart border convexity due to enlarged right atrium
- Marked left border convexity due to enlarged infundibulum
- Narrow hilum—aortic shadow not made out
- Pulmonary trunk is not forming the left border.

PROSTHETIC VALVE

Types of Prosthetic Valves

- Mechanical valve
- Bio-prosthetic valve.

Mechanical prosthetic valves are of 3 types
- Bileaflet valve
- Tilting disc type.
- Ball and cage type.

Bileaflet is the most commonly used mechanical valve
- Durability of mechanical prosthetic valve: Up to 25 to 40 years.
- All mechanical prosthetic valve requires lifelong anticoagulation.

Complications of mechanical prosthetic valve
- Thromboembolic disease.
- Occlusion of the valve by the clot.
- Infective endocarditis.
- Paravalvular leak

Thromboembolic risk is more with mechanical mitral valve than mechanical aortic valve.

Bioprosthetic Valve

- Least risk of thromboembolism.
- Thromboembolism can occur in 1st to 3rd postoperative months.
- Produces heart sounds similar to normal heart sounds.

Indications for Bioprosthetic Valve

- Older patients
- Not compliant with oral anticoagulation
- Persons with contraindications for oral anticoagulation.
- Normal sinus rhythm.
- Young females want to have pregnancy.

Patient of mitral valve disease with atrial fibrillation on anticoagulation—mechanical valve is ideal as the patient is already on anticoagulation.

Prosthetic Valve (Mechanical) Sounds

Mitral Prosthetic Sounds

Opening sound: Corresponds to opening snap.
Closing sound: Corresponds to first heart sound.

Aortic Prosthetic Sounds

Opening sound: Corresponds to ejection click.
Closing sound: Corresponds to 2nd heart sound.

CARDIOMYOPATHY

Chronic disease of the cardiac muscle characterized by thickening, enlargement, stiffening of cardiac muscle with decreased function and diminished ability to pump the blood.

Different Types of Cardiomyopathies

- Dilated cardiomyopathy
- Hypertrophic cardiomyopathy
- Restrictive cardiomyopathy.

Idiopathic cardiomyopathy: Cardiomyopathy without a known cause (HT, IHD and valvular heart disease are not present).

Other Less Common Varieties

- Arrhythmogenic right ventricular dysplasia.
- Peripartum cardiomyopathy
- Cardiomyopathy of unknown aetiology.

Dilated Cardiomyopathy

Pathophysiology

- There is enlargement and dilatation of cavities of the ventricles.
- There is decreased systolic function with decreased diastolic function.
- LV ejection fraction is reduced.
- There is tendency for formation of blood clots in the ventricles.

Causes

- Infective: Viral, diphtheria, toxoplasmosis, Chagas disease.
- Toxins: Alcohol and heavy metals
- Coronary artery disease.
- Peripartum cardiomyopathy

Clinical Features

- Massive cardiomegaly
- Presence of murmur:
  - Mitral regurgitation and tricuspid regurgitation
  - Cardiac failure: Biventricular failure
  - Intraventricular clot formation
  - Presence of cardiac arrhythmias

ECG: Biventricular/biatrial hypertrophy with high voltage of QRS in precordial leads.
- LBBB
- VPCs and ventricular arrhythmias
- Left axis deviation

Chest X-ray: Massive cardiomegaly, biventricular enlargement and evidence of pulmonary venous congestion.

Restrictive Cardiomyopathy

Characterised by stiffening and rigidity of cardiac muscle affecting the diastolic function of the heart.

Causes

- Idiopathic
- Amyloidosis
- Sarcoidosis
- Hemochromatosis
- Radiation
- Endomyocardial fibrosis.

Pathophysiology

- Ventricular diastolic function is severely abnormal with normal systolic function.
- Atrium is significantly dilated with moderate dilatation of the left ventricle.

Clinical Features

- Exertional fatigue and dyspnea
- Right hypochondrial pain
- Edema feet
- Enlarged liver
- Ascites
- JVP-rapid Y-descent
- Presence of Kussmaul's sign
- Cardiomegaly with prominent cardiac apex
- There will be presence of 4th heart sound.

Differential diagnosis: Constrictive pericarditis.

Hypertrophic Obstructive Cardiomyopathy

Disease of the myocardium: Inherited with mutation in the gene in the heart muscle protein.

Pathophysiology

- Enlargement of muscle mass of the heart. There is marked hypertrophy of left ventricle without known cause.
- Hypertrophy is asymmetrical with septal hypertrophy.

- There will be obstruction to the outflow tract of left ventricle during systole. Obstruction is dynamic with increased obstruction during increased contractility of the ventricle.

Clinical Features

- Exercise intolerance/dyspnea.
- Chest pain due to coronary ischemia.
- There is deficient coronary supply due to increased oxygen demand by the hypertrophied myocardium.
- Associated anatomical abnormality of coronary artery can occur.
- Palpitation due to atrial/ventricular arrhythmias.
- Exertional syncope/postexertional syncope.
- Ventricular tachycardia/fibrillation can cause sudden cardiac death.

Signs

Carotid pulse: Brisk.

Apical impulse: LV apex—double apex—due to palpable S4.

Auscultation: Left-sided fourth heart sound (due to decreased LV compliance).

Murmurs: Due to LV outflow tract obstruction—ejection systolic murmur at left sternal border not conducted to carotids.

Murmur of HOCM: Murmur increases when LV cavity size decreases, e.g. Valsalva, standing.

Murmur decrease: LV volume increases, e.g. handgrip, squatting.

CONGENITAL COMPLETE HEART BLOCK

May be asymptomatic.

Clinical Features

Pulse: Bradycardia heart rate—around 40–50/minute.

 Note

In acquired complete heart block, heart rate will be lower than congenital heart block.

Wide Pulse Pressure

High systolic pressure

- Normal LV with large volume of ventricular ejection
- No sinus arrhythmia

JVP: Irregular cannon 'a' wave

- Right atrium contracts against closed tricuspid valve.

Precordium

Auscultation

Bradycardia

First heart sound

- Varying in intensity due to varying PR interval
- Louder 1st heart sound can occur: Cannon sound
- 2nd heart sound—normal split
- 3rd and 4th heart sound can be heard

Murmur: ESM at the aortic area—due to large volume of blood ejected from the left ventricle.

ECG changes: In complete heart block

- P waves are more than QRS complexes, there is no relationship between P wave and QRS complexes (AV dissociation)
- P wave rate (atrial rate) is around 60 to 100/minute
- QRS rate (ventricular rate) is around 30 to 40/minute

Morphology of QRS in complete heart block: If the escape rhythm is from AV node: Narrow QRS.

If the escape rhythm is from lower conducting system: Wide QRS.

CARDIOVASCULAR SYSTEM

Differential Diagnosis of Cardiac Disease

1st and 2nd decade of life

- Cardiac symptoms: Consider congenital/rheumatic heart disease.
- If childhood onset of symptoms—possible congenital heart disease.

- History of cyanosis, squatting episodes—possible cyanotic heart disease.
- History of progressive dyspnea and palpitation since childhood later on development of cyanosis—possible VSD/PDA.
- Predominantly presents with palpitation after 4th decade of life—type of congenital heart disease—ASD
- 2nd and 3rd decades of life with cardiac symptoms like dyspnea and PND—consider possible rheumatic heart disease like mitral stenosis.
- 2nd and 3rd decades of life predominant palpitation and fatigue with later on dyspnea—consider mitral regurgitation.
- 4th and 5th decades of life—with cardiac symptoms:
  - Like syncope, palpitation chest pain—consider aortic stenosis/IHD.
  - Predominant palpitation and chest pain at 4th and 5th decades of life—consider AR/IHD/hypertension.
- If there is history of fever with cardiac symptoms—consider infective endocarditis/rheumatic fever.

If there is pre-existing cardiac disease with development of fever

Consider

- Infective endocarditis
- Rheumatic fever
- Systemic infection like pneumonia.

Cardiac conditions associated with fever

- Rheumatic fever
- Endocarditis—infective/noninfective
- Atrial myxoma
- Pericarditis
- Systemic illness

If there is sudden deterioration in cardiac symptoms in a pre-existing cardiac disease

Consider

- Volume overload
- Stopping of cardiac medications like diuretics
- Atrial fibrillation
- Infective endocarditis
- Systemic infection
- Attack of rheumatic fever
- Pulmonary embolism
- Acute coronary event

Gradual deterioration in a chronic cardiac disease

Consider

- Aggravation of basic cardiac disease.
- Severe anemia
- Thyroid dysfunction
- Development of hypertension/IHD

Consider following cardiac disease 6th decade onwards

- Hypertensive heart disease
- Ischemic heart disease
- Consider MVP with MR
- ASD
- RHD with possible aortic valve disease.

Consider following cardiac disease above 60 years of age

- IHD
- Hypertensive heart disease.
- Degenerative aortic valve disease.
- Bicuspid aortic valve with dysfunction.

📝 *Note*

- *Always consider cardiomyopathy after ruling out other cardiac disease.*
- *Patient presenting with ascites and swelling of feet—rule out constrictive pericarditis.*
- *Always rule out atrial fibrillation in an embolic CVA.*

Respiratory System

Important Clinical Aspects

Major Interlobar Fissure

Draw a line starting at T2 spine along the medial border of scapula and continue the line along the axilla till it joins the costo-chondral junction of 6th rib (line crosses the 5th rib at mid-axillary line).

Minor Interlobar Fissure

- Draw a line starting from the level of 4th costal cartilage to meet the major inter-lobar fissure at the axilla.
- Apex of the lung lies 2–3 cm above the level of clavicle.

Lymphatic drainage of the lung and pleura

- Chest wall and parietal pleura—drain to axillary lymph nodes.
- Right lung and left lower lobe—right supraclavicular lymph node.
- Left upper lobe—left supraclavicular lymph node.

Examination of Respiratory System

Muscles of Inspiration

Primary muscles

- External intercostals
- Diaphragm

Accessory muscles

Strap muscles of neck
- Sternomastoids
- Scalenus anterior
- Trapezius and pectoralis

Muscle of Expiration

Primary muscles

- Internal intercostals
- Subcostals

Accessory muscles: Abdominal muscles.

Inspiratory dyspnea: Difficulty in breathing due to pathological obstruction in the larynx, trachea and bronchi.

For example, major airway obstruction.

Expiratory dyspnea: Difficulty in breathing due to pulmonary parenchymal disease, medium and small airway disease.

Example: Bronchial asthma, chronic emphysema.

Paradoxical movement of abdomen: Normally during inspiration—abdomen moves outwards. If it moves outwards during expiration, it is called paradoxical movement of abdomen—indicates diaphragm paralysis.

Bucket handle movement of chest

- This is the name given to the normal movement of ribs of 7–10.
- Movement occurs in the anteroposterior axis resulting in raising and lowering of middle parts of ribs: This is called bucket handle movement.
- During elevation of ribs—there is increase in the transverse diameter of the thorax.

Pump handle movement of ribs

Movement of upper ribs and sternum during normal respiration moving upwards increases the AP diameter of the thorax mimics pump handle movement.

Respiratory Centers

Pontine respiratory center
- Pneumotaxic center
- Apneustic center

Medullary respiratory center
- Dorsal neurons group—center for inspiration
- Ventral respiratory neurons—center for expiration.

Abnormal Respiratory Patterns

Kussmaul's breathing
Occurs in patients with metabolic acidosis. There is increased rate and depth of respiration (air hunger).

Cheyne-Stokes respiration
- Waxing and waning of breathing.
- There is gradual increase in the depth and frequency of respiration followed by decrease in the depth and frequency with a brief period of 10–30 sec of cessation of breathing (apnea).
- For example, patient with low cardiac output with decrease blood supply to the respiratory center.

Biot's breathing: There is rapid and shallow breathing associated with periods of apnea (regular or irregular).

Apneustic breathing
- Occurs in patients with pontine pathology.
- There is sudden stoppage of respiration.

Central neurogenic hyperventilation
- Occurs in: Head injury, cerebral hypoxia—damage to mid-brain and pons.
- There is persisting hyperventilation.

Central neurogenic hypoventilation
- Causes—as for neurogenic hyperventilation
- There is persisting hypoventilation.

Important Clinical Points While Examining Respiratory System

Spinoscapular distance
- Distance of angle of the scapula from the spine.
- It is decreased in conditions with volume loss on the affected side.

Spino-acromion distance: Distance of acromion from the thoracic spine. It is increased in patients with volume loss on the affected side with drooping of shoulder.

Grocco's triangle: A triangular area posteriorly from side of the vertebral spine—opposite to the side of pleural effusion—due to bulging of posterior mediastinal pleura into the opposite hemithorax—producing an area of dullness.

Percussion

Upward Shift of Traube's Space

Causes
Due to volume loss on the left side
- Pulmonary fibrosis on the left side
- Pulmonary collapse on the left side
- Diaphragm paralysis on the left side.

Cracked pot resonance (ref)
- Percussion over a pulmonary cavity that communicates with the bronchus.
- Sound resembling—striking over a cracked pot.

Auscultation

Whispering pectoriloquy
- Hallmark of consolidation due to turbulence of airflow across glottis and trachea heard through consolidation.
- As such vocal cords do not vibrate and vocal cords are held closer while whispering.

Hamman's sign
- Also called mediastinal crunch
- Heard in patients with pneumomediastinum
- Crunching/rasping sound
- Heard with each heart beat

- Due to beating of heart against tissues filled with air.

Amphoric breathing: Low-pitched bronchial breathing with high-pitched metallic overtones.

Causes: Open and tension pneumothorax, large superficial cavity with patent bronchus.

Bronchovesicular breathing

- Intermediate between vesicular and bronchial breathing.
- Normally heard over 1st and 2nd intercostal space anteriorly and between scapulae posteriorly.

Causes of Tubular Breathing

- Consolidation
- Pulled trachea syndrome
- At or just above the level of massive pleural effusion.
- Upper lobe mass lesion in contact with the main bronchus.
- Left interscapular area near the spine in a patient of massive pericardial effusion (Ewart's sign).
- In patients with d'Espine's sign positivity.

COUGH AND HEMOPTYSIS

Important Clinical Aspects

Hemoptysis

- Massive hemoptysis may occur if there is bleeding from bronchial arteries because of high pressure (systemic pressure) in bronchial arteries.
- If the pulmonary capillaries bleed which can produce alveolar hemorrhage: They are under lower pressure.
- In patients with bronchiectasis—due to repeated infection and long standing inflammatory pathology—along with abnormalities in the bronchus—bronchial vessels become closer to the surface and can produce massive hemoptysis.

- Pulmonary tuberculosis can produce hemoptysis due to active disease, cavity bleed and aspergilloma.
- Massive hemoptysis is called when more than 200–600 ml/day.

Different Causes of Cough with Normal Chest Radiology

- Post-nasal dripping
- Cough variant asthma
- Patient on ACE inhibitor treatment
- Gastroesophageal reflux disease
- Allergic respiratory disorder.

PULMONARY FUNCTION TESTS

Lung Volumes

Tidal volume: This is the amount of air which is inhaled or exhaled while the person is breathing normally (normally around …500 ml).

Minute volume: This is the total amount of air which is exhaled/minute.

Residual volume: Person is exhaling as much as possible—it is the amount of air that is remaining in the lungs after exhaling as much as possible.

Forced expiratory volume: FEV1

- Patient is asked to expire during the test.
- This is the amount of air which is expired during the first second.

Inspiratory reserve volume: Person is asked to inhale the normal volume of air (tidal volume). Person is asked to forcibly inhale additional volume of air—usually around 3000 ml.

Expiratory reserve volume

- Patient is asked to expire a normal tidal volume (around 500 ml).
- Person is asked to expire by effort further volume of air (around 1200 ml) after normal expiration.

Lung Capacities

Vital capacity: This is the total amount of air that can be exhaled after inhaling as much air the person can inhale—around 4800 ml.

Forced vital capacity (FVC): This is the amount of air that can be forcibly exhaled as much as possible.

Total lung capacity (TLC): This is the total volume of lungs when filled with as much air as possible (around 6000 ml).

Functional residual capacity: Person is asked to exhale normally. This is the amount of air in the lungs after normal exhalation (2400 ml).

Inspiratory capacity: This is the amount of air that can be inspired maximally (around 3600 ml).

Peak expiratory flow rate
- This is the amount of air which can be expelled from the lungs at the highiest rate
- This is measured by the peak flowmeter and measured as litres/minute.
- PEFR tests the capacity of the person how fast the person can breath out.

Measurement of PEFR: Person is asked to take breath in as deeply as possible and then breath out or blow out as fast and as hard as possible into the mouthpiece of the *peak flowmeter*.

DLCO—carbon monoxide—diffusion coefficient: This is the measurement of transfer of carbon monoxide molecules from alveolar gas to the hemoglobin of RBCs in the pulmonary circulation (decreased in obstructive and restrictive lung disease).

PFT in Obstructive Airway Disease

Suggestive of airflow obstruction: FEV1/FVC is less than 70% of predicted value (FEV1 is significantly reduced).

Advanced disease: ↑Total lung capacity, ↑Functional residual capacity and ↑Residual volume.

Emphysema
- Significant increase in total lung capacity
- ↓ of CO diffusion coefficient

Assessment of reversibility of airways: Increase of at least of 12% of FVC, PEFR and FEV1 after 10–15 minutes of therapeutic doses of bronchodilator agent (inhaled or nebulised).

Restrictive lung disease
- Both FEV1 and FVC are reduced
- FEV1/FVC ratio is either normal or increased.
- Residual volume, functional residual capacity and total lung capacity is reduced.
- Decrease in the carbon monoxide diffusion coefficient.

INTERSTITIAL LUNG DISEASE

Type of disease: Inflammatory or granulomatous disease.

Structures involved
- Interstitium of the lung
- Blood vessels
- Lymphatics
- Alveolar epithelium

Pathologically: Absence of infection or malignancy.

Common Causes of ILD
- Idiopathic pulmonary fibrosis
- Pulmonary fibrosis secondary to connective tissue disorders
- Occupational and environmental related ILDs
- Sarcoidosis

Symptoms and Signs
Common symptoms
- Progressive dyspnea
- Dry cough
- Occasionally wheeze

Rare symptoms
- Chest pain
- Hemoptysis

Dyspnea: Progressive dyspnea over months to years and is the most common manifestation of ILD (not associated with PND).

Dry cough: May be a manifestation of ILD without significant sputum.

Wheezing: Associated with conditions like-Churg-Strauss syndrome, chronic eosinophilic pneumonia and respiratory bronchiolitis.

Chest pain
- Not common
- May be due to pneumothorax

Hemoptysis: Unusual except in patients with vasculitis/alveolar hemorrhage.

Easy fatigability: Common to all ILDs.

Age group involved
Less than 40 years
- ILD with connective tissue disorders
- Sarcoidosis

Between 40–60 years: Idiopathic pulmonary fibrosis.

Sex distribution
ILD predominantly in men
- ILD with rheumatoid arthritis
- Idiopathic pulmonary fibrosis
- ILD with occupational lung disease.

ILD predominantly in women
- Due to connective tissue diseases (except rheumatoid lung)
- Churg-Strauss disease.

History of smoking
Smoking is more likely to be associated with
- Idiopathic pulmonary fibrosis
- Langerhans cell histiocytosis
- Farmer's lung

Occupational history
History of exposure to allergen, dust, chemicals, e.g. hypersensitivity pnuemonitis, Farmer's lung.

Family history: Positive family history is present in disorders like sarcoidosis.

Recurrent attack of breathlessness in ILD
- For example, Churg-Strauss disease
- Eosinophilic pneumonia

Different types of ILDs depending on the duration of symptoms
Days to weeks
- Allergy to drugs, fungi, helminthiasis
- Acute interstitial pneumonia

Weeks to months: Cryptogenic organising pneumonia, sarcoidosis, SLE polymyositis.

Duration in years
- ILD associated with connective tissue disorders
- Sarcoidosis
- Idiopathic pulmonary fibrosis

Past history in a patient of ILD
- History of parasitic infestation—in case of pulmonary eosinophilia
- History of exposure to HIV infection—patients with organizing pneumonia.
- History of drugs, allergens and exposure to pets.

Signs: In a patient of ILD
- Central cyanosis
- Clubbing
- Chest expansion—decreased
- Bilateral late inspiratory crackles called Velcro rales
- Wheeze in Churg-Strauss syndrome.

 Note

Crepitations are common with inflammatory types of ILDs.

Inspiratory squeaks: Characteristic of bronchiolitis-rhonchi which are high pitched.

Look for: Evidence of pulmonary hypertension, CCF, respiratory failure.

Complications of ILD
1. Progressive respiratory failure type I
2. Pneumothorax
3. Recurrent pulmonary infection
4. Pulmonary hypertension

Investigations in ILD
Chest X-ray
- Volume of the lung is decreased
- Reticulonodular pattern
- Upper lobe nodules in ILD
  - Rheumatoid lung
  - Sarcoidosis
  - Langerhans cell histiocytosis
  - Silicosis

- Honey combing—cystic spaces with fibrosis
- CT scan HRCT
  - Ideal investigation
  - To look for extent of lung involvement
  - Involvement of alveoli and alveolitis
  - Evidence of mediastinal adenopathy
  - Emphysema

 Note

Hilar adenopathy in ILD.

- Patients of ILD like idiopathic pulmonary fibrosis can have bilateral hilar adenopathy which are less than 2 cm.
- If bilateral hilar adenopathy is >2 cm, it is more likely to be associated with sarcoidosis.

Pulmonary function tests in ILD
- Total lung capacity and residual volume is decreased.
- FEV1/FVC ratio is almost equal to 1 (both FEV1 and FVC are decreased)
- Carbon monoxide diffusion coefficient is reduced.

Arterial blood gas
- Oxygenation is decreased
- Respiratory alkalosis

Bronchoalveolar lavage: Fluid can be examined for type of cells, bacteria, malignant cells, CD4/CD8 ratio.

Bronchoscopy/bronchoalveolar lavage
Look for
- Neutrophilia
- Eosinophilia in pulmonary eosinophilia
- Lymphocytosis: Occur in sarcoidosis, connective tissue disease, hypersensitive pneumonia.
- In sarcoidosis: CD4/CD 8 ratio is > 3.5
- Look for fungi, viruses (CMV) and pneumocystis
- BAL fluid: For malignant cells in lymphangitis carcinomatosis

Lung biopsy—for confirmation of histopathological diagnosis
- Risk of pneumothorax is more after lung biopsy in patients with ILDs.
- Rheumatoid factor, ANA and ANCA can be positive in corresponding disorders
- Above factors can also be false positive in idiopathic pulmonary fibrosis.

Usual Interstitial Pneumonia (UIP)
Most common form of interstitial fibrosis.

Features
- Patchy areas of interstitial fibrosis with alternating areas of normal lung.
- Can have chronic scarring of lung or honeycomb changes.
- Can include—collagen disease, drug induced, chronic hypersensitivity pneumonitis.

PNEUMONIC CONSOLIDATION
What is consolidation?
- Radiological sign
- Air space opacity of the chest

Consolidation can occur due to
- In heart failure: Lung parenchyma is filled with fluid.
- In pneumonia: Lung parenchyma is filled with inflammatory exudates.
- In lung abscess: Filled with necrotic material/pus
- Filled with blood: In pulmonary hemorrhage.
- Filled with cells: Pulmonary malignancy.

Pneumonic consolidation: Region or part of lung filled with inflammatory exudates.

Classification of pneumonia: Depending on the anatomical part involved: Segmental/lobar/bronchopneumonia.

Host factors: Community acquired: Acquired in community without other risk factors.

Hospital acquired (after 48 hours after hospital admission)
- Health care associated (HAP)

- Ventilator associated (VAP): After 48 hours on ventilator.

Aspiration pneumonia: Occurs due to aspiration of stomach contents/secretions.

Depending on the aetiological agent
- Bacterial
- Viral
- Fungal
- Parasitic
- Chemical

Risk factors for pneumonia
- Smoking
- Alcoholism
- Dysphagia
- COPD
- Immune suppression
- Viral infection of the lung
- Extremes of ages.

Bronchopneumonia (lobular pneumonia)
- Bilateral patchy involvement
- Inflammation of lung and bronchioles.

Clinical signs of acute bacterial pneumonia
- Febrile
- Presence of herpes labialis

Signs of consolidation
- Chest: Movement decreased on the affected side
- Mediastinum central
- Dull note on percussion
- VF and VR increased
- Tubular bronchial breathing
- Whispering pectoriloquy (hallmark of consolidation).
- Crepitations:
  - Early stage: Fine (late inspiratory)
  - Late stage: Coarse crepitations
- Presence of pleural rub due to associated pleuritis.

Radiological signs
- Dense homogenous opacity with air bronchogram.
- Opacity corresponds to lobe/segment.

LUNG ABSCESS

Definition

Microbial infection of the lung tissue causing liquefaction and necrosis of the lung with formation of cavities > 2 cm (radiologically).

Risk factors for the development of lung abscess
Common
- Alcoholism
- Diabetes mellitus
- HIV infection
- COPD
- Altered sensorium.

Less common risk factors
- Gastroesophageal reflux disease
- CVA
- Malnutrition
- Immune suppression.

Source of infection from outside the lung and factors in the lung which can cause lung abscess
- Anaerobic bacteria from oral cavity
- Infection of bulla in the lung
- Infection distal to bronchial obstruction
- Tricuspid valve endocarditis
- Metastatic abscess from hematogenous spread.

Lung abscess due to aspiration of oropharyngeal contents can occur due to
- Periodontal disease
- Seizure disorder
- Alcohol
- Dysphagia
- General anesthesia.

Organisms causing lung abscess
- *Gram-positive bacteria*
  - *Staphylococcus aureus*
  - *Streptococcus pyogenes.*
- *Gram-negative bacteria*: Klebsiella and Pseudomonas
- *Rarer organisms*
  - *Mycobacterium tuberculosis*
  - *Meliodosis*
  - *Nocardia*

- Fungal infection
- Actinomycosis

Parts of lung involved in aspiration lung abscess

- Apical segment of right lower lobe/occasionally left side.
- Posterior segment of right upper lobe
- Middle lobe on the right side.

Types of lung abscess

- Acute—less than 6 weeks
- Chronic—more than 6 weeks
- Primary—aspiration of bacteria into the lungs without pre-existing lung disease.
- Secondary—due to pre-existing lung condition
  - Bronchiectasis
  - COPD
  - Obstruction to the bronchus.

Clinical Features

History

- Fever with chills and rigors.
- Cough with large amount of sputum with postural variation.
- Hemoptysis.
- Foul smelling sputum in anaerobic infection.

Signs

- Fever and toxemia
- Evidence of gingivitis/periodontal disease/halitosis
- Clubbing
- Signs of pulmonary consolidation/cavity.
- May be associated with empyema, pyo-pneumothorax.
- Necrotising pneumonia: Evidence of pneumonia/liquefaction of lung tissue—without chest X-ray evidence of definite cavity (cavity <2 cm).
- Lung abscess: Evidence of lung abscess with cavity size > 2 cm in the X-ray.

Infective causes of cavity in the lung

- Bacterial including tuberculosis
- Fungal infection

- Infection of bulla/cyst
- Cavitating lung infarct.

Noninfectious causes of cavity in the lung

- Cavitating bronchogenic carcinoma
- Nodular silicosis
- Cavitating rheumatoid nodule
- Granulomatosis with angiitis (Wegener's granulomatosis).

Complications of lung abscess

- Infection of lung segments with destruction of parenchyma and fibrosis
- Bronchiectasis
- Empyema thoracis
- Pyopericardium
- Metastatic brain abscess

Investigations

- Complete blood picture: Leucocytosis
- Blood culture and sensitivity
- Chest X-ray/CT scan
- Sputum: Gram stain/culture sensitivity
- Bronchoscopy—if suspected obstruction
- Analysis of empyema fluid.

PULMONARY CAVITY

- Pulmonary cavity occurs due to destruction of lung parenchyma.
- Occurs as a radiolucency within the pulmonary parenchyma in the following conditions
  - Within consolidation
  - Within the mass
  - Within the nodule

Characteristic Features of Different Pulmonary Cavities

Cavity due to lung abscess

- Either due to aspiration or necrotizing pneumonia
- Aspiration lung abscess: Either superior segment of lower lobe or anterior and posterior segment of upper lobe.
- Necrotising pneumonia: Cavity size <2 cm
- Lung abscess: Cavity size >2 cm.

Complications of lung abscess cavity
- Can rupture into pleura resulting in pyo-pneumothorax
- Can cause massive hemoptysis
- Dissemination of infection resulting in systemic sepsis.

Tuberculous cavity
- Location
  - Upper lobe—apical and posterior segments
  - Lower lobe—superior segments
- Can be thin walled or thick walled
- More likely to be infectious

Open negative syndrome
- Occurs in a patient of pulmonary tuberculous
- Persistence of cavity after full course of chemotherapy for TB
- There will be epithelialisation of cavity preventing the cavity to collapse
- Sputum AFB is negative.

Complications of TB cavity
- Secondary bacterial infection
- Hemoptysis (due to Rasmussen aneurysm)
- Aspergilloma
- Pneumothorax
- Dissemination of TB due to erosion into a blood vessel.
- Scar carcinoma (usually adenocarcinoma)

Cavity due to malignant disorder
- Usually cavitating squamous cell carcinoma of lung
- Also metastasizing gastrointestinal malignancy or sarcomas.
- Irregular thick-walled cavity.

Clinical aspects of cavity in the lung
- Multiple cavities in the lung occurs due to pulmonary tuberculosis, lung abscess or cavitating metastases.
- Airfluid level inside of cavity in the chest—ray occurs in lung abscess/rarely malignancy.

- Fungal ball like inside a cavity can occur in aspergillosis/blood clots.
- Floating water lily like appearance occurs in patients—due to collapsed membrane of a ruptured hydatid cyst.

Thin-walled cavities occur due to
- Lung abscess.
- Pneumatocoele (Staphylococcal lung abscess)
- Pulmonary TB
- Cystic disease of the lung

Thick-walled cavities in the lung
- Lung abscess
- Squamous cell carcinoma
- Wegener's granulomatosis
- Pulmonary TB.

Causes of cavities in the lung
Infective causes
- Pulmonary tuberculosis
- Necrotising pneumonia
- Pneumatocele
- Septic pulmonary emboli

Rare
- Fungal infection
- Nocardiosis
- Meliodosis

Non-infective causes
- Rheumatoid nodule
- Granulomatous disorder

Vascular causes: Pulmonary infarction
Congenital: Cystic disease of lung.
Malignant disorder
- Cavitating squamous cell carcinoma of lung
- Cavitating secondaries

Causes of upper lobe cavity
- Pulmonary tuberculosis
- Lung abscess
- Cavitating malignancy
- Wegener's granulomatosis
- Rheumatoid nodule

Clinical signs of pulmonary cavity

- Presence of bronchial breathing of cavernous type
- Occasionally amphoric type of bronchial breathing
- Increased vocal fremitus and vocal resonance, bronchophony and whispering pectoriloquy
- Crepitations.

Post-tussive suction in a cavity

- Present in a patient with thin-walled collapsible cavity communicating with the bronchus.
- Appearance of suction sound during inspiration after coughing.

Cracked-pot resonance

- Tympanic resonant percussion note over the chest.
- Occurs in a patient of pulmonary cavity communicating with the bronchus.

 Note

Lung abscess cavity and cavitating malignancy are associated with clubbing.

- Tuberculous cavity is usually associated with evidence of volume loss due to fibrosis.

PULMONARY TUBERCULOSIS

Aetiological agent: Mycobacterium tuberculosis.

Mycobacterium tuberculosis

- Aerobic bacterium: Rod-shaped
- Neutral on gram staining
- Cannot be decolorized by acid and alcohol (acid and alcohol fast).
- Acid fastness is due to cell wall lipids like
  - Mycolic acid
  - Mycostearic acid.
- Because of the characteristic cell wall structures containing lipids and peptidoglycans—they are not sensitive to most antibiotics.

Other examples of organisms which are acid-fast

- *Mycobacterium leprae*
- Cryptosporidium
- Isospora
- Nocardia
- Rhodococcus

Route of spread: Respiratory.

Clinical Features

Primary tuberculosis: Occurs in the early phase of infection with mycobacterium TB.

Primary pulmonary tuberculosis

- Common in children
- Presents as fever and pleuritic chest pain. Usually involves lower part of the upper lobe or upper part of the lower lobe. Initial tuberculous focus is called Ghon's focus.

Ghon's focus: Subpleural caseating granulomatous lesion.

Site: Lower part of the upper lobe or upper part of the lower lobe.

Associated features

- Hilar and paratracheal lymphadenopathy.
- Erythema nodosum—in the lower extremities.
- Phlyctenular conjunctivitis.

Course: Usually heals spontaneously. Remains as a calcified focus in the chest X-ray.

Ghon's complex

- Presence of Ghon's focus
- Local lymphadenopathy
- Presence of thickening of pleura.

Progressive primary tuberculosis

- Manifests in persons with impaired immunity.
- For example, infection with retrovirus
- Primary lesion progresses to clinical manifestations.

Manifestations

- Necrosis and cavity formation or primary focus with increase in the size.

- Lymphatic spread of mycobacterium TB causes hilar and paratracheal lymphadenopathy causing obstruction to bronchi.
- Development of pneumonia due to rupture of lymph node into bronchus.
- Development of bronchiectasis either due to
    - Pneumonia causing necrosis and destruction of bronchus.
    - Bronchial obstruction by lymph node
- For example, middle lobe bronchiectasis (Brock's syndrome).

Development of pleural effusion due to
- Rupture of subpleural focus containing bacilli of mycobacterium TB into the pleura.
- Hypersensitivity reaction to tubercular protein.
- There can be dissemination of primary infection causing military tuberculosis/disseminated tuberculosis.
- Primary lesion can spread causing focus of tuberculosis into other organs like bone and meninges and can manifest as tuberculous meningitis.

Postprimary tuberculosis
Occurs in adults: Occurs due to reactivation of latent previous infection/reinfection.

Manifestations
- *Site of involvement*: Upper lobe: Apical and posterior segment (due to high O_2 tension in the upper lobe—high oxygen tension is required for the growth of *Mycobacterium tuberculosis*.)
- Lower lobe—superior segment.

Types of lesions
- Small tubercular infiltrates.
- Pneumonic form of tuberculosis
- Development of pulmonary cavity
- Multiple small lesions throughout the lung due to bronchogenic spread.

Consequences of the lesion (if not treated)
- Death—due to intensive pulmonary involvement.

- Development of fibrosis and cavity with extensive parenchymal destruction.
- Rarely spontaneous resolution.

Symptoms
- Significant weight loss.
- Fever—evening raise of temperature with night sweats

 Note

Tubercular pneumonia, disseminated TB can have high grade fever.

- Elderly debilitated may not have high grade fever.
- Tuberculosis can manifest as PUO.

Cough: Can be severe, dry and occasionally purulent.

Hemoptysis
- Can be scanty/life-threatening.
- Hemoptysis is due to
    - Secondary bacterial infection of the cavity.
    - Endobronchial lesion:
    - Erosion of vessel of a cavity.
    - Dilated vessel rupture: Rasmussen's aneurysm.
    - Aspergilloma
    - Scar carcinoma

Chest pain: Due to pleural involvement.

Dyspnea: Due to pleural effusion/due to extensive parenchymal involvement.

Signs
- Severe anemia
- Clubbing: Rarely due to extensive involvement.
- Presence of crepitations, rhonchi, consolidation, cavity, pleural effusion.

Investigations
- Very high ESR (may be > 100/hour)
- Anemia
- High lymphocyte count
- Myelophthisic anemia: Due to marrow involvement.

Chest X-ray: Infiltration, cavity, fibrosis, pleural effusion, pneumothorax.

Mantoux test

A form of skin test: Substance most commonly used; purified protein derivative (PPD) derived from culture of *Mycobacterium tuberculosis*.

It is a form of delayed hypersensitivity reaction.

Dose administered

- 5 tuberculin units (0.1 ml) intradermal injection—read after 48 to 72 hours.
- Persons with tuberculin hypersensitivity develop an induration.

Site of administration: Left forearm.

Type of reaction

- Erythema
- Induration (usually around 5 to 10 mm)
- Rarely vesicle and necrosis can occur.

Reaction more than 5 mm

- Old-healed TB
- Recent contact with TB
- HIV-positive individuals (can have less than 5 mm reaction)

False positive reaction

- Nontubercular mycobacteria
- Previous BCG vaccination

False negative reaction

- Severely immune suppressed (anergy)
- Sarcoidosis
- Severe or disseminated TB
- Very old tubercular infection
- Less than 6 months of age

Mantoux not recommended in the following situations: Recently undergone Mantoux testing.

 Note

Mantoux test has presently not recommended and is replaced by other specific tests like QuantiFERON gamma assay.

Sputum test

- Staining for mycobacterium TB in the sputum sample.
- 2 or 3 sputum samples—better morning samples.
- Ziehl-Neelsen stain—less sensitive but cheaper.
- Auramine rhodamine staining and fluorescence staining more sensitive but costlier.

Nucleic acid amplification technique: Rapidly detects pulmonary/extra pulmonary tuberculosis.

Present test available

- Real time nucleic acid amplification test—gene Xpert MTB/RIF (called CBNAAT in India—detects tuberculosis and rifampicin resistance within 2 hours).
- It is used as initial lab test.
- Very useful in tuberculous meningitis in detecting TB in CSF.

 Note

CBNAAT: Cartridge-based nucleic acid amplification test.

Culture of Mycobacterium

- Culture by Lowenstein-Jensen or Middlebrook medium—requires 6–8 weeks for bacterial growth.
- Present technique: By molecular methods—mycolic acid high pressure liquid chromatography detection of growth by fluorescent technology can detect growth 2–3 weeks.

Drug sensitivity testing: All cases isolated for mycobacterium should be tested for INH and rifampicin resistance. Second line drugs testing should be conducted including for Quinalones and injectable drugs if MDR-TB is suspected.

TB in HIV-positive patient

- Tuberculosis can manifest at any level of CD count and at any stage of HIV infection. There is an annual risk of around 10% of developing TB in a patient of HIV with positive Mantoux test.

- With higher CD4 count pulmonary tuberculosis manifests as typical pattern with involvement of upper lobe with infiltration and cavity. With lower CD4—less of cavitation, and more of pleural effusion and hilar and paratracheal lymphadenopathy and lower lobe involvement.
- Extra pulmonary tuberculosis is more common in HIV-positive patients.
- Rate of sputum positivity is less common in patients with HIV with pulmonary tuberculosis.
- Immune reconstitution inflammatory syndrome (IRIS) is more common in patient with TB with HIV infection after starting antiretroviral therapy especially in patient with lower CD4 count and extrapulmonary TB.
- Around 30% of mortality in HIV infection is due to tuberculosis related.
- Infection with atypical mycobacterium is lower in a patient of HIV infection who is infected with *Mycobacterium tuberculosis*.

Important Clinical Definitions in Tuberculosis

Clinical tuberculosis: Diagnosis of TB is on clinical basis. Decided to give treatment for pulmonary tuberculosis. Bacteriological confirmation of TB is not present.

Bacteriologically confirmed TB: Bacteriological specimen is positive for TB—either sputum smear is positive or culture is positive.

Relapse: Treated for tuberculosis on the previous occasion. Disease was cleared and treatment was completed. Newer episode of TB is diagnosed. It is either true relapse or may be a newer infection.

Cured TB: Confirmed TB-bacteriologically at the beginning of treatment and either smear or culture has become negative at the last month of treatment or at least once previous.

Treatment failure: Diagnosed as tuberculosis where in smear or culture is still positive after 5 months or later of treatment—consider drug resistance.

Drug resistance: Resistance to one of the main drugs either INH or rifampicin.

Disseminated TB: Tuberculosis involving 2 or more distant sites.

Miliary TB: Presence of miliary opacities of 1 to 2 mm (millet seed shaped) in the chest X-ray and can also involve other organs.

Cryptic TB
- Occurs in middle aged and elderly.
- Usually presents as fever, weight loss, loss of appetite/PUO.
- Typical features of TB are absent
- Can involve multiorgan systems
- Direct evidence for TB is absent
- Should be considered in the DD of PUO in the elderly.

MDR-TB: Resistance to INH and rifampicin with or without resistant to any other drugs.

XDR-TB (Extensively drug resistant TB): Mycobacteria have become resistant to INH and rifampicin and also to most of the alternative drugs used for treatment for TB (include fluoroquinalones and one of the injectable drugs: Amikacin and Capreomycin).

Total drug resistant: Resistance to all the first line drugs and all the 2nd line drugs tested.

Defaulter: Patient where in treatment was interrupted for 2 consecutive months or more.

PCR-based assays: Detect MTB and also the drug resistance and mutation in the target resistance gene regions.

DESTROYED LUNG

Severe destruction of lung parenchyma by infection
- Large area of lung is destroyed.
- There will be fibrosis and cavity formation of lung parenchyma and formation of bronchiectasis.
- Most common cause is pulmonary tuberculosis.
- Destroyed lung is more common on the left side.

Left-sided involvement causing destroyed lung
- May be due to left main bronchus is more narrower and lengthier than the right.
- More likely to be compressed by lymph nodes.
- Drainage of secretions may be affected due to narrower left main bronchus.

BRONCHIECTASIS
- Bronchiectasis is defined as abnormal permanent dilatation of bronchi with thickening of the wall with superadded infection.
- Bronchiectasis usually involves airway of >2 mm in diameter.

Pathological Types

Cystic type/saccular type: Cystic dilatation of bronchi with air fluid level.

Cylindrical type: Bronchi were dilated and straight.

Varicose: Irregularly dilated bronchi.

> **Key Points:**
> - Bronchiectasis is a form of suppurative lung disease.
> - Bronchiectasis is also a form of chronic obstructive pulmonary disease.

Causes

Congenital disorders
- Cystic fibrosis
- Primary ciliary dyskinesia
- Hypogammaglobulinemia
- Bronchomalacia
- Bronchial cartilage deficiency: Williams-Campbell syndrome.
- Alpha-one anti-trypsin deficiency.

Acquired
- Infective lung disease
- Sequelae of necrotizing pneumonia
- *Mycobacterium tuberculosis*
- Bronchopulmonary aspergillosis
- As a sequelae of whooping cough/measles.

Due to bronchial obstruction due to foreign body
- Middle lobe syndrome
- Bronchial stenosis
- COPD
- Rarely autoimmune disorders.

Tractional bronchiectasis: Due to fibrosis of pulmonary parenchyma causing mechanical traction of bronchi.

Causes
- Radiation
- Sarcoidosis
- Interstitial lung disease.

Bronchiectasis sicca
- Occurs as a sequelae of pulmonary tuberculosis
- Predominantly affects upper lobe with good drainage, so less collection of secretions (sicca).
- Presents as recurrent dry cough with episodes of hemoptysis.
- Hemoptysis can be life-threatening as bleeding is from bronchial vessels under systemic pressure

Proximal/central bronchiectasis
- Occurs in patients with bronchopulmonary aspergillosis.
- Affects upper lobe involving lobar segmental bronchi which are central in location.
- Bronchi are dilated with obstruction due to mucus plug.

Pseudobronchiectasis
- Occurs as a consequence of acute infection of pulmonary parenchyma.
- There is no destruction of bronchial walls.
- Can occur after an attack of pertussis/mycoplasma infection (reversible and permanent abnormality not occurring due to effective therapy and without recurrence).
- May represent early stage of bronchiectasis.

Clinical Manifestations

Symptoms: Recurrent attacks of cough with expectoration.

Sputum
- Large quantity
- 3-layered sputum
  - mucoid
  - mucopurulent
  - purulent thick
- Postural variation
- Foul smelling

Hemoptysis in a patient of bronchiectasis
- Occurs due to secondary infection
- Due to repeated inflammation, bronchial arteries become dilated and tortuous and bleed at systemic pressure.

Other manifestations
- Breathlessness
- Pleuritis with chest pain
- Fever
- Wheezing
- Fatigability and weight loss.

Signs
- Halitosis
- Clubbing
- Sinusitis
- Hypertrophic pulmonary OA
- Cyanosis.

Respiratory
- Rhonchi
- Coarse leathery crepitations
- Evidence of obstruction to the airflow.

Due to complications: Evidence of lung abscess. For other details of bronchiectasis: Refer to *Manipal Manual of Clinical Medicine*.

PLEURAL EFFUSION

Collection of fluid in the pleural cavity is called pleural effusion.

Normal pleural space
- Potential space between parietal and visceral pleura.
- Normal intrapleural pressure is negative (around minus 7.5 cm of H_2O) and it becomes further negative during inspiration.

Pathogenesis of pleural effusion
- Normal pleural cavity is having negative intrathoracic pressure
- There is small amount of fluid in the pleural cavity acts as a lubricant.
- Osmotic pressure, hydrostatic pressure and lymphatic drainage decide the amount of fluid in the pleural cavity.
- Fluid from the capillaries in the parietal pleura enters into the pleural cavity and is normally cleared by lymphatics. If the fluid accumulation exceeds the capacity of lymphatics to absorb, then fluid accumulates in the pleural cavity.

Pathogenesis of TB pleural effusion
- Pleuritis and pleural effusion in tuberculosis occurs due to:
  - Delayed hypersensitivity reaction for tubercular proteins causing inflammatory reaction.
  - Rupture of subpleural caseous tubercular focus from the lung with direct infection of pleura with antigen-induced reaction.
- Above mechanisms increase the permeability of capillaries causing exudation of fluid exceeding the capacity of lymphatics to absorb (lymphatic obstruction can occur due to inflammation).

Pathogenesis of pleural effusion
Different mechanisms for the development of pleural effusion.

Due to increase in the hydrostatic pressure
- SVC obstruction
- CCF

Due to altered permeability of pleural capillaries
- Infection
- Inflammation
- Malignancy

Due to lymphatic obstruction: Malignancy.

Due to primary disease of pleura: Mesothelioma.

Peritoneal fluid reaching the pleural cavity: Ascites.

Due to decreased osmotic pressure

- Cirrhosis of liver
- Nephrotic syndrome.

Clinical Features

Symptoms/signs: Refer to *Manipal Manual of Clinical Medicine.*

Causes of pleural effusion without mediastinal shift

- Loculated pleural effusion
- Minimal pleural effusion
- Associated with mass lesion causing collapse of the upper lobe on the same side of pleural effusion.
- Mesothelioma of pleura
- Due to mediastinal fibrosis
- Mass lesion causing mediastinal fixation.

Synpneumonic effusion: Effusion due to pneumonia without isolation of organism.

Parapneumonic effusion: Effusion due to pneumonia with same organism isolated.

Sympathetic effusion: Effusion due to inflammation of surronding structures. For example, pericarditis, pneumonia, liver abscess.

Analysis of pleural fluid

Pleural fluid glucose—very low

- Empyema
- Rheumatoid arthritis

Pleural fluid pH < 7.1: Occurs with empyema and requires drainage.

Pleural fluid lymphocytosis

- Tuberculosis
- Lymphoma
- Sarcoidosis
- Rheumatoid arthritis

Eosinophilia in the pleural fluid

- Presence of air in the pleural cavity
- Asbestosis and helminthiasis
- Fungal infection.

Mesothelial cells in the pleural fluid

- If mesothelial cells >5% of total cells—less likely to be tuberculosis
- (Tuberculosis causes fibrotic reaction rather than mesothelial reaction).

  Pleural fluid ADA >43 U/ml suggestive of TB

  Pleural fluid gamma interferon >140 pg/ml: s/o: Tuberculosis

  Pleural fluid amylase: Increased in
  - Pancreatic effusion
  - Ruptured esophagus
  - Malignancy
- Pleural fluid amylase: Isoenzyme—salivary amylase is increased: Likely to be bronchogenic carcinoma.

Hydropneumothorax

- Presence of air and fluid in the pleural cavity
- *Causes*
  - Chest trauma
  - Tuberculosis
  - Thoracocentesis
  - Bronchopleural fistula.
- *Signs*
  - Hyperresonant note above the level of fluid.
  - Stony dull note below
  - Horizontal level of dull note
- Presence of shifting dullness over the chest
- Coin test positive at the level of hyperresonant note
- Presence of succussion splash.

HEMOTHORAX

Presence of blood in the pleural cavity

- Commonly caused by trauma.
- Bleeding disorders, diagnostic/therapeutic procedures in the pleural cavity can cause hemothorax.
- Hematocrit of the pleural fluid is more than 50% of circulating blood hematocrit is suggestive of hemothorax.

Chylothorax

- Accumulation of chyle in the pleural cavity
- Commonly occurs due to trauma to the chest/mediastinal tumors.
- Triglyceride level in the pleural fluid is more than 100 mg/dl.

Cholesterol effusion

- Occurs in patients with chronic pleural effusion.
- Pleural fluid contains high concentrations of cholesterol
- Mimics chylothorax: For example, TB pleural effusion, rheumatoid arthritis.

Important clinical points with pleural effusion

- If the pleural fluid BNP is > 1500 pg/100 ml is suggestive of CCF causing pleural effusion.
- In a patient of synpneumonic pleural effusion if the thickness of the fluid is 1 cm in depth from chest wall to the lung in the chest X-ray, paracentesis of the fluid is required.
- Malignant pleural effusion is commonly caused by carcinoma of breast, lung and lymphoma.

PULMONARY COLLAPSE (Atelectasis)

Collapse or atelectasis

- There is absence of gas exchange in the lungs with closure of lungs.
- There is absence of lung volume with alveoli become deflated.

Types of pulmonary collapse

- Passive or relaxation collapse (the intrapleural pressure becomes positive with underlying lung becomes relaxed):
  - Causes: Pleural effusion
  - Pneumothorax
- Obstructive collapse (resorption or absorptive collapse): Oxygen is resorbed from the alveoli and volume of the alveoli is decreased and alveoli become gas less and collapse.

- Obstructive collapse occurs due to blockage of airways (intraluminal lesions)
- Compressive collapse: Due to mass compressing the airway/lung.
- Cicatrisation collapse: Fibrosis or scar tissue of the lung parenchyma causes decrease in the lung expansion.

 Note

Occasionally lower part of the lung alveoli become collapsed—gravity dependent.

Types of collapse depending on the part of the lung involved

- Linear/plate atelectasis/subsegmental collapse.
- Segmental collapse
- Lobar collapse

Signs of pulmonary collapse

- Signs of volume loss on the affected side
- Decreased movement on the affected side
- Mediastinum shifted to the same side
- Impaired percussion note
- Absence of breath sounds.
- Right lower lobe collapse: Shifting of liver dullness upwards (difficult to delineate from dullness due to pulmonary collapse)
- Left lower lobe collapse: Shifting of Traube's space upwards.

Chest X-ray

- Evidence of volume loss (narrowing of intercostal spaces)
- Dense homogenous opacity corresponding to lobe/segment.
- Mediastinum shifted to the same side.
- Lower lobe collapse: Pulling up of diaphragm on the affected side.

Causes of pulmonary collapse

Collapse can occur due to

- Airway obstruction—due to intrinsic cause
- Extrinsic obstruction.
- Compression of lung tissue
- Collapse of alveoli

Collapse due to intrabronchial causes
- Mucus plug
- Intrabronchial growth
- Foreign body obstruction

Collapse due to extrinsic compression of bronchus
- Lymphoma
- Mass lesion
- Enlarged lymph nodes.

Collapse due to compression of the lung
- Pleural effusion
- Pneumothorax
- Mass lesion in the lung.
- Collapse of the alveoli—due to alveolar disease.

Right middle lobe syndrome
- Middle lobe bronchus is having narrow orifice.
- Middle lobe bronchus is surrounded by lymph node tissues.
- Can be compressed by enlarged lymph node—collapse of right middle lobe— right middle lobe syndrome—Brocke's syndrome, e.g. tuberculosis.
- Collapse of the right middle lobe is usually associated with recurrent infection and bronchiectasis.

PNEUMOTHORAX
- Presence of air/gas in the pleural cavity is called pneumothorax.
- Pneumothorax causes collapse of the underlying lung. Symptoms and signs depend on the degree of collapse.
- Can impair ventilation and oxygenation.

Types of Pneumothorax
- Primary pneumothorax occurs without pre-existing lung disease.
- Spontaneous pneumothorax: Primary— no inciting event (no pre-existing lung disease)
- May have subpleural blebs
- Secondary pneumothorax: Due to coexisting lung disease—like emphysema.

- Traumatic pneumothorax is due to trauma to the chest wall.
- Depending on the pathophysiologic mechanism pneumothorax is divided into closed, open and tension pneumothorax.

Tension pneumothorax
- Air is trapped in the pleural cavity with increase in the intrapleural pressure.
- Mediastinum is pushed to the opposite side.
- There will be disturbance in the hemodynamics with interference in the cardio-pulmonary function.

Pathophysiology of tension pneumothorax
- Occurs due to discontinuation of tracheo-bronchial tree.
- Parenchymal tissue of the lung forms a one-way valve allowing air to enter into the pleural cavity during inspiration and preventing the air to escape during expiration. This leads to accumulation of air in the pleural cavity and increase in the intrapleural pressure with compromise in the hemodynamic function.

Consequences of tension pneumothorax
- Collapse of the ipsilateral lung with shift of mediastinum to opposite side.
- Can lead to compression of contralateral lung.
- Impairs the venous return to right atrium.
- Can lead to hypoxia, respiratory failure and cardiovascular collapse.

Clinical features of tension pneumothorax
History: Sudden onset of chest pain and dyspnea.

Signs
- Tachycardia
- Tachypnea
- Hypotension.
- R.S: Decreased chest expansion on the affected side
- Mediastinum shifted to the opposite side
- Hyperresonant percussion note on the affected side.

- Breath sound absent on the affected side.
- No added sounds.

Risk factors for spontaneous primary pneumothorax
- Chronic smoking
- Tall and thin body habitus
- Marfan's syndrome

Secondary—pneumothorax
- Emphysema and chronic bronchitis
- Bronchial asthma
- Pulmonary TB
- Cavity of lung abscess rupturing producing pyopneumothorax.
- Cystic fibrosis
- Idiopathic pulmonary fibrosis

Catamenial pneumothorax
- Recurrent pneumothorax
- Usually within 48 hours of menstruation
- In patients with thoracic endometriosis.

Iatrogenic
- During diagnostic or therapeutic procedure in the lung or pleura-like thoracentesis.
- Needle aspiration or lung biopsy.
- CVP catheter
- Thoracotomy

Pneumomediastinum
- Due to increased alveolar pressure, alveoli can rupture and air can escape into the mediastinum.
- Air also can occupy subcutaneous spaces of neck and other fascial planes.
- Air also can escape into the pleura causing pneumothorax.

Risk factors for pneumomediastinum
- Acute severe asthma
- Severe coughing
- Mechanical ventilation with high PEEP
- Respiratory infection
- Rarely seizures
- During childbirth.

Clinical features of pneumomediastinum
- Sudden onset of precordial pain
- Can have subcutaneous emphysema

- Hamman's mediastinal crunch; Crunching sound occurs along with the heart beat and increases during expiration—occurs with pneumomediastinum.

Differential Diagnosis of Pneumothorax

Common
- Acute coronary syndrome/acute MI
- Pulmonary embolism
- Rib fracture
- Cardiac failure
- Pleuropericarditis

Less common
- Aortic dissection
- Rupture oesophagus

Clinical Features of Pneumothorax in General

Spontaneous pneumothorax
- May not have any clinical features.
- May be detected on routine radiological evaluation.
- If coexisting lung disease, dyspnea becomes exacerbated.

Can present with acute onset of chest pain and dyspnea
- Sudden onset of unilateral chest pain—pleuritic type.
- Radiates to shoulder on the same side.
- Associated with sudden onset of dyspnea.

Secondary pneumothorax: Sudden onset of exacerbation of dyspnea due to coexisting lung disease.

Signs of pneumothorax
- Unilateral decrease of chest expansion and chest movement.
- Mediastinum shifted to opposite side (if small pneumothorax mediastinum will not be shifted).
- Hyperresonant percussion note on the affected side.
- Absent breath sounds on the affected side.
- Bell Tympany—tympanitic percussion note heard over massive pneumothorax.

Closed pneumothorax: Air escapes into the pleura and the communication between the pleura and the lung is sealed off. May resolve spontaneously.

Open pneumothorax: Communication between the pleura and lung persists. There will be development of pyopneumothorax. Requires surgical correction.

PULMONARY FIBROSIS

Pulmonary fibrosis occurs due to damage to the pulmonary parenchyma with scarring of lung tissue.

Types and Causes of Pulmonary Fibrosis

Replacement fibrosis: Occurs due to
- Pneumonia
- Tuberculosis
- Pulmonary infarct.

Focal fibrosis: Due to pneumoconiosis (coal workers/silica).

Interstitial (diffuse) fibrosis
- Interstitial lung disease
- Drugs like bleomycin, busulphan, methotrexate and asbestos exposure can also cause pulmonary fibrosis.

Clinical signs
- On the affected side
- Signs of volume loss (hollowing, flattening and drooping of shoulder)
- Mediastinal shift to the same side.
- Chest movement and expansion decreased
- Impaired/dull percussion note
- Breath sound intensity decreased except in upper lobe fibrosis, breath sound intensity is increased with bronchial breathing.
- Crepitations.

Upper lobe fibrosis—pulled trachea syndrome (usually on the right side): Due to tracheal shift to the same side—there can be increased VF/VR with the presence of tubular breathing (heard in the infraclavicular area)—on the affected side but not in the axilla.

 Note

In a patient of upper lobe cavity—cavernous bronchial breathing is heard both in the axilla as well as in the infraclavicular area.

- Pulled trachea syndrome is more likely to occur on the right side—due to anatomy of the right main bronchus (straighter compared to the left).

Lower lobe fibrosis
Right side: Liver dullness will be felt above the 5th intercostal space and may not be able to differentiate from dullness due to fibrosis.

Lower lobe fibrosis
Left side: Resonance of Traube's space will be percussed above the normal location (due to pulling up of diaphragm).

Interstitial fibrosis
There will be presence of Velcro rales.

Table 2.1: Differences between pulmonary and pleural fibrosis		
	Pulmonary fibrosis	Pleural fibrosis
Signs of volume loss	+	++
Rib crowding	+	++
Mediastinal shift to same side	+	Usually not present
Percussion note	Impaired/dull	Dull
Auscultation	Breath sound intensity ↓ (UL fibrosis—it is ↑ with bronchial breathing)	Breath sound Intensity severely decreased
Added sounds	Crepitations—present	No added sounds

Causes of upper lobe fibrosis
- Pulmonary tuberculosis
- Necrotising pneumonia
- Rheumatoid lung
- Silicosis
- Ankylosing spondylitis
- Radiation.

PLEURAL FIBROSIS

- Fibrosis of parietal and visceral pleura
- Architecture of pleural tissue is lost
- It may be localized part of pleura like pleural plaques or diffuse fibrosis of pleura with pleural thickening.
- Visceral pleural fibrosis can extend into the lung parenchyma.

Causes of pleural fibrosis: Occurs due to severe inflammation of pleura with exudative pleural effusion.

Causes: Common
- Parapneumonic effusion/empyema thoracis
- Tuberculosis
- Asbestosis
- Hemothorax

Less common
- Radiation
- Rheumatoid pleural effusion
- Chemical pleurodesis

Clinical features
- Massive pleural fibrosis causes severe restrictive lung disease.
- There will be fusion of parietal and visceral pleura.

Clinical signs
On the affected side
- Volume loss—affected side
- Decreased chest expansion
- Mediastinum not shifted except apical pleural fibrosis.
- Crowding of ribs on the affected side
- Dull percussion note
- Breath sounds decreased
- No added sounds

Fibrothorax
- This is a severe form of pleural fibrosis.
- Pleural surfaces are deposited by thick fibrotic tissues. Both pleural layers are involved. There will be adhesion of 2 layers of pleura.
- Causes severe volume loss.

MASS LESION IN THE LUNG

Nodule in the lung: Lesion less than 3 cm in diameter.

Mass lesion in the lung: Lesion >3 cm in diameter.

Solitary pulmonary nodule: Lung lesion less than 3 cm in diameter with normal aerated lung, pleura and mediastinum.

Characteristic features of benign pulmonary nodule
- Occurs in persons with less than 40 years of age.
- Nonsmokers
- Nodule size is smaller
- Deposition of calcium is present inside the nodule
- Size of the nodule does not double at least for 2 years.

Causes of benign nodular lesions in the lung
Infectious cause
- Pneumonia/lung abscess
- Tuberculosis
- Fungal infection

Non-infectious causes
- Sarcoidosis
- Wegener's granulomatosis
- Rheumatoid arthritis
- Bronchial adenoma
- Hamartoma of lung

Hamartoma: Arise from epithelium of the lung containing fat and cartilage.

Causes of malignant lung mass
- Bronchogenic carcinoma
- Lymphoma
- Secondary deposits in the lung.

Bronchogenic carcinoma
- Chronic smokers have got 10 times more chance of developing bronchogenic carcinoma.
- Chronic smoking causes squamous cell carcinoma, small cell carcinoma and anaplastic carcinoma.

- Adenocarcinoma is more likely to occur in females and in nonsmokers. Squamous cell carcinoma and small cell carcinoma- are usually centrally situated.
- Adenocarcinomas are usually peripherally located.
- Clubbing is a feature of nonsmall cell carcinomas.
- Hypertrophic pulmonary osteoarthropathy is usually associated with adenocarcinomas.

Features of bronchogenic carcinoma
Centrally situated tumors
- Severe intractable cough
- Hemoptysis—may be massive
- Bronchial obstruction
  - Dyspnea, wheeze
  - Recurrent pneumonia not resolving
- Cavity formation.

Peripheral lesions
- Causes pleuritic chest pain
- Skeletal pain due to chest wall invasion
- Pleural effusion.
- Both central and peripheral lesions can cause recurrent lower respiratory infection.

Features due to local spread of the tumor
- Mediastinal mass with SVC obstruction.
- Horner's syndrome.
- Elevation of hemidiaphragm due to phrenic nerve palsy
- Hoarseness of voice—recurrent laryngeal nerve palsy.
- Features of Pancoast's tumor
- Extension can occur into pericardium, cardia and regional lymph nodes.

Can present with paraneoplastic syndrome:

Pancoast tumor (superior pulmonary sulcus tumor)
Features
- Pain in the distribution of C8-T1 and pain over the shoulder.
- Atrophy and weakness of small muscles of hand.
- Pain and tenderness over the 1st and 2nd rib.

Upper lobe—mass
Features
- Fullness of the upper part of chest.
- Dullness over the infraclavicular and supraclavicular area.
- Signs of mediastinal mass.
- Can cause upper lobe collapse
- If the mass is in contact with the upper lobe, bronchus can result in bronchial breathing.
- Supraclavicular lymphadenopathy
- Horner's syndrome
- Phrenic nerve palsy
- SVC obstruction

Adenocarcinoma
- Common type of bronchogenic carcinoma.
- Common in women and in nonsmokers.
- Peripherally located.

Squamous cell carcinoma
- Strongly associated with smoking
- Common carcinoma to cavitate
- Carries bad prognosis.

Small cell carcinoma
- Common in smokers
- Metastasis occurs early
- Paraneoplastic syndrome common
- Carries worst prognosis.

APPROACH TO A PATIENT OF MEDIASTINAL MASS

Parts of mediastinum
- *Anterior mediastinum*: From sternum to pericardium and brachiocephalic vessels
- *Middle mediastinum*: Between anterior and posterior mediastinum.
- *Posterior mediastinum*: From posterior part of pericardium and trachea anteriorly and vertebral column posteriorly.
- *Superior mediastinum*: Boundaries:
  - Above, thoracic inlet
  - Below: Thoracic plane at the level of sternal angle.
  - Lateral: Mediastinal pleura.
  - Posterior: Borders of upper thoracic vertebra.

Structures in the superior mediastinum

Vascular structures

- Veins: Upper part of SVC
- Arteries: Aortic arch and great vessels
- Nerves: Vagus nerve
- Left recurrent laryngeal nerve
- Cardiac nerves.

Lymph nodes

- Brachiocephalic
- Tracheobronchial
- Paratracheal.

Other structures

- Trachea
- Oesophagus
- Thymus
- Thoracic duct

Common cause of mediastinal mass

Anterior mediastinum

- Thymoma
- Lymphoma

Middle mediastinum

- Lymph node masses
- Vascular masses
- Pleuropericardial cyst
- Bronchial tumors

Posterior mediastinum

- Neurogenic tumors
- Oesophageal abnormality
- Aortic aneurysm
- Bronchogenic tumor
- Lymph node mass

Superior mediastinum

- Retrosternal goiter
- Aortic arch aneurysm
- Lymph node mass—from bronchogenic carcinoma
- Metastasis
- Lymphoma

Clinical features of mediastinal mass: May not have any symptoms and can be detected on routine examination.

Common symptoms of mediastinal mass

- Depend on the site and nature of mass
- Can present with fever, weight loss.

Specific symptoms due to mass effect over the structures

- Dyspnea, orthopnea
- Dysphagia
- Hoarseness of voice
- Airway obstruction
- SVC obstruction
- Stridor
- Hemoptysis.

Signs

- Depend on the cause of mediastinal mass.
- If due to enlarged lymph nodes or mass in the mediastinum:
  - Signs of SVC obstruction
- Signs of mediastinal widening (dullness on either side of the sternum and over the manubrium and upper part of the sternum).
- Enlarged lymph nodes in the neck
- If mediastinal widening is due to aortic aneurysm: Signs of aortic aneurysm will be present.
- Possible other signs: Depend on the side of involvement:
  - Diaphragm palsy
  - Horner's syndrome
  - Signs due to compression of right or left main bronchus
  - d' Espine's sign—posterior mediastinal mass.

 Note

There will be other signs of causing the mediastinal mass like carcinoma lung, lymphoma, etc.

SUPERIOR VENA CAVAL (SVC) OBSTRUCTION

Anatomical aspects

- Superior vena cava is located in the middle mediastinum.
- It originates from the junction of right and left innominate veins and joins the right atrium.

- SVC is the major draining vessel from head and neck, upper extremities and upper thorax.

Causes of SVC obstruction

Pressure effect on SVC
- Bronchogenic carcinoma
- Mediastinal mass/lymph node enlargement.

Thrombosis of SVC
- Related to central venous catheter
- Intravascular device.

Other causes
- Aortic aneurysm
- Tuberculosis/syphilis
- Thymoma

Malignant invasion/mass pressing on SVC
- 80% of the masses are malignant
- *Usual causes*
  - Bronchogenic carcinoma
  - Lymphoma
  - Metastatic carcinoma
  - Hypercoagulable state

Effect of SVC obstruction
- There will be opening of collateral circulation.
- Azygos, hemiazygos and connecting intercostal veins play important connection.
- Internal mammary veins and tributaries communicate with superior and inferior epigastric veins.
- Long thoracic veins communicate with femoral and vertebral veins.

Clinical features

Symptoms
- Puffiness of face
- Headache
- Distended nonpulsatile neck veins
- Swelling of upper extremities

Symptoms due to involvement and compression of other mediastinal structures
- Dysphagia
- Stridor

- Dyspnea
- Hoarseness of voice

Signs
- Non-pulsatile distended neck veins
- Distended chest wall veins
- Puffiness of face and swelling of upper extremities (Fig. 2.1)
- Cyanosis
- Papilledema
- Stupor/coma.

Due to involvement of other mediastinal structures and pleura
- Horner's syndrome
- Diaphragm palsy
- Pleural effusion

Different levels of SVC obstruction

SVC obstruction—above the level of joining of azygos
- Distended arm and neck veins
- Edema of neck, face and arm
- Dilated veins over the upper extremities
- Less prominent chest wall veins.

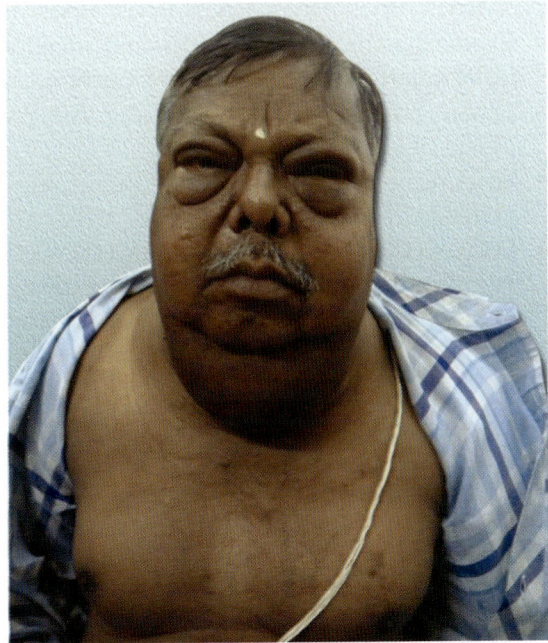

Fig. 2.1: SVC obstruction (facial puffiness and prominent chest wall veins)

SVC obstruction at the level of azygos or below azygos
- More severe symptoms
- Veins over the abdominal wall, anterior and posterior aspect of abdomen with flow downwards to IVC.
- More prominent chest wall veins.

CHRONIC OBSTRUCTIVE PULMONARY DISEASE

🔑 Key Points:

- In COPD airflow obstruction is not fully reversible.
- Obstruction to the airflow is more during exhalation.
- Obstruction to the airflow is more likely in smaller airways with trapping of air.
- Trapping of air and hyperinflation of alveoli and pushing down of diaphragm result in interfering of lung function.

Disorders which are catogorised as COPD
- Chronic obstructive bronchitis
- Emphysema
- Bronchiectasis

Consequence of chronic bronchitis and emphysema
- Excess production of mucus and airway inflammation with recurrent infection.
- Severe obstruction to the airflow, hyperplasia of goblet cells.
- Squamous cell metaplasia with carcinogenesis.
- Disturbance in the gas exchange with ventilation/perfusion mismatch resulting in hypoxia and CO_2 retention causing development of pulmonary hypertension.

Obstruction to the airflow occurs due to
- Edema of airways
- Inflammation of airways
- Fibrosis
- Smooth muscle hypertrophy (less common than bronchial asthma).

Clinical findings
- Chronic cough, dyspnea and wheeze
- Recurrent infective exacerbations

- Use of accessory muscles of respiration
- Tripod position of the patient (Fig. 2.2).

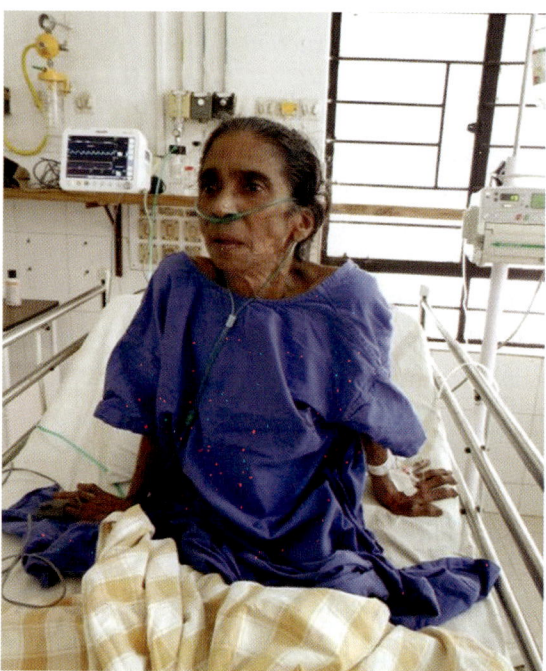

Fig. 2.2: Tripod position in advanced COPD

Patients with emphysema are significantly emaciated
- Due to increase of tumor necrosis factor alpha (↑TNF alpha)
- Decreased consumption of calories.

Hoover's sign: Inward movement of rib cage during inspiration (due to low flat diaphragm and altered diaphragmatic contraction) in patients with severe airflow obstruction.

Look for following signs in a patient of COPD
- Look for signs of chronic bronchitis (crepitations and rhonchi).
- Look for emphysema
- Signs of airflow obstruction (decreased breath sounds, rhonchi and prolonged expiration)
- Signs of pulmonary hypertension
- Signs of type 2 respiratory failure.

Different Types of Emphysema (Clinical)

COPD with Emphysema

Subcutaneous emphysema (surgical emphysema)
Presence of air in the skin/subcutaneous tissue. Air can escape from respiratory or gastrointestinal tract. Air usually spreads to the chest wall, face and neck. Air is felt as crackles to touch and present as subcutaneous crepitus or crepitations. Usual causes are trauma to the chest/neck/insertion of intercostal tube.

Compensatory emphysema: Hyperinflation of the lung occurs due to damage to the some portion of the same lung or significant damage to the opposition lung. There is no destruction of interalveolar septa.

Localised emphysema
- Occurs in partial fixed obstruction to the bronchus. There will be trapping of air.
- In the localized part of the lung with fixed monophonic wheeze.

Mediastinal emphysema (pneumomediastinum)
Presence of air in the mediastinum. Air can escape from the lungs, airways or from GIT. Can present as precordial pain, dyspnea and subcutaneous emphysema. May be associated with mediastinal crunch (Hamman's sign). Can mimic cardiac tamponade.

RESPIRATORY FAILURE

Mechanisms of oxygenation of lung and removal of carbon dioxide can become defective resulting in decreased oxygen concentration of blood with retention of carbon dioxide causing respiratory failure.

Types of Respiratory Failure

Type I Respiratory Failure
- Due to hypoxia and oxygenation failure
- Arterial blood gas shows very low pO_2 (<60 mm of Hg) with pCO_2 decrease.

Acute type I respiratory failure
Causes
- Acute pulmonary edema
- ARDS
- Pneumonic consolidation
- Pneumothorax
- Acute pulmonary embolism
- CNS cause brainstem dysfunction

Chronic type I respiratory failure
Causes
- Interstitial lung disease
- Emphysema

Type 2 Respiratory Failure
- There is decreased oxygenation with ventilatory failure.
- ABG shows ↓ pO_2 with ↑ pCO_2

Causes of acute type 2 respiratory failure
- Acute severe asthma
- Tension pneumothorax
- Acute brainstem injury
- Narcotic overdosage
- GB syndrome

Chronic type 2 respiratory failure
Causes
- COPD with exacerbation
- Chronic ILD
- Neuromuscular disorders

Features
- CO_2 retention causing vasodilation:
  - High volume bounding pulse
  - Warm extremities
  - Palmar erythema
  - Central cyanosis
  - Polycythemia
  - Papilledema
  - Flapping tremor
- CO_2 narcosis
  - Drowsiness
  - Altered sensorium
  - Unconsciousness

Type 3 respiratory pulmonary failure
- Occurs due to atelectasis of parenchyma of lung.
- Commonly occurs postoperatively.
- Administration of general anesthesia can lead to atelectasis of dependent part of the lungs. This can be overcome by chest

physiotherapy, change of position and noninvasive ventilation.

Type 4 respiratory failure

- Occurs due to decreased perfusion of muscles of respiration.
- Occurs in patients with hypotension and shock.

ACUTE SEVERE ASTHMA

Exacerbation of symptoms of asthma in spite of taking regular asthma medications.

Features

- Severe form of dyspnea
- Not able to complete sentences
- Severe wheeze
- Tachycardia
- Pulsus paradoxus
- Central cyanosis
- Chest examination—may reveal bilateral rhonchi and can become silent chest.

Silent chest: Due to severe airflow obstruction with significant reduction in breath sounds.

To look for following abnormalities in a patient of acute severe asthma

- Respiratory infection
- Upper airway obstruction
- Collapse lobe/segment
- Pneumothorax
- Cardiac disease.

Investigations

Pulmonary function tests: Peak expiratory flow rate—severely decreased with evidence of airflow obstruction.

Arterial blood gas

- pO_2 is decreased
- Initially pCO_2 is decreased due to hyperventilation.
- If normal pCO_2 in acute severe asthma suggestive of decreased washing out of CO_2.
- ↑ pCO_2 suggestive of type 2 respiratory failure.

Chest X-ray look for

- Hyperinflation
- Pneumothorax

- Collapse segment
- Consolidation.

Refractory asthma: Symptoms of asthma is persisting with recurrent attacks of asthma with significant defect in the lung function.

Mechanisms

- Cytokine regulations become abnormal.
- Glucocorticoid receptor inhibition by cytokines.

Steroid resistant asthma: Symptoms of asthma not responding in spite of taking prednisolone 40 mg BD × 2 weeks.

Brittle asthma: Significant variation/fluctuation in the symptoms of asthma.

Aspirin sensitive asthma

Features

- Clinical features of bronchial asthma.
- Symptoms are exacerbated by administration of aspirin.
- Usually associated with nasal and ethmoidal polyps.
- Combination of above features is called Samter's triad.
- Any NSAID can exacerbate asthma, may be due to the blockage of protective prostaglandins.

Complications of bronchial asthma

Acute severe asthma

- Acute respiratory failure and respiratory arrest
- Hypoxic cardiac arrest
- Tension pneumothorax
- Segmental pulmonary collapse due to mucus plug

Chronic complications

- Chronic type I respiratory failure
- Recurrent exacerbations
- Pneumothorax
- Recurrent pulmonary infections
- Polycythemia
- Complications due to medications

Gastrointestinal Tract including Liver and Pancreas

INVESTIGATIONS OF LIVER DISEASE

Biochemical Tests

Liver Function Test

- Serum bilirubin
- Liver enzymes
- Serum albumin
- Serum globulin
- Coagulation factors

Serum bilirubin

Normal: 0.2–0.9 (up to 1 mg/dl)

Direct: 30% of total bilirubin (around 0.3 mg/dl).

> **Key Points: Regarding serum bilirubin**
>
> Transport of bilirubin—conjugation is the rate limiting step in the hepatocyte metabolism (early affected in hepatic disorders).
>
> - Increase of conjugated bilirubin is always pathological.
> - Bilirubin level does not always correlate with severity of liver disease.
> - Unconjugated bilirubin raise may be because of other factors apart from liver disease.

Liver enzymes

- AST (aspartate aminotransferase)–SGOT: Serum glutamic-oxaloacetic transaminase.
- ALT (alanine aminotransferase)–SGPT: Serum glutamic-pyruvate transaminase.
- ALP: Alkaline phosphatase—from liver: (Other sources—bone, neutrophil, intestine and placenta).

- 5' Nucleotidase
- ALP and 5' nucleotidase—secreted from liver cell biliary canalicular membrane.
- GGTP: Gamma glutamil transpeptidase. Secreted from hepatocyte endoplasmic reticulum and epithelial cells of bile duct.

AST and ALT

- ALT—produced in the liver. Any parenchymal damage to the liver—there will be leaking of ALT into the circulation (normal level—5 to 56 u/l).
- AST—produced in the liver and also skeletal muscles (normal level—5 to 40 u/l).
- ALT and AST increase indicate damage to the liver cells.

Causes of liver enzyme raise

- Viral, ischemic and drug-induced liver disease (usually more than 10 times the normal).
- Alcoholic and leptospira hepatitis—enzyme raise up to 5 times
- Cirrhosis of liver—not significant liver enzyme raise (around 2 to 5 times).
- Liver enzyme raise can also occur in non-alcoholic steatohepatitis (NASH).
- Paracetamol overdosage causes very high raise in liver enzymes.
- In parenchymal liver disease—viral hepatitis—there is significant increase of ALT > AST.
- In alcoholic hepatitis—there is raise of AST compared to ALT in ratio of AST: ALT—

2:1 (if the ratio is 3:1—it is more suggestive of alcoholic hepatitis).
- Pyridoxal phosphate deficiency in alcoholics causes decrease in ALT synthesis.
- ALT and AST are not increased in biliary tract obstruction.

Alkaline phosphatase
- Alkaline phosphatase is produced by the liver and also by bone, intestine, placenta and neutrophils.
- Alkaline phosphatase can be elevated in obstructive biliary disease (> 4 times)

Causes of alkaline phosphatase raise
- Obstructive biliary disease—intrahepatic/ extrahepatic obstruction
- Causes of isolated increase in alkaline phosphatase in elderly—consider infiltrations of the liver by malignant conditions.
- Occasionally disorders like disseminated TB and other granulomatous conditions can cause isolated increase in ALP.

5'-Nucleotidase
- It is a membrane glycoprotein of liver cells.
- Likely to be elevated in cholestatic disorders, hepatitis, primary liver malignancy and biliary cirrhosis.
- Normal value: 5–17 IU/liter
- Helps to identify the cause of ALP raise as liver disease
- GGTP: Gamma glutamyltranspeptidase
- Parenchymal liver enzyme. Normal level: 9–35 IU/L
- Raises within 24 hours of alcohol consumption.
- 30 days may be required to return to normal level after stopping alcohol consumption.
- Also raised in intrahepatic and extrahepatic obstruction.

Serum albumin
- Albumin is synthesized by the liver.
- Normal level of serum albumin: 3.5 gm– 5.5 gm/dl.
- Half life of serum albumin: Around 3 weeks.
- Decrease of serum albumin is usually indicative of chronic liver disease.

Serum globulin
- Normal liver clears the antigen produced by the bacteria in the intestine which reaches the liver. Cirrhotic liver is not able to clear the antigens which reach the systemic circulation producing antibodies with increase in globulin.
- Liver disorders associated with raise in certain immunoglobulins:
  - Alcoholic liver disease: Increase IgA level
  - Autoimmune liver disease: Increase in IgG level
  - Primary biliary cirrhosis: IgM increase.

Alpha-Fetoprotein
- It is produced by yolk sac and liver during fetal development.
- It is elevated in hepatocellular carcinoma.
- It can also get elevated in germ cell tumors
- In hepatocellular carcinoma values will be >500 ng/ml.

Prothrombin time and other coagulation factors
Prothrombin time depends on vitamin K dependent coagulation factors (factor III, V, VII and X), prolongation of prothrombin time is suggestive of liver disease and indicates bad prognosis.

 Note

Most of the coagulation factors are produced by the liver. Only factor VIII is not synthesized by the liver (synthesized by vascular endothelium).

Blood Ammonia
- Raise in serum ammonia level may be indicative of liver disease.
- Normally ammonia is produced by the protein metabolism and by the bacteria of intestine and liver converts it to urea.
- Serum ammonia level may not correlate with the degree of hepatic encephalopathy.

 Note

Blood urea level may be significantly low in severe liver disease.

Urine Examination

Conjugated bilirubin gets filtered through the glomerulus and appears in the urine. Appearance of bilirubin in the urine is suggestive of conjugated hyperbilirubinemia and possible liver disease. In hemolytic anemia there will be presence of urobilinogen in the urine.

Anti-Liver Kidney Microsomal (LKM) Abs

Auto-antibodies against the cytochrome P-450–206 system.
- *Type 1 Abs*: Found in patients with type 2 autoimmune hepatitis
- *Type 2 Abs*: In patients with drug-induced liver disease (Tienilic acid induced)
- *Type 3 Abs*: In patients with chronic delta hepatitis.

Imaging Studies in Liver Disease

Ultrasound

- In obstructive jaundice—can detect biliary tract dilatation
- Can detect fatty liver and gall stones
- Can detect architecture of liver and nodularity.

CT Scan Abdomen MRI

- For obstructive biliary disease
- For detecting dilatation of biliary tract
- For fatty liver and hepatic masses
- ERCP—for detection of cause of obstructive jaundice.
- Can detect periampullary lesion and sclerosing cholangitis.
- ERCP is also helpful for introducing stents into the biliary tract, removal of biliary stones and also for sphincterotomy.
- MRCP—more safer than ERCP.
- Advantages of MRCP
  - No radiation risk
  - No pancreatitis risk
  - Faster development of images.

For evidence of cirrhosis: Investigations are available for measuring degree of fibrosis like ultrasound-based elastography which can also be used for monitoring the progress of cirrhosis.

In hepatic malignancy: Techniques are available for embolization of the malignant lesion with chemotherapy drugs and also for radio-frequency ablation.

Biopsy of the liver: For histopathological diagnosis of liver disease.

JAUNDICE

Sources of Bilirubin

- Main sources of bilirubin is from RBCs and hemoglobin breaking down.
- Other sources: Due to ineffective erythropoiesis.
- Due to premature erythroid cells which are destroyed in the marrow.
- Other sources: From tissues: Myoglobin and cytochromes.

Metabolism of Bilirubin

- In the blood bilirubin is bound to albumin and is transported to liver by binding to albumin.
- In the liver: Bilirubin is conjugated and excreted into the bile and then to the duodenum.
- In the distal ileum and colon-hydrolysed to unconjugated bilirubin.
- Bacteria in the gut → unconjugated bilirubin → urobilinogen—excreted in the feces (as urobilins or sterocobilins).
- 10–20% of urobilinogen—absorbed into the portal system and re-excreted by the liver (enterohepatic circulation).

Delta Bilirubin

- This is the albumin bound fraction of direct bilirubin.
- Due to significant cholestasis and hepatobiliary disease: There will be impairment of bilirubin excretion from the liver and small fraction will be bound to albumin.

Significance of Delta Bilirubin

- As it is tightly bound to albumin—not excreted by the kidney.
- Because it is bound to albumin its half life is that of albumin (12–14 days.)
- Because it is not excreted in the urine, urine becomes negative for bilirubin in spite of conjugated hyperbilirubinemia.
- Even though patient is clinically improving, serum bilirubin is slowly decreasing because of prolonged half life of delta bilirubin.

Normal serum bilirubin level 0.2–1 mg/dl: Normal direct bilirubin—up to 30% of total bilirubin.

Direct hyperbilirubinemia: Direct bilirubin > 20% of total bilirubin

Indirect bilirubinemia: Direct bilirubin less than 15% of total bilirubin or indirect bilirubin = Total bilirubin – direct bilirubin.

Urine bilirubin

- Direct/conjugated bilirubin appears in the urine.
- Indirect bilirubin (bound to albumin)—not excreted by the kidney.
- Delta bilirubin (direct bilirubin bound to albumin)—not excreted by the kidney.
- Proximal tubules absorb the bilirubin which is excreted by the kidney.

Clinical aspects of jaundice

- Sclera is the first structure to become yellow and usually becomes yellow when bilirubin level is around 3 mg/dl.
- Sclera has got increased affinity for bilirubin due to high elastic tissue.
- Tongue—undersurface and oral cavity can become yellow but later than sclera.

Other causes of yellowish discoloration of the body

- Hypercarotenemia—sclera not involved.
- Excessive quinacrine exposure.

Unconjugated hyperbilirubinemia

- Commonly caused by hemolysis

- Bilirubin level does not exceed more than 5–6 mg/dl in a patient of hemolysis due to the normal functioning of the liver.

Causes of very high bilirubin in a patient of hemolysis

- Severe hemolysis—like sickle cell crisis.
- Associated liver disease.
- Obstructive jaundice due to pigment gall stones.

APPROACH TO PATIENT OF JAUNDICE

CAUSES OF JAUNDICE

Acute Causes (2 to 4 Weeks)

Acute Hepatitis

Infective

- Viral hepatitis
- Acute attack of malaria
- Enteric fever
- Leptospirosis
- Acute cholecystitis
- Acute pancreatitis
- Systemic sepsis

Drug-induced hepatitis (INH, rifampicin, pyrizinamide)
Alcoholic hepatitis
Ischemic hepatitis

Other causes of acute jaundice

Acute hemolysis: Acute malaria, drug induced, hemolytic crises of chronic hemolytic anemia.

Drug induced: Paracetamol overdosage.

Acute hepatic congestion

- CCF
- Acute Budd-Chiari syndrome

Chronic causes of jaundice

Unconjugated hyperbilirubinemia

- Chronic hemolytic anemias
- Familial hyperbilirubinemias: Gilbert's syndrome, Crigler-Najjar syndrome

Conjugated hyperbilirubinemia
- Chronic parenchymal liver disease
  - Cirrhosis of liver, chronic hepatitis, hepatic malignancies
  - Hepatic veno occlusive disease
- Obstructive biliary disease: Gall stone disease, carcinoma—head of pancreas, secondaries in the porta hepatis.

HISTORY IN A PATIENT OF JAUNDICE

Fever: Infective disorder of the liver/gall bladder or secondary involvement of liver due to sepsis.

Right hypochondrial pain
- Liver or gall bladder disease
- Recurrent right hypochondrial pain, jaundice and fever: Cholecystitis

Systemic symptoms: Arthralgia, myalgia. Rash: Viral/leptospira/connective tissue disorders. History of travel to endemic area: Viral hepatitis, malaria, etc.

Drug intake
- Hepatotoxic drugs
- Anabolic steroids
  Transfusion of blood products, drug abuse, needle sharing: Viral hepatitis B, C, retroviral infection
- Exposure to commercial sex workers: Hepatitis B and C/retroviral infection
- History of alcohol and hepatotoxins consumption: Parenchymal liver disease
- Bleeding tendency, hemetemesis and malena: Portal hypertension or parenchymal liver disease.
- Itching and clay colored stool; obstructive jaundice
- History of abdominal pain, alcoholism and jaundice: Possible pancreatitis.
- Painless progressive jaundice: Extrahepatic obstruction like carcinoma head of the pancreas/secondaries in the porta hepatis.

Family history of jaundice
- Possible viral hepatitis
- Occasional Wilson's disease

- Familial hyperbilirubinemias
- Hemolytic anemias

Neurological involvement with jaundice
- Chronic hepatic encephalopathy
- Wilson's disease
- Alcohol-induced CNS involvement.

Clinical Examination in a Patient of Jaundice

Clinical Signs

Severe emaciation and anemia
- Cirrhosis of liver
- Malignant disorder

Signs of CCF: Cardiac cirrhosis.

Lymphadenopathy
- Virchow's node: GI malignancy
- Sister Joseph nodule: Abdominal malignancy
- Systemic disease including lymphoma
- Look for signs of liver cell failure: For parenchymal liver disease.

Systemic Examination

Hepatosplenomegaly
- Liver disease
- Systemic illness: Malaria, viral illness, leptospirosis, tuberculosis, HIV infection
- Hemolytic anemia
- Hematological malignancy

Ascites with jaundice
- Liver disease
- Malignancy
- Systemic illness like disseminated TB.
- Murphy's sign: Cholecystitis
- Enlarged gall bladder: Carcinoma head of pancreas.

CHOLESTASIS

Condition Characterised by Inability of the Bile to Drain into the Bile Duct

Occurs either due to impaired secretion of the bile by the liver cells (intrahepatic) or obstruction to the bile flow outside the liver (extrahepatic).

Obstruction to the bile flow
- Intrahepatic
- Extrahepatic.

Causes

Intrahepatic
- Hepatic (intrahepatic)
- Hepatitis—viral
- Drug-induced: Cholestasis
- Inborn errors of bile acid synthesis

Extrahepatic
- Stricture bile duct
- Cholelithiasis
- Primary sclerosing cholangitis
- Occlusion of bile ducts:
  - Carcinoma of head of pancreas
  - Lymph node—at porta hepatis

Features of cholestasis
- High-colored urine
- Icterus: Sclera may become greenish yellow (due to biliverdin)
- Pruritis
- Clay-colored stools
- Evidence of liver disease
- Xanthoma/Xanthelasma
- Carcinoma head of pancreas—presence of enlarged gall bladder.
- Features of other causes of obstruction to bile ducts.
- High-colored urine and icterus: Due to increase of conjugated bilirubin.
- Pruritis—due to increased level of circulating bile salts
- Xanthoma/Xanthelasma—due to altered metabolism of cholesterol.
- Bleeding, bony pain: Malabsorption of fat soluble vitamins like vitamins K, D, and A.

Investigations

For cholestasis
- LFT: Higher level of conjugated bilirubin.
- Alkaline phosphatase is significantly raised.
- Serum cholesterol is increased. Prothrombin time is prolonged.

- Evidence of hepatocellular disease
  - Liver enzymes—increased
  - 5-nucleotidase and GGTP are increased.
  - Viral markers may be positive.

For extrahepatic obstruction
- Ultrasound abdomen
- CT scan abdomen
- ERCP.

VIRAL HEPATITIS

Main Viral Pathogens (Hepatotropic) Causing Viral Hepatitis
- Viral hepatitis A
- Viral hepatitis B
- Viral hepatitis C
- Viral hepatitis D
- Viral hepatitis E and occasionally viral hepatitis G.
- Epstein-Barr, herpes, CMV viruses can also cause viral hepatitis.

Features—common to all viral hepatitis
- Fever
- Jaundice
- Soft, tender enlarged liver
- Phase of cholestasis
- Elevated liver enzymes.

Viral hepatitis A
- RNA virus
- Faeco-oral transmission
- Incubation period 15–45 days
- Chronicity—not present
- Viral markers:
  - Initial 3 months—anti-hepatitis A IgM antibody
  - After 3 months—anti-hepatitis A IgG antibody.

Viral hepatitis B
- DNA virus
- Parenteral transmission
- Incubation period 30–180 days
- Rash and polyarthritis may be associated.

- Can have severe fulminant course.
- Chronic carrier state, cirrhosis and hepatocellular carcinoma can occur.
- Evidence of chronic carrier state: HBsAg +ve
- Evidence of recent infection within 3 months: Anti-HBcAb (anti-hepatitis B core antibody) IgM +ve
- Evidence of past infection: Anti-HBcAg—IgG +ve
- Evidence of active replication—HbeAg (hepatitis B e-antigen) and quantitative estimation of viral DNA load.
- Evidence of resolved infection: Anti-hepatitis B surface antibody (anti-HBsAg antibody).
- Evidence of vaccination against hepatitis B—anti-HBsAg Ab positive but anti-HBcAb negative.

Hepatitis C
- RNA virus
- Parenteral transmission
- Incubation period 15–50 days
- Acute presentation—rare
- Chronic infection—causes
  - Chronic hepatitis
  - Cirrhosis of liver
  - Hepatocellular carcinoma.
- Hepatocellular carcinoma—risk increases in patients with hepatitis C with alcoholism.
- Hepatic C can be associated with vasculitis, Cryoglobulinemia and lichen planus.
- Viral markers: Anti-hepatic C antibody: IgM (3 months).
- Anti-hepatitis C antibody: IgG (after 3 months)
- Estimation of viral RNA load with genotyping.

Hepatitis D
- Features are similar to hepatitis B
- Viral markers—anti-hepatitis D antibody-IgM/IgG

Hepatitis E
- RNA virus

- Faeco-oral route of transmission
- Incubation period 15–60 days
- Presentation—acute hepatitis (mild)
- Fulminant hepatic failure: Can occur in pregnancy
- Chronicity—very unlikely—rarely in immune compromised individuals.
- Viral markers—anti-hepatitis E antibody IgM/IgG.

Complications of Viral Hepatitis

Acute
- Fulminant hepatic failure
- Cholestatic hepatitis
- Relapsing hepatitis
- Rarely acute pancreatitis, myocarditis and GB syndrome.

Chronic
- Chronic hepatitis and cirrhosis of liver (hepatitis B, C and D)
- Aplastic anemia (with hepatitis A)
- Polyarteritis nodosa (hepatitis B)
- Cryoglogulinemia: Chronic hepatitis C
- Glomerulonephritis: Chronic hepatitis B.

CHRONIC HEPATITIS

Inflammation and necrosis of liver occurring over 6 months characterized by biochemical, clinical, immunological and histopathological evidence of hepatitis.

Classification

Aetiological
- *Viral hepatitis*: B, C, D, rarely hepatitis E in immune compromised individuals and also CMV and EB virus
- *Drug induced*: Amiodarone, methotrexate, INH.
- Cryptogenic
- *Others*
  - Alcohol
  - Non-alcoholic steatohepatitis
  - Wilson's disease
  - Hemochromatosis
  - Alpha-1 antitrypsin deficiency

– Autoimmune disorders including sclerosing cholangitis.

Classification by grading: Mild, moderate and severe.

Classification by staging
Stage 0: No fibrosis
Stage 1: Mild fibrosis
Stage 2: Moderate fibrosis
Stage 3: Severe fibrosis
Stage 4: Cirrhosis

Typical histological evidence of chronic hepatitis
- Portal triaditis with lymphocytic infiltration
- Piecemeal necrosis in the parenchyma.

Bridging hepatic necrosis: Fibrosis of portal areas extending into adjacent vascular structures.
   Can form regenerating nodules of cirrhosis.

 Note

- *Acute hepatitis A can trigger autoimmune disorders.*
- *Hepatitis E virus can result in chronic hepatitis in immunosuppressed patients.*

Clinical Features of Chronic Hepatitis

In general
- Fatigability
- Loss of appetite
- Jaundice—fluctuating with recurrent worsening

Features of chronic liver disease: Jaundice, bleeding tendency, edema, ascites, hepatomegaly, hepatic encephalopathy, coagulopathy, hypersplenism.

Chronic Hepatitis B

Features
- Arthralgia/arthritis
- Leucocytoclastic vasculitis.
- Immune complex glomerulonephritis
- Polyarteritis nodosa (20% HBsAg positive).

Chronic Hepatitis C

Features
- 85–90% of hepatitis C: Develop chronic hepatitis

- 50% of hepatitis C develop cirrhosis
- Immune complex mediated complications are less compared to hepatitis B
- Can develop
  - Mixed cryoglobulinemia
  - B cell lymphoma
  - Type 2 diabetes mellitus, lichen planus.

Autoimmune hepatitis
Features
- Women middle aged
- Features similar to chronic hepatitis B
- Recurrent jaundice
- Features of vasculitis
- Erythema nodosum
- Colitis, pleuritis, sicca syndrome
- Maculopapular eruptions
- High titer of ANA.

Complications of chronic hepatitis
- Hepatic encephalopathy
- Portal hypertension
- Cirrhosis
- Hepatocellular carcinoma

Investigations
- CBP—can have pancytopenia
- LFT—elevated liver enzymes
- Prolonged prothrombin time
- Decrease level of albumin
- RFT: Can be abnormal
- Work up for auto-immune aetiology
- Investigation for viral aetiology
- Investigation for Wilson's disease, hemochromatosis and alpha-1 anti-trypsin deficiency
- Imaging studies like CT scan, MRI and upper GI endoscopy.
- Liver biopsy

DIFFERENTIAL DIAGNOSIS OF HEPATOMEGALY

Clinical Aspects

Surface Markings of Liver

Upper border: Line joining a point about 1 cm below the right nipple to a point about 2 cm below the left nipple.

Lower border: Runs obliquely from 9th right to 8th left costal margin crossing the midline about half way between the base of Xiphoid cartilage and umbilicus.

Caudate lobe of the liver

- Independent portion of the liver.
- Supplied by right and left hepatic vein and portal vein
- Blood from caudate lobe drains directly into the IVC

Significance: Caudate lobe becomes enlarged in hepatic outflow obstruction.

Acute enlargement of liver

Common causes

- Acute hepatitis
- Liver abscess
- Congestive cardiac failure

Less common causes: Acute Budd-Chiari syndrome.

Causes of acute hepatitis

- Acute viral hepatitis
- Drug-induced hepatitis
- Acute alcoholic hepatitis
- Acute attack of malaria, typhoid fever, leptospirosis, endocarditis can also cause acute hepatitis.

Acute Hepatitis

Acute viral hepatitis

- History of fever, nausea, vomiting
- High colored urine at the end of 1st week.
- Presence of jaundice
- Soft enlarged tender liver.
- LFT: Elevation of ALT > AST (more than 10 times)
- Viral markers are positive
- Leukopenia.

Alcoholic hepatitis

- History of alcohol intake prior to the onset of jaundice.
- Fever and abdominal pain after alcohol intake along with appearance of jaundice (no prodromal phase)

- Soft tender enlarged liver
- LFT: Increase in the liver enzymes (not more than 5 to 10 times)
- Increased AST > ALT-ratio of 2:1
- GGTP is increased
- Leucocytosis.
- Drug-induced and ischemic hepatitis can also present as acute liver enlargement.

Typhoid fever (*enteric hepatitis*)

- High grade fever
- Enlarged liver—soft and tender
- Splenomegaly (at the end of 1st week)
- Relative bradycardia, rose spots
- Bone marrow/blood culture: *Salmonella typhi* positive
- Widal test: O antigen—1:160 with raising titer—in the 2nd week.

Acute attack of malaria

- History of fever with chills and rigors with typical malarial paroxysms
- No rash or lymphadenopathy
- Presence of hepatosplenomegaly
- Peripheral smear is positive for malarial parasite.

Acute Budd-Chiari syndrome

- Sudden onset of right hypochondrial pain, swelling of feet with distention of abdomen.
- Enlarged tender liver, jaundice, ascites and distended back veins.
- Ascitic fluid: Increase in the protein without much cellular response.
- Ultrasound abdomen and CT angiogram demonstrates the occlusion of the major hepatic veins.

Acute liver abscess

- History of fever with chills and rigors
- Right hypochondrial pain
- Tender enlarged liver
- Amoebic liver abscess
  - Common in alcoholics, previous history of amoebic dysentery—rare
  - Single abscess—posterosuperior aspect of the liver

- Pyogenic liver abscess: Multiple abscess, source of infection may be a pelvic abscess

Congestive cardiac failure

- History of dyspnea, swelling of feet, abdominal distension.
- Raised JVP, enlarged tender liver, pitting edema.
- Abnormal cardiac findings
- Echocardiogram—abnormal
- Other acute febrile illness like, leptospirosis, infectious mononucleosis, infective endocarditis can also present as acute hepatomegaly.

Chronic Hepatomegaly

Causes

- Fatty liver
- Chronic hepatitis
- Cirrhosis of liver
- Primary liver malignancy
- Secondaries in the liver
- Chronic Budd-Chiari syndrome

Fatty liver

- History of alcoholism, diabetes mellitus, obesity, and evidence of metabolic syndrome (nonalcoholic steatohepatitis).
- Firm enlarged liver.
- LFT: Minimum raise of liver enzyme may be present
- Ultrasound; Demonstrates fatty liver.

Chronic hepatitis

- History of fever, jaundice, pain right hypochondrium and weight loss for 6 months.
- Presence of jaundice, firm enlarged liver and may be tender.
- LFT: Raised liver enzymes
- Liver biopsy—diagnostic.

Cirrhosis of liver

- Typical history of cirrhosis and portal hypertension.
- Signs of liver cell failure present.
- Presence of ascites
- Firm liver—may be nodular and enlarged.

- Splenomegaly present
- LFT minimal raise of liver enzyme and bilirubin.
- Serum albumin low and PT prolonged.
- US abdomen and upper GI endoscopy for evidence of oesophageal varices
- US abdomen: Altered liver architecture with nodularity.

Primary liver malignancy: (Hepatocellular carcinoma)

- Hard nodular liver (may be single nodule).
- Presence of icterus
- Ascites may be present
- Presence of hepatic bruit: Feature of cirrhosis may be present.
- Serum alpha-fetoprotein is increased (>500 IU)
- Ultrasound of liver: Demonstrates the malignant lesion.

Secondaries in the liver

- Multiple hard nodules in the liver.
- No bruit over the liver (umbilication may be present over the nodule)
- Icterus present
- Ascites may be present
- Left supraclavicular lymphadenopathy.
- Ultrasound liver—multiple nodules.
- LFT—significant increase in the alkaline phosphatase.
- Evidence of primary malignancy.

Causes of Multiple Hepatic Secondaries

Primary malignancy: Stomach, colon, breast, lung.

Chronic Budd-Chiari syndrome

- Presents as cirrhosis of liver.
- Presence of hepatomegaly, ascites, prominent venous collaterals and back veins.
- Ultrasound—demonstrates enlarged liver—IVC, hepatic veins thrombosed.
- Other causes of chronic hepatomegaly like lymphoma, leukemia, etc. are discussed in corresponding chapters.

Tender Enlarged Liver

Causes

- Acute hepatitis
- CCF/TR
- Amoebic liver abscess
- Pyogenic liver abscess
- Acute Budd-Chiari syndrome
- Hepatic malignancy.

Acute hepatitis (see above)

Congestive cardiac failure

- History of dyspnea, swelling of feet
- JVP ↑, tender enlarged liver with pedal edema.
- Icterus, ascites may be present.
- Presence of TR murmur and pulsatile liver.
- Echocardiogram abnormal.

Liver abscess

- History of fever with chills and rigors.
- Soft, tender, enlarged liver.
- Jaundice may or may not be present.

Amoebic liver abscess

- Common in persons with alcohol intake.
- Single abscess: Right posterosuperior aspect of liver.
- Fever with chills and rigors.
- Intercostal tenderness with enlarged tender liver.
- Amoebic serology is positive in 95% of cases.

Pyogenic liver abscess

- Multiple abscess in the liver
- Blood culture positive for bacteria.

Causes of massive enlargement of liver

- Fatty liver
- CCF
- Liver abscess
- Malignancy of the liver
- Budd-Chiari syndrome
- Amyloidosis
- Storage disorders.

Causes of hepatomegaly with jaundice

Acute

1. Acute hepatitis: Viral, alcohol, drug induced
2. Acute infectious disorders
   - Leptospirosis
   - Acute malaria
   - Rickettsial fever
   - Endocarditis.
3. CCF
4. Acute liver abscess
5. Acute Budd-Chiari syndrome.

Chronic

- Chronic hepatitis
- Cirrhosis of liver
- Chronic Budd-Chiari syndrome
- Hemolytic anemias
- Disseminated tuberculosis
- Lymphomas
- Malignancy of the liver.

CIRRHOSIS OF LIVER

Alcohol Induced

Features

- H/o consumption of alcohol
- Signs of liver cell failure
- Hepatosplenomegaly with ascites
- Investigations evidence of cirrhosis and portal hypertension.

Post-Necrotic Cirrhosis (Viral Hepatitis, B and C)

Hepatitis B

- May be a known case of hepatitis B positive.
- Macronodular cirrhosis.
- HBsAg positive with anti-HBc IgG positivity and HBeAg positivity.
- 1–5% of HBsAg positive will develop chronic hepatitis B and of these 20–25% will develop cirrhosis.

Hepatitis C

- Persons with contact with hepatitis C— 70–80% will develop chronic hepatitis and quarter of these will develop cirrhosis.

- Signs of cirrhosis
- Small shrunken liver
- Antibodies to HCV will be present.

Autoimmune hepatitis and cirrhosis
- Common in females
- Features of autoimmune disease and cirrhosis.
- Positive autoantibodies, positive ANA and antismooth muscle antibody.

Non-alcoholic steatohepatitis
- Evidence of obesity and other features of metabolic syndrome.
- Absent of history of alcoholism and viral markers.
- Evidence of cirrhosis.

Primary biliary cirrhosis
- Present as fatigue and pruritis
- Hyperpigmentation, xanthelasma and xanthoma can be present.
- Evidence of cirrhosis
- ALP can be significantly raised
- Increase in the level of IgM
- Anti-mitochondrial antibody present.

Cardiac cirrhosis
- Signs and symptoms of long standing right-sided cardiac failure.
- Liver becomes firm and enlarged
- Signs of RV failure
- Less chance of variceal hemorrhage and encephalopathy.

Wilson's disease
- Presents as liver disease in young (2nd or 3rd decade).
- Presence of KF ring, extra pyramidal involvement.
- Evidence of cirrhosis.
- Serum ceruloplasmin level is low and 24 hours urinary copper is increased (>100 microgram).
- Liver biopsy diagnostic; more than 200 microgram of copper/1 gm of dry weight of liver tissue.
- ATP7B gene mutation is associated with Wilson's disease.

Features of decompensated cirrhosis
Presence of
- Jaundice
- Ascites
- Variceal hemorrhage
- Hepatic encephalopathy.

HEPATIC ENCEPHALOPATHY

Hepatic encephalopathy is neuropsychiatric and behavioral disturbances occurring in patients with liver cell failure.
- Liver cell failure may be
  Acute: Fulminant hepatic failure.
  Chronic
  – Chronic hepatitis
  – Cirrhosis with portosystemic shunting.
  – Hepatocellular carcinoma
- There is no preexisting brain disease.

Pathogenesis and Pathology

- Manifestations are thought to be due to toxic substances—which are not cleared by the liver. Toxic substances reach the brain causing the manifestations.
- Following substances may be responsible for the manifestations of hepatic encephalopathy
  – Ammonia
  – GABA
  – Octopamine
  – Manganese.
- There is significant astrocyte dysfunction with cerebral edema (in patients with acute liver cell failure).

Precipitating Factors

- Intake of sedatives and hypnotics.
- High protein intake
- Hepatotoxic drugs
- Hypokalemia
- Systemic infection/spontaneous bacterial peritonitis.
- GI bleed/constipation
- Surgical procedures.

Clinical Features

- Altered sleep rhythm
- Altered sensorium
- Constructional apraxia
- Asterixis
- Cerebral edema (common with acute liver cell failure)
- Convulsions
- Fetor hepaticus

Neurological features (due to porta systemic shunting) in chronic encephalopathy

- Myelopathy
- Extrapyramidal features
  - Tremor
  - Rigidity
  - Bradykinesia
- Chronic hepatocerebral dysfunction
  - Occurs in patients with chronic liver disease like cirrhosis. It is a form of sub-clinical encephalopathy.
  - Person can have neuropsychiatric manifestations, movement disorders and cognitive dysfunction.

Grades of Hepatic Encephalopathy

Grades

I: Altered sleep rhythm

Minimal confusion and minimal dysfunction of higher mental function.

II: Disturbed higher mental function.

Presence of Asterixis

III: Drowsy

Disoriented

Asterixis

IV: Coma

Investigations

- EEG characteristic slow frequency, high amplitude triphasic waves.
- CT/MRT: Globus pallidus shows hyper-intensity.
- Cerebral edema
- LFT—abnormal
- Serum—ammonia may be raised.

Differential diagnosis of hepatic encephalopathy

Due to alcohol: Intoxication/withdrawal

- Sedative intake
- Metabolic encephalopathy—hypoglycemia, hyponatremia, uremia
- Intracranial infection
- Subdural hematoma
- CVA
- Intracranial tumor.

Fulminant Hepatic Failure

Manifestations of hepatic encephalopathy occurring within 8 weeks of development of signs and symptoms of liver disease with normal functioning of the liver before.

Subacute Hepatic Failure

Abnormality of liver function like presence of jaundice, elevated liver enzymes after 8 weeks and up to 24 weeks of onset of liver disease.

Features of Fulminant Hepatic Failure

- Jaundice
- Ascites
- Hepatic encephalopathy
- Upper GI bleed and systemic bleed
- Cerebral edema
- Hypotension
- Tachycardia.
- There will be decrease in the liver span.

Causes of Fulminant Hepatic Failure

Acute hepatitis

- Viral, drugs, ischemic hepatitis
- Paracetamol overdosage
- Autoimmune hepatitis.

Rare

- Wilson's disease
- Acute fatty liver of pregnancy
- HELLP syndrome
- Acute Budd-Chiari syndrome
- Hepatic malignancy.

Pediatric age group
- Galactosemia
- Fructose intolerance
- Reye's syndrome.

Complications of hepatic encephalopathy
- Metabolic acidosis
- Systemic bleed
- Cerebral edema
- Systemic infection
- Renal failure
- Convulsions.

Investigations
LFT
- Serum bilirubin increased
- Liver enzymes increased
- Serum ammonia is increased
- Blood glucose is decreased
- Platelet count is decreased
- Prothrombin time is prolonged
- Serum lactate is increased.

PORTAL HYPERTENSION

Formation of Portal Vein
- Portal vein is formed by the joining of superior mesenteric vein and splenic vein.
- Splenic vein is also joined by the inferior mesenteric vein. Drains blood from most of the GIT spleen, pancreas and gall bladder.

Portal vein pressure and portal hypertension
- Normal portal pressure: 5 to 10 mm of Hg
- Portal hypertension: Portal pressure > 12 mm of Hg (can present with variceal bleed)

Portocaval anastamotic sites
- Lower end of oesophagus
- Anorectal junction
- Bare area of liver
- Around the umbillicus
- Peritoneum.

Classification of portal hypertension
Presinusoidal
- Thrombosis of portal vein
- Thrombosis of splenic vein

- Compression of splenic or portal vein
- Schistosomiasis
- Congenital atresia of portal vein/congenital hepatic fibrosis.

Sinusoidal
- Cirrhosis of liver
- Alcoholic hepatitis

Postsinusoidal
- Budd-Chiari syndrome.
- IVC obstruction
- Severe TR
- Constrictive pericarditis
- Restrictive cardiomyopathy.

Pathogenesis
Portal hypertension develops whenever there is
1. Obstruction to the portal blood flow
2. Increase in the splanchnic blood flow.
- Obstruction to the portal blood flow occur due to hepatic fibrosis, occlusion of the portal vein tributaries and regenerating nodules in cirrhosis.
- Portal blood flow increases due to splanchnic vasodilatation.
- Portal hypertension results in hemorrhage into the GIT. This bleed is likely to occur whenever portal pressure is more than 12 mm of Hg and systemic infection.

Clinical features of portal hypertension
- Gastrointestinal bleed
- Splenomegaly
- Dilated tortuous veins over the abdomen.
- Ascites
- Hypersplenism

Complications of portal hypertension
- GIT hemorrhage
- Chronic portal hypertensive gastropathy.
- Formation of ascites
- Portal pulmonary hypertension
- Pancytopenia due to hypersplenism.

Investigations
- Ultrasound/CT scan/MRI of the abdomen
- Upper GI endoscopy

- For aetiology of portal hypertension:
  - Rule out hypercoagulable state
  - Rule out cirrhosis of liver
  - Rule out IVC obstruction by angiogram: Echocardiogram.

Factors which increases the risk of variceal bleed
- Increase in the variceal size
- Endoscopic red sign in upper GI scopy
- Presence of ascites
- Acute alcohol consumption
- GERD
- Infection/inflammatory endotoxins.

HEPATORENAL SYNDROME

What is Hepatorenal Syndrome

Renal function deterioration which is occurring in the background of cirrhosis of liver or fulminant hepatic failure.

Conditions associated
- Cirrhosis of liver
- Fulminant hepatic failure
- Severe alcoholic hepatitis

Common precipitating factors
- Gastrointestinal bleeding
- Systemic infection
- Diuretic overdosage
- Removal or large volume of ascitic fluid without proper volume replacement.

Pathogenesis: There is decrease in the blood flow to the kidney with increase in splanchnic blood flow. Decrease blood flow occurs due to vasoconstrictions including renin and angiotensin.

Types of HR syndrome
Type 1
- Rapidly progressive renal failure
- Serum creatinine >2.5 mg/dl raises within a period of less than 2 weeks.

Type 2
- Slowly progressive renal failure
- It is associated with diuretic resistant ascites

Prognosis: Bad except for liver transplantation.

Treatment: TIPS (transjugular intrahepatic portocaval shunt)/hemodialysis.

PORTOPULMONARY HYPERTENSION

There is development of pulmonary hypertension in a patient of portal hypertension.

Pulmonary hypertension occurs due to: Pulmonary vasoconstriction and pulmonary vascular remodeling resulting in increased pulmonary vascular resistance.

Pathogenesis: There is increased cardiac output, hyperdynamic status, increased pulmonary vascular shear stress, pulmonary vasoconstriction and thrombosis are responsible for pulmonary hypertension.

Pathology
- Plexogenic arteriopathy
- Endothelial cell proliferation
- Proliferation of smooth muscle cells
- Thrombosis of pulmonary vessels.

Clinical features
- Exertional dyspnea
- Chest pain
- Syncope
- Signs of pulmonary artery hypertension
- Signs of portal hypertension.
- Pulmonary artery pressure > 25 mm of Hg
- Pulmonary capillary wedge pressure is not increased
- Pulmonary vascular resistance is increased.
- Investigations, complications and treatment are same as that of pulmonary hypertension.

📄 *Note*

- *Female sex and autoimmune hepatitis are risk factors for the development of portopulmonary hypertension.*
- *Vasoactive substances (endothelin I, thromboxane A2, vasoactive intestinal peptide, etc.) reach the pulmonary circulation through the portosystemic shunt resulting in pulmonary hypertension.*

Non-cirrhotic Portal Fibrosis and Portal Hypertension

Development of intrahepatic portal hypertension without evidence of cirrhosis or other liver disease.

Characteristic features

- Presence of portal hypertension
- Absence of evidence for cirrhosis
- There will be phlebosclerosis of portal venous system.

Possible aetiological factors

- Intraabdominal infection chronic → Embolization into the portal vein → Thrombophlebitis sclerosis.
- Chronic consumption of arsenic
- Genetic, immunologic factors and increased hepatic and splanchnic blood flow may also be responsible for the development of portal hypertension.

Pathology: Dilatation, sclerosis, fibrosis of portal venous system with occasional thrombosis with normal hepatic parenchymal histology (thrombosis of major hepatic and portal veins is usually absent).

Clinical features

- Young individuals presenting with recurrent hematemesis.
- Mass in the left hypochondrium due to massive splenomegaly .
- No evidence of signs of liver cell failure
- Absence of ascites
- No development of hepatic encephalopathy in spite of upper GI bleed.

Investigations

- Pancytopenia due to hypersplenism
- LFT normal with normal prothombin time
- Presence of oesophageal varices
- Dilatation of portal vein and splenic vein collaterals

EXTRAHEPATIC PORTAL HYPERTENSION

Due to the obstruction to the portal blood flow outside the liver—leading to development of portal hypertension.

Caused by

- Thrombosis of portal veins
- Malignant obstruction to the portal vein.
- Pancreatic pathology like pancreatitis.

Aetiology of portal vein occlusion

In children

- Umbilical sepsis
- Intra-abdominal infection.
- Congenital anomaly of portal vein.

Adults

- Oral contraceptive pills
- Hypercoagulable state
- Intra-abdominal infection
- Myeloproliferative disorder
- Cirrhosis of liver
- Inflammatory bowel disease.
- Tumors—obstruction due to:
  - Hepatocellular carcinoma
  - Pancreatic carcinoma
  - Lymph node at porta hepatis
- Tumor can also directly invade the portal vein.

Manifestations

Acute onset

- Sudden onset of upper abdominal pain (in acute portal vein thrombosis)
- Nausea and vomiting
- Signs and symptoms of primary disease
- Progressive ascites.

Chronic

- Signs and symptoms of portal hypertension.
- There will be sudden worsening of ascites in a patient of cirrhosis.

Signs

- Splenomegaly
- Occasionally—ascites
- Signs of primary disease.

Rule out

- Other causes of portal hypertension
- Budd-Chiari syndrome
- Cirrhosis of liver
- Granulomatous disorders.

HEPATOPULMONARY SYNDROME

Hepatopulmonary syndrome consists of triad of features

- Liver disease (acute/chronic)
- Intrapulmonary vascular dilatation
- AV gradient—hypoxemia.

Pathophysiology of hepatopulmonary syndrome: In patient with both acute and chronic liver cell failure. There will be formation of intrapulmonary arteriovenous communications and dilatations.

Pathogenesis

- Substances like nitric oxide, TNF-alpha and endothelin I are not cleared by the liver produce vasodilatation.
- This causes hypoxemia due to ventilation perfusion mismatch
- Proposed pathological mechanisms
  - Pulmonary A-V shunting
  - Portopulmonary venous anastamosis
  - Angiogenesis.

Clinical manifestations

- Background of liver disease (signs of liver disease including spider angiomas)
- Insidious onset of dyspnea.
- Patient will have platypnea, orthodeoxia (due to increased blood flow to the lung bases while in sitting or standing position).
- Cyanosis, clubbing
- Pulse oximetry—demonstrates hypoxia (PaO$_2$↓ of 5% or more or 4 mm Hg more from supine to upright).
- Pulmonary angiogram will demonstrate diffuse fine vascular anastamotic channels.
- Contrast transthoracic echo to demonstrate intrapulmonary vascular dilatation.

BUDD-CHIARI SYNDROME

Occlusion of outflow tract of hepatic veins—either due to thrombosis or non-thrombotic occlusion. IVC may also be involved.

Aetiology

- Infective disorder: TB, syphilis

- Neoplastic disorder: Hepatocellular carcinoma/renal cell carcinoma, involving the hepatic veins/IVC.
- Inherited disorders with prothrombotic state: Protein C and S deficiency.
- Hematological disorders
  - Polycythemia vera
  - Paroxysmal nocturnal hemoglobinuria
  - APLA syndrome.
- Oral contraceptive pills
- Pregnancy.

Pathophysiology

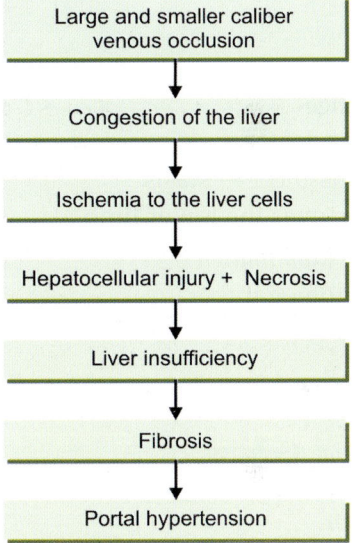

Large and smaller caliber venous occlusion
↓
Congestion of the liver
↓
Ischemia to the liver cells
↓
Hepatocellular injury + Necrosis
↓
Liver insufficiency
↓
Fibrosis
↓
Portal hypertension

Caudate lobe enlargement

- Independent connection to IVC. Becomes enlarged in hepatic outflow obstruction.
- Blood is shunted through it to IVC. Caudate lobe is supplied by right and left hepatic artery and portal vein.

Clinical features of Budd-Chiari syndrome

Classical triad of features

- Abdominal pain
- Massive hepatomegaly
- Ascites

Different types of presentation

Acute presentation

- Acute right hypochondrial pain.

- Rapid development of jaundice and ascites
- Acute rapid enlargement of liver
- Can develop renal failure.

Chronic presentation
- Most common presentation
- Patient presents with progressive abdominal distention with ascites.
- Development of progressive jaundice and hepatomegaly.
- Ultimately develop cirrhosis of liver.

Fulminant form of presentation: Can have severe liver dysfunction.

Clinical signs
General examination
- Jaundice
- Pedal edema
- Venous ulcers—stasis
- Ulcers over the lower limb

Systemic examination
- Hepatomegaly
- Splenomegaly
- Ascites
- Collaterals—veins over the back and flanks.

Differential diagnosis
- Other conditions associated with cirrhosis of liver.
- Congestive cardiac failure
- Constrictive pericarditis.

Complications
- Cirrhosis of liver
- Can develop encephalopathy, portal hypertension and oesophageal varices and hepatorenal syndrome.

Hepatic outflow obstruction
- Can also involve IVC—can have collaterals over the back and flanks
- Hepatojugular reflux is absent.

Venous collaterals develop between: Superficial inferior epigastric veins (IVC territory) communicate with superior epigastric veins (SVC territory).

Investigations
Ascitic fluid analysis
- High protein content of the fluid >2 gm/dl
- Cells < 500 cells/cum.

Imaging
- CT scan to demonstrate the obstruction.
- Work up for aetiology of venous obstruction.

HEPATIC VENO-OCCLUSIVE DISEASE

Characteristics and pathogenesis
- Obliteration of small venules in the liver.
- Occurs due to endothelial injury causing non-thrombotic occlusion of terminal hepatic venules and sinusoids.
- There will be venous congestion causing necrosis of liver cells ultimately leading to cirrhosis.

Aetiological factors
- High dose chemotherapy, e.g. before bone marrow transplantation like azathioprine.
- Irradiation
- Pyrrolizidine alkaloids (herbal tea)
- Aflatoxins

Presentation: Ascites, hepatomegaly 2–3 weeks after chemotherapy. Occasionally manifests as: Fulminant hepatic failure. Can eventually develop cirrhosis with portal hypertension.

HEPATOCELLULAR CARCINOMA

Etiologies contributing to hepatocellular carcinoma
- Chronic hepatitis B and C
- Alcoholic cirrhosis
- Non-alcoholic steatohepatitis (NASH)
- Toxins: Aflatoxins
- Drugs: Anabolic steroids, contraceptives and arsenic.

Cirrhosis which are less likely to be associated with hepatocellular carcinoma
- Biliary cirrhosis
- Cardiac cirrhosis
- Wilson's disease
- Alpha-1 antitrypsin deficiency.

Clinical features

Symptoms

- Fatigue
- Abdominal pain—right hypochondrium
- Abdominal distension (due to hepatic mass/ascites)
- Jaundice (obstruction to intrahepatic ducts)
- Ascites
- Symptoms of portal hypertension.

Signs

- Hard enlarged liver with bruit
- Other signs of chronic liver disease
- Ascites: Hemorrhagic
- Other—manifestations
- Fever, Budd-Chiari syndrome.

Paraneoplastic manifestations

- Hypoglycemia
- Hypercalcemia
- Erythrocytosis
- Gynecomastia
- Porphyria cutanea tarda

Investigations

- Ultrasound, CT scan, PET scan
- Ascitic fluid—hemorrhagic—for malignant cytology
- Alfa-fetoprotein
- Liver biopsy
- Investigations for etiological factors.

ASCITES

Different Causes of Abdominal Distension

- Fluid—ascites
- Fecal matter
- Flatus
- Fetus
- Fat accumulation

Fluid causing abdominal distension

- May be associated with edema, puffiness of face, dyspnea and decreased urine output.
- If only ascites without edema—local abdominal cause.

- If distension of the abdomen with pain = possible peritonitis, intestinal obstruction and pancreatitis.

If distension of abdomen without pain

- Fat accumulation
- Due to flatus
- Slow development of ascites

Fat accumulation occurs in

- Cushing's syndrome
- Obesity
- Insulin resistance.

Fecal matter

- Associated with constipation and vomiting
- May be due to intestinal obstruction.

Slowly developing abdominal distension can also occur due to

- Intra-abdominal mass
- Hepatosplenomegaly.

Approach to a Patient of Ascites

History: Rapid distension of abdomen associated with abdominal pain and fever:

- Acute peritonitis
- Acute pancreatitis
- Other intra-abdominal infection.

Slow development of distension abdomen with ascites

Causes

Fever, weight loss, altered bowel habits

- Intra-abdominal tuberculosis
- Lymphomas
- Connective tissue disease
- Malignancy

History of jaundice, hematemesis malena, pedal edema

- Chronic liver disease/cirrhosis of liver.
- History of puffiness of face, swelling of feet and history of hypertension—renal disease like nephritic syndrome/nephrotic syndrome.
- History of breathlessness, swelling of feet, decreased urine output—cardiac failure.

- History of distension of abdomen, pedal edema, distended neck veins: Constrictive pericarditis.
- History of sudden onset right hypochondrial pain, distension of abdomen, presence of prominent back veins—acute/chronic Budd-Chiari syndrome.

Clinical examination
Look for
- JVP ↑ (CCF, constrictive pericarditis)
- Kussmaul's sign—constrictive pericarditis
- Signs of liver cell failure along with splenomegaly—cirrhosis of liver.
- Pedal edema and puffiness of face—renal cause
- For evidence of hypothyroidism
- For evidence of collagen disease
- Hard liver with bruit—hepatocellular carcinoma
- Multiple nodules in the liver—secondaries in the liver
- Venous hum—over the umbilicus—in portal hypertension.
- Pulsatile liver: Tricuspid regurgitation
- Splenomegaly—portal hypertension, lymphoma and TB
- Look also for: Tenderness over the abdomen—peritonitis/malignancy.
- Look for—doughy feeling of the abdomen—TB peritoneum
- Look for—mass/intra-abdominal lymphadenopathy.
- Look for—testicular mass

Per rectal examination
- Look for—hemorrhoids—may be suggestive of portal hypertension/colonic malignancy.
- Look for—mass/malignant deposit—in the rectum.

Grades of ascites
- Grade I—can be detected on abdominal ultrasound.
- Grade II—shifting dullness present.
- Grade III—abdominal distension with fluid thrill.

Cirrhotic ascites
Characteristics
- Transudative ascites
- High SAAG ascites.

Mechanism of ascites in cirrhosis of liver
- ↑Hydrostatic pressure—in splanchnic circulation
  - due to hepatic fibrosis and nodularity causing resistance to blood flow.
  - Splanchnic vasodilatation occurs due to
    - increase nitric oxide production
    - increase tumor necrosis factor
- ↓ Osmotic pressure in the portal circulation due to decrease of albumin.
- There is decrease in the effective circulating volume with decrease of renal perfusion leading on to
  - Increase in the ADH
  - Stimulation of renin angiotensin system causing salt and water retention.

Causes of ascites
Transudative
- Nephrotic syndrome
- CCF
- Hypoproteinemic states.

Exudative
- Peritonitis of any cause
- Peritoneal secondaries
- Pancreatic disease
- Lymphoma
- Connective tissue disease.

Causes of high SAAG ascites
- Cardiac failure
- Cirrhosis of liver
- Hepatic veno-occlusive disease.

Causes of low SAAG ascites
- Peritonitis
- TB
- Hepatic metastasis
- Pancreatitis.

Spontaneous bacterial peritonitis
- Infection of ascites in the absence of any other cause.
- Culture of ascitic fluid—grows one organism.
- Polymorphs in the ascitic fluid >250 cells/cmm.

Secondary bacterial peritonitis
- Multiple pathogens in the culture of ascitic fluid.
- Fluid glucose is markedly reduced (<50 mg/dl).
- Significant increase in the polymorphs in ascitic fluid.
- Can occur in bowel perforation and intra-abdominal/pelvic abscess.

Spontaneous bacterial peritonitis occurs in
- Cirrhosis of liver
- CCF
- Acute hepatic failure
- Nephrotic syndrome

Effect of massive ascites—chronic—due to chronic raised intra-abdominal pressure
- Umbilical herniation
- Divarication of recti with fatty hernia of linea alba.
- Stretch marks: Pleural effusion.

REFRACTORY ASCITES

Definition

In a patient of cirrhosis—ascites is said to be refractory—when it is not responding to dose of diuretics: Spironolactone 400 mg + Frusemide 160 mg for 1 week along with salt restriction.

Features of refractory ascites
- Rapidly re-accumulates within 4 weeks of response.
- Patient does not loose significant weight.
- Urinary sodium secretion is less.

Types of refractory ascites
1. Resistant to diuretics: Ascites which is not responding to diuretics along with salt restriction.
2. Diuretics is not possible to be used because of complications caused by diuretics.

Rule out the following conditions in a patient of refractory ascites
- Portal vein thrombosis
- Spontaneous bacterial peritonitis
- Hepatocellular carcinoma in a patient of refractory ascites
- Advanced liver disease.

Therapeutic options in a refractory ascites due to cirrhosis
- Massive paracentesis with volume replacement.
- Intravenous albumin infusion
- Le Veen shunt
- Hepatic transplant.

FATTY LIVER: HEPATIC STEATOSIS AND NASH (Non-alcoholic steatohepatitis)

Causes of Fatty Liver

Chronic Alcoholism

Non-alcohol causes
- *Drug-induced*
  - Corticosteroids
  - Tetracyclines
  - Amiodarone
- *Metabolic*
  - Wilson's disease
  - Storage disease
  - Metabolic syndrome
- *Systemic diseases*
  - Inflammatory bowel disease.
  - Gastrojejunal bypass
- *Pregnancy*: Acute fatty liver of pregnancy.

NON-ALCOHOLIC STEATOHEPATITIS (NASH)

Features

Absence of Alcoholism

Lobular hepatitis
Consequences
- Steatohepatitis
- Liver cell injury
- Fibrosis

Etiopathogenesis

Factors responsible for hepatocyte injury

- Insulin resistance
- Hepatic triglyceride accumulation
- Oxidative stress and excess cytokine production

Above factors result in inflammation and fibrosis. Oxidative stress, mitochondrial dysfunction and apoptosis along with stimulation of transforming growth factor beta cause significant hepatocyte damage. There will be stimulation of stellate cells resulting in collagen synthesis.

Risk factors involved

- Central obesity
- Hyperglycemia
- Hypertension
- Hypertriglyceredemia

Clinical features

- May be asymptomatic
- May have enlarged liver (fatty liver) or may have only elevated liver enzymes and increased ALP.
- Can present with cirrhosis and occasionally hepatocellular carcinoma

Differential Diagnosis

Other causes of hepatomegaly and cirrhosis.

Investigations

- Ultrasound abdomen
- Hepatic elastography
- CT/MRI of liver
- Liver biopsy
- Scan for estimating liver fibrosis and fat accumulation

Hepatic Histology in NASH

- Hepatic steatosis
- Ballooning degeneration of hepatocytes
- Lobular inflammation
- Mallory bodies in the liver cells
- Inflammatory cell infiltration
- End result: Hepatic fibrosis

Disorders of Pancreas

Investigations for Pancreatic Disease

Pancreatic function tests

Pancreatic enzymes: Amylase and lipase levels.
Pancreatic—amylase in pancreatitis: More than 3 times the normal is suggestive of pancreatitis.

Amylase can be normal in the following circumstances in pancreatitis:

- Chronic pancreatitis.
- Resolving acute pancreatitis (after 3–5 days)
- Hypertriglyceredemia induced pancreatitis.
- In acute pancreatitis pancreatic amylase level usually returns to normal within 7 days.

Persistence raise of amylase level in acute pancreatitis

- Pseudocyst formation
- Ductal obstruction or disruption of pancreatic duct.

Other causes of serum amylase raise apart from pancreatic disorders

- Salivary amylase increase: Parotitis
- Neoplastic disorders: Carcinoma of lung
- Head injury
- *Abdominal disorders*
  - Peptic ulcer perforation
  - Intestinal obstruction
  - Peritonitis

Amylase in other body fluids

- Pleural fluid amylase increase due to:
  - Pancreatitis
  - Oesophageal rupture
  - Carcinoma lung

 Note

In carcinoma lung causing pleural effusion—salivary isoenzyme of amylase is increased.

Ascitic fluid amylase is increased in

- Pancreatic ascites
- Pseudocyst and leakage
- Main pancreatic duct disruption.

Serum lipase level: Serum lipase level is a better test for pancreatitis especially in patients with renal dysfunction.

Exocrine Pancreatic Function Tests

Measurement of fecal pancreatic elastase: Stool elastase amount directly reflects output of this enzyme by the pancreas.

Secretin infusion: IV infusion of secretin—causes pancreatic stimulation—duodenal contents can be collected for bicarbonate estimation.

For Detection of Diffuse Pancreatic Disease

Radiological investigations

- Plain X-ray abdomen—to detect pancreatic calcification.
- US abdomen—can detect
  - Acute pancreatitis and its abdominal complication.
  - Pancreatic calcification and gall stones.
- CT abdomen
  - For acute pancreatitis
  - For chronic pancreatitis
  - Complications of pancreatitis
  - Calcification of pancreas.
- Routine CT is not recommended in acute pancreatitis except while suspecting complications.
- Endoscopic ultrasound (EUS)
  - For visualization of pancreatic duct and parenchyma of pancreas
  - For gall stones in acute pancreatitis.
  - In chronic pancreatitis.
- MRI/MRCP/ERCP
  - For the pathology in the pancreatic duct, bile duct and parenchyma of pancreas.
  - ERCP—for the lesions of the pancreas and bile duct.
- Biopsy of the pancreas: For parenchymal lesions of the pancreas—malignancy/mass lesion.

ACUTE PANCREATITIS

Acute inflammation of the pancreas

Common causes

- Alcoholism
- Gall stone disease
- ERCP
- Hypertriglyceredemia.

Rare causes

- Infection—viral—mumps
- Renal failure
- Vasculitis
- Connective tissue disorder
- Hypercalcemia

Clinical features

Abdominal pain

- Site—around the umbilicus—minimal or may be severe.
- Radiation—to back, retrosternal area
- Relieved by—stooping forward.
- Other features
  - Vomiting
  - Jaundice
  - Abdominal distension
  - Hypotension

Clinical signs

- Tachycardia and hypotension.
- Skin discoloration of abdomen
- Abdominal distention due to
  - Pancreatic ascites
  - Paralytic ileus
- Jaundice due to obstruction of the bile duct:
  - Edema of head of pancreas
  - Due to gall stones.
- Hypotension—due to
  - Loss of fluid into the abdomen—due to inflammation of the pancreas.
  - Vasodilation produced by release of kinins
- Skin discoloration
  - Cullen's sign—occurrence of hemoperitoneum causing bluish discoloration around the umbilicus.

    – Turner's sign—discoloration of flanks—red/blue—indicates hemorrhagic pancreatitis with hemoglobin catabolism.

Systemic examination

Abdomen

- Tenderness and rigidity
- Ascites
- Epigastric mass due to pseudocyst
- There may be bilateral basal crepitations and left-sided pleural effusion.

Complications of acute pancreatitis

Abdominal

- Obstructive jaundice
- Pseudocyst/ascites
- Portal vein/splenic vein/thrombosis.

Systemic

- GI bleed
- Renal failure
- ARDS
- Shock
- Hypocalcemia
- Hyperglycemia
- Sepsis

Differential Diagnosis

Other causes of acute abdomen

- Peptic ulcer perforation
- Acute intestinal obstruction
- Acute cholecystitis
- Inferior wall myocardial infarction
- Mesenteric ischemia
- Diabetic ketoacidosis and basal pneumonia can mimic pancreatitis.

Chronic Pancreatitis

Chronic inflammation of the pancreas leading onto irreversible damage to the pancreatic structure and functions.

Common causes

- Alcoholism
- Hyperlipidemia
- Hypercalcemia
- Idiopathic

Rare causes

- CRF
- Tropical pancreatitis
- Genetic disorder
- Autoimmune pancreatitis.

Clinical features

- Recurrent abdominal pain
- Weight loss
- Steatorrhea
- Malabsorption
- Glucose intolerance
- Recurrent exacerbations.

Investigations

- Serum amylase, lipase may be normal
- Bilirubin level increase—may be due to bile duct stricture
- Hyperglycemia
- Stool-elastase level is decreased.
- Evidence of pancreatic exocrine or endocrine deficiency
- CT abdomen/MRI
- Endoscopic ultrasound

Complications

- Steatorrhea and malabsorption
- Glucose intolerance
- Recurrent abdominal pain—severe
- Obstructive jaundice
- Rarely—biliary structure
- Cirrhosis.
- Carcinoma pancreas

CHRONIC DIARRHEA

Chronic diarrhea: Diarrhea persisting for more than 4 weeks.

Causes

- Irriitable bowel syndrome
- Infective
  - HIV related
  - Amoebiasis
  - Giardisis
  - Helminthiasis
  - Cryptosporidiosis
  - Tuberculosis

Endocrine disorders

- Thyrotoxicosis
- Addison's disease
- Diabetes mellitus
- Pancreatic vipomas

Previous GI surgeries

Drugs and alcohol: Laxatives, antibiotics and NSAIDs.

Pancreatic

- Cystic fibrosis
- Chronic pancreatitis
- Carcinoma pancreas

Intestinal

- Inflammatory bowel disease
- Malabsorption syndrome
- Bacterial overgrowth
- Ischemia
- Radiation
- Diverticula
- Malignancy/lymphoma

Different Mechanisms of Chronic Diarrhea

Secretory diarrhea

- Characterised by large volume of stool which is watery and abdominal pain is absent.
- Due to secretion of large amount of water with electrolytes (chloride) due to defective fluid and electrolyte transport across the intestinal mucosa.
- Malabsorption is not a feature of secretory diarrhea
- For example, laxative abuse
- Chronic alcoholism
- Chronic bacterial infection.

Steatorrhea: Passing of large amount of stool— greasy/oily, foul smelling with difficulty in flushing—due to fat malabsorption

Associated features

- Weight loss
- Deficiency of vitamins, proteins

Causes

- Alcohol intake
- Laxative abuse
- Carcinoid syndrome
- Pancreatic pathology
- Obstructive biliary disease

Osmotic diarrhea

- Due to the presence of osmotically active solutes which are absorbed poorly in the intestine. They drag large amount of fluid into the intestinal mucosa.
- For example, antacids which are magnesium containing.
  - Carbohydrate malabsorption.
  - Chronic laxative abuse.

Inflammatory diarrhea

- Due to inflammation of intestinal mucosa
- There will be excretion of blood and mucus from the intestinal mucosa

Associated features

- Abdominal pain, fever, blood and mucus in the stool
  - For example, inflammatory bowel disease
  - Chronic GIT infection.

Diarrhea due to abnormal intestinal motility

Due to altered motility of the intestine:

- There will be rapid intestinal transit.
  - For example, hyperthyroidism
  - Carcinoid syndrome
  - Diabetic autonomic neuropathy
  - Irritable bowel syndrome

Differences between large bowel and small bowel diarrhea

Small bowel diarrhea	Large bowel diarrhea
• Large amount of watery diarrhea	Less amount of watery diarrhea
• Less frequent loose stools	More frequent loose stools
• Abdominal pain around the umbilicus	Abdominal pain—lower abdomen
• Tenesmus not present	Tenesmus present

Approach to a Patient of Chronic Diarrhea

History

- Enquire—onset and duration
- Stool characteristics
- Presence of blood and mucus
- Abdominal pain and character
- Fever and weight loss
- Intake of medications and laxatives.

Other systemic manifestations

- Cough and fever (possible tuberculosis)
- Fatigue + pigmentation (possible Addison's disease/B_{12} deficiency)
- Flushing episodes (carcinoid syndrome).
- Ask for extra intestinal manifestations associated with inflammatory bowel disease.
- History of diabetes mellitus, thyrotoxicosis and Addison's disease.
- History of alcoholism, laxative and drugs (Antacids, NSAIDs, antibiotics, etc.)
- Family history of inflammatory bowel disease/sprue/IBS.

Clinical examination

Look for

- Severe anemia: Due to
  - Malabsorption
  - Inflammatory bowel disease
  - Malignancy
- Clubbing
  - IBD
  - Malabsorption.
- Edema: Hypoalbuminemia
- Lymphadenopathy: Systemic disease
- Jaundice: Pancreatic disease, obstructive jaundice.
- Oral candidiasis: HIV-related diarrhea.
- Pigmentation of creases and oral cavity:
  - Addison's disease
  - Vitamin B_{12} deficiency.

Look for

- Erythema nodosum—inflammatory bowel disease.
- Evidence of extra-articular manifestations—inflammatory bowel disease.

- Evidence of collagen disease
  - Joint involvement
  - Oral ulcers
- Dermatitis herpetiformis—coeliac disease
- Evidence of thyrotoxicosis, carcinoid flush, autonomic neuropathy.

On examination of the abdomen

Tenderness over the abdomen

- Periumbilical—small intestinal pathology
- Tenderness over the left iliac fossa/hypogastrium—large bowel disease.

Mass per abdomen

- Intra-abdominal malignancy
- Lymph node mass
- Abdominal tuberculosis

Ascites

- Malignancy/TB
- Hypoalbuminemia

Per rectal examination look for

- Rectal bleed
- Mucosal abnormality/secondary deposit
- Anal sphincter tone

Conditions which mimic diarrhea

- Fecal incontinence:
  - Due to defect in the anal sphincter, defect in the rectum or may be due to:
  - Neuromuscular disorder
  - Frequent passage of rectal contents mimicking diarrhea

Pseudodiarrhea

- Increased frequency of stool
- Stool is small in amount
- Feeling of evacuation incomplete e.g. irritable bowel syndrome.
- Inflammation of terminal rectum.

TUBERCULOSIS OF THE ABDOMEN

Abdominal Sites Involved in Abdominal Tuberculosis

- Terminal ileum, caecum, peritoneum and lymph nodes.
- Other parts involved: Oesophagus, large intestine and rectum.

Pathogenesis

Involvement of gastrointestinal tract by tuberculosis

- Spread of mycobacterium TB by hematogenous route.
- Swallowing of sputum with AFB reaching the GIT directly.
- Possibility of spread through drinking cow's milk containing bovine TB bacilli.

Pathological types

Ulcerative type: May involve the intestine circumferentially (likely to produce stricture) (typhoid ulcer—vertical corresponding to Peyer's patches).

Hypertrophic type: Usually at Ileocecal junction: Presents as mass in the right iliac fossa and can cause obstruction to the intestine.

Lymph node involvement

- Involves mesenteric lymph nodes
- Presents as intra-abdominal lymph node mass (tabes mesenterica)

TB peritoneum

- Presents as ascites due to peritonitis
- Patient will have abdominal tenderness with doughy feeling of the abdomen with thickening of the omentum and fibrous adhesions. Peritoneal involvement is due to direct spread of bacilli from ruptured lymph node.

Clinical manifestations

- Fever, weight loss
- Abdominal pain
- Ascites
- Mass per abdomen
- Lower GI bleed
- Intestinal obstruction
- Fistula in the anal region (can mimic Crohn's disease).

Investigations

- ESR is increased
- Ascitic fluid analysis: Lymphocyte dominant and exudative.

- CT scan abdomen—for visualizing lymph nodes, peritoneum and ileocaecal region.
- Laparoscopic peritoneal biopsy.

 Note

Occasionally cirrhosis of liver and tuberculosis abdomen can coexist together.

HAEMOCHROMATOSIS

- Hereditary disorder of iron metabolism.
- Increased absorption of iron from the gastrointestinal tract with iron deposition in the parenchymal cells of liver.
- Hemosiderosis—term used to describe detection of iron in the tissue which is stainable.

Clinical manifestations of hemochromatosis

- Dermatological pigmentation of skin described as slate gray (Bronze-like).
- Hepatic: Cirrhosis of liver and hepatocellular carcinoma.
- Cardiac: Restrictive cardiomyopathy and cardiac arrhythmias.
- Endocrine: Diabetes mellitus (due to pancreatic pathology).
- Pituitary involvement: Hypogonadotropic hypogonadism.
- Joint involvement: Arthropathy.

Investigations

- Serum iron, ferritin and percent transferring saturation
- Liver biopsy.
- CT/MRI liver: Hepatic iron concentration.

Clinical significance of Wilson's disease and hemochromatosis regarding liver disease

- Suspect Wilson's disease if unexplained liver disease occurs in young especially if the person has neurological manifestations.
- Suspect hemochromatosis of liver: In young along with skin pigmentation and cardiac involvement.

INFERIOR VENA CAVAL OBSTRUCTION

Causes

- Thrombosis of interior vena cava.
- Budd-Chiari syndrome.
- Extrinsic compression by
  - Amass/neoplasm
  - Aortic aneurysm
  - Abdominal mass
  - Pregnant uterus.
- Due to tumor invasion
  - Renal cell carcinoma
  - Hepatocellular carcinoma
- Iatrogenic cause: Vascular/dialysis catheter.

Clinical Features of IVC Obstruction

- Swelling of feet and pedal edema
- Collaterals veins over the abdomen and back
- Hepatic and renal involvement
- Ascites
- Venous ulcer over the lower extremities.

Collaterals in IVC Obstruction

Anterior abdominal collaterals

- Superficial epigastric vein arises from the femoral vein (below) anastomoses with thoracoepigastric vein (above) which connects with lateral thoracic vein and axillary vein.
- Inferior epigastric vein (below) from external iliac vein anastomoses with superior epigastric vein which anastamoses with internal thoracic (mammary) vein.

Lateral abdominal collaterals: Superficial epigastric, superficial circumflex iliac vein below communicates with lateral thoracic vein which connects with axillary vein.

 Note

Superficial epigastric vein also communicates with para umbillical vein and can form caput medusa in patients with portal hypertension.

Direction of blood flow in a vein

- Select a vein of 3 cm free from branches
- 2 fingers are placed close together over the middle of the venous segment. Both fingers are moved in opposite direction.
- Milking the underlying vein—complete the emptying of vein.
- Finally one of the fingers is released and direction and speed of filing can be observed. Procedure is repeated in the other direction.

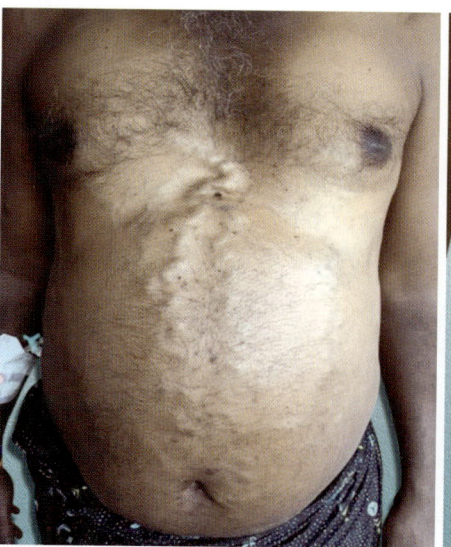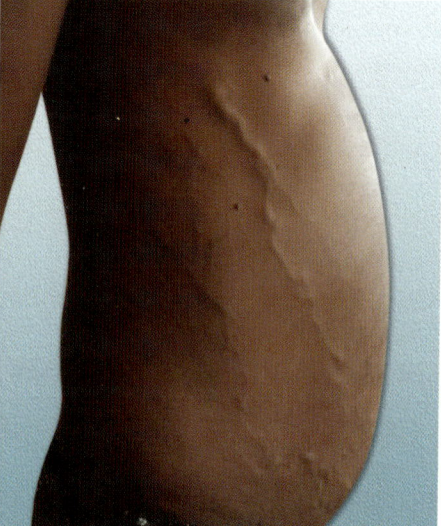

Fig. 3.1: Dilated abdominal veins in IVC obstruction

DIFFERENTIAL DIAGNOSIS OF ABDOMINAL PAIN

Different Types of Abdominal Pain

- Hollow viscus pain—colicky pain.
- Solid organ enlargement—dull aching pain.

Pain of abdominal wall origin

- Pain is usually of aching type which increases on movement of abdomen and is constantly present.
- Pain of hollow viscus origin
  - Obstruction to the hollow viscera causes colicky pain
  - Distention of the hollow viscus causes steady pain.
- Pain of gall bladder origin
  - Present in the right hypochondrium.
  - Can be felt in the lower part of thorax tip of scapula.
  - Common bile duct obstruction, causes pain in the epigastrium and felt in the right lumbar region.
- Dilatation of pancreatic duct
  - Pain is present in the epigastric region.
  - Pain is more in the lying down position and decreases on sitting up and stooping forward.

- Pain of intestinal origin: Obstruction to the small intestine: Colicky abdominal pain. Pain is felt around the umbillicus.
- Obstruction to the colon
  - Pain is felt below the level of umbillicus.
  - Less severe colicky/steady pain.
- Pain of urinary tract obstruction
- Pain of distended urinary bladder
  - Suprapubic pain
  - Dull aching pain
  - Patient can become restless.
- Ureter colic—severe colicky pain. Radiating from loin to groin with sweating and vomiting.
- Pain of upper ureteric obstruction: Colicky pain
- Pain in the renal angle
- Pain of peritoneal origin
- Peritoneal irritation causes spasm of abdominal muscles
- There will be guarding and rigidity.
- Leaking of gastric and pancreatic juices into the peritoneal cavity causes severe pain.
- Superior mesenteric artery occlusion produces severe continuous pain.

Central Nervous System

GENERAL PHYSICAL EXAMINATION

- Pallor
- Icterus
- Cyanosis
- Clubbing
- Lymphadenopathy
- Edema

Vital signs

- Pulse
- BP
- Respiratory rate
- Temperature

Pallor

- Suggestive of anemia with neurological involvement
- Causes of anemia with neurological involvement
  - B12 deficiency
  - Nutritional disorders like niacin deficiency, B6 deficiency
  - Anemia of systemic disease
- Polycythemia—may be a risk factor for CVA, cortical venous sinus thrombosis.

Icterus: Associated systemic illness.

Cyanosis: Due to

- Systemic conditions
- Respiratory paralysis, e.g. respiratory muscle paralysis due to neuronal disease.

Clubbing

- Associated systemic conditions

- Associated with malignancy with paraneoplastic syndrome of CNS.

Lymphadenopathy: Associated systemic illness.

Edema

- Associated systemic illness.
- Venous stasis due to paralysed limbs/DVT.
- Look for thyroid swelling, for thyroid myopathy/thyrotoxic paralysis
- Pulse rate: Bradycardia may be due to raised intracranial pressure
- Tachycardia: Systemic illness/tachy arrhythmias
- Rate—variation can occur in autonomic neuropathy, e.g. GB syndrome
- Rhythm—irregular rhythm may be due to atrial fibrillation—causes embolic CVA
- Volume and character alteration occurs with cardiac disease
- Thickening of vessel wall with atherosclerotic vascular disease

Blood pressure—variation

- May be hypertensive
- May be due to autonomic neuropathy/ AIDP/porphyria
- Reactionary hypertension in acute CVA
- Due to raised intracranial pressure

Respiratory rate and rhythm

- Abnormality of respiratory rate and rhythm can occur due to
  - Paralysis/respiratory muscle paralysis due to AIDP/muscle paralysis.

- Brainstem dysfunction results in respiratory rhythm abnormality.

Temperature: Raise in temperature can be associated with febrile illness and neurological involvement.

Hyperpyrexia can be associated with
- Pontine hemorrhage
- Heat stroke
- Neuroleptic malignant syndrome
- Cerebral malaria

Specific General Examination Features in Certain Neurological Disorders

- In CVA: Xanthelasma, xanthoma, Hollenhorst plaques in the retina (cholesterol emboli).
- Look for neurocutaneous markers—in certain neurological disorders.

Hollenhorst Plaque

- Appears as refractile bright yellow plaque in the retinal.
- Artery indicates retinal artery embolization.

Source of Embolization

Atherosclerotic plaque in the ipsilateral internal carotid artery.

Neurocutaneous Markers

Adenoma sebaceum
- Angiofibromas over the face/nasolabial fold. Reddish/pinkish papules/nodules.
- Associated with tuberous sclerosis.

Telangiectasia
- Presence of telangiectasia (in the eye)
- Ataxia telangiectasia associated with cerebellar disturbance

Port vein stain
- Vascular anomaly of the skin—color of the skin resembles fortified red wine. Part of Sturge-Weber syndrome.

Sturge-Weber syndrome: Port vein stain of the skin and associated with encephalotrigeminal angiomatosis.

Café-lait spot: Hyperpigmented (light brown to dark brown) macular lesions of around 0.5 cm in diameter. If more than 6 in number—associated with neurofibromatosis type-I.

Lisch nodules: Doom-shaped yellowish nodules projecting from the surface of the iris. Associated with neurofibromatosis type-I.

Phakomatosis: Syndrome characterised by involvement of nervous system, skin and ocular structures arising from ectoderm, e.g. neurofibromatosis.

GENERAL PHYSICAL EXAMINATION IN NERVOUS SYSTEM DISORDER

Different Types of Facial Appearances

Parkinsonism—masked facies.
Pseudobulbar palsy—involuntary laughter/crying.
Ptosis—unilateral/bilateral occurs in
- 3rd nerve palsy
- Myasthenia gravis
- Horner's syndrome
Weakness of facial muscles—myopathies/facial palsy.
Temporal wasting—Vth nerve palsy/myotonic dystrophy.
Hatchet facies—myotonic dystrophy
Angle of mouth deviation—7th nerve palsy
Other disorders with typical appearance of face with nervous system involvement
- Myxedema/cretinism
- Down's syndrome
- Acromegaly.

Dermatological Examination in Nervous System Disorder

Adenoma sebaceum—tuberous sclerosis
Cutaneous angiomas: Sturge-Weber syndrome
Septic focus over the skin—spinal epidural abscess.
Subcutaneous nodules
- Neurofibromatosis
- Secondary malignant deposits

Photosensitive eruptions—Porphyria
Rashes over the skin

- Viral exanthema
- SLE
- Dermatomyositis
- Herpes zoster and herpes simplex

Greasy skin: Seborrheic dermatitis in Parkinsonism.

Café au lait spots: Neurofibromatosis.

 Note

Observe also for the presence of bed sores.

Examination of Eyes: Related to CNS Disorders

Proptosis: Thyroid disease (usually bilateral). Caroticocavernous fistula (usually unilateral).

Lisch nodule—neurofibromatosis

Dry eye—collagen disease/Sjögren's syndrome

KF ring—Wilson's disease

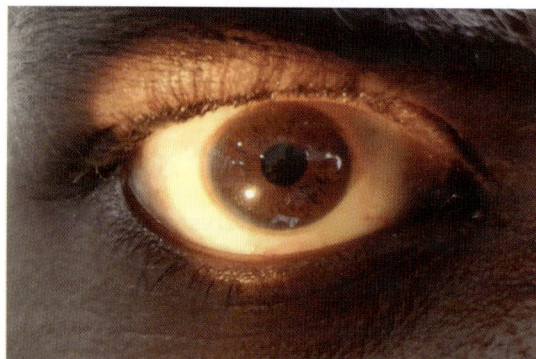

Fig. 4.1: KF ring in Wilson's disease

Herpes zoster ophthalmicus: Vth nerve involvement

Tortuous conjunctival vessels: Ataxia telangiectasia

Ophthalmic fundus examination for

- Papilledema
- Optic atrophy
- Choroid tubercles
- Cytoid bodies (SLE/neuroretinitis)
- Subhyaloid hemorrhage (in subarachnoid hemorrhage)

- Diabetic and hypertensive retinopathy
- Hollenhorst plaques

Ear Examination

- Ear discharge—associated with otitis media and CNS infection.
- Vesicles over the ear: In Ramsay Hunt syndrome.

Oral Cavity Examination

Glossitis: B12 deficiency

- Peripheral neuropathy
- Subacute combined degeneration of spinal cord

Macroglossia

- Amyloidosis
- Myxedema
- Down's syndrome

Blue line over the gum: Lead toxicity

Dry mouth: Sjögren's syndrome

Mouth ulcers: Behçet's syndrome

Notched teeth: Congenital syphilis

Oral candidiasis: HIV infection

Presence of icterus, bleeding in the oral cavity, gum hypertrophy (phenytoin usage) also should be observed.

Examination of Neck (of CNS Importance)

Observe for the following abnormalities

- Low hair line
- Short neck } Craniovertebral anomaly
- Deformity of neck—torticollis—disease of cervical spine
- For thyroid swelling
- Palpation and auscultation of carotid for thrill and bruit

Examination of Back (of CNS Importance)

Kyphoscoliosis

- Friedreich's ataxia
- Muscular dystrophy
- Syringomyelia
- Tuft of hair over the spine—spina bifida occulta

Examination of Feet

Pescavus	Bilateral	Idiopathic
		Friedreich's ataxia
		Charcot-Marie-Tooth disease
		Hereditary spastic paraplegia
Unilateral	Syringomyelia	Poliomyelitis
Foot drop: *See later.*		

Auscultation Over the Head and Spine

- For bruit—over the temporal region/eye ball/mastoid/spine.
- *Occurs in*
  - Angiomas
  - Aneurysms
  - AV fistula

Orbital Bruit

Occurs at the site contralateral to the carotid stenosis due to increased flow across the non-occluded carotid artery. It can also indicate significant intracranial occlusive disease.

Nose, Mouth and Throat

Saddle nose deformity: Congenital syphilis.
Bacterial infection over the nose: Cavernous sinus thrombosis.
Watery discharge from the nose: CSF rhinorrhea.
Blackish discharge with discoloration of palate: Rhinocerebral mucormycosis.

Hand Examination

Healed scars/Burns over the terminal phalanges
- In syringomyelia
- Leprosy
- Hereditary sensory motor neuropathy

Nails
Transverse ridges and discoloration: Arsenic/thallium poisoning (Mees' lines)
Genitalia—Ulcers
- Syphilis
- Behçet's syndrome
- Vesicular eruption: Herpes genitalis.

CEREBRAL BLOOD SUPPLY

Arterial supply of the brain is mainly carried out by
- Internal carotid artery and its branches
- Vertebral artery and its branches.

Branches of internal carotid artery
Important intracranial branches
- Ophthalmic artery
- Superior hypophyseal artery
- Posterior communicating artery
- Anterior choroidal artery
- Middle cerebral artery
- Anterior cerebral artery

Branches of anterior cerebral artery
Lenticulo striate arteries
- Anterior communicating artery
- Recurrent artery of Heubner

Branches of middle cerebral artery
- Divides into upper and lower divisions
- Gives rise to lenticulo striate arteries

Branches of vertebral artery
Originates from subclavian artery and terminates as basilar artery.
Branches
- Anterior spinal artery
- Posterior spinal artery.

Posterior inferior cerebellar artery
Two vertebral arteries terminate as basilar artery.

Basilar artery
- Formed by joining of two vertebral arteries.
- Divides to form two posterior cerebral arteries.

Main branches
- Anterior inferior cerebellar arteries
- Pontine arteries
- Labyrynthine arteries
- Superior cerebellar artery

Middle cerebral artery (MCA) supplies
Lateral surface of cerebral hemisphere except area supplied by anterior cerebral artery.

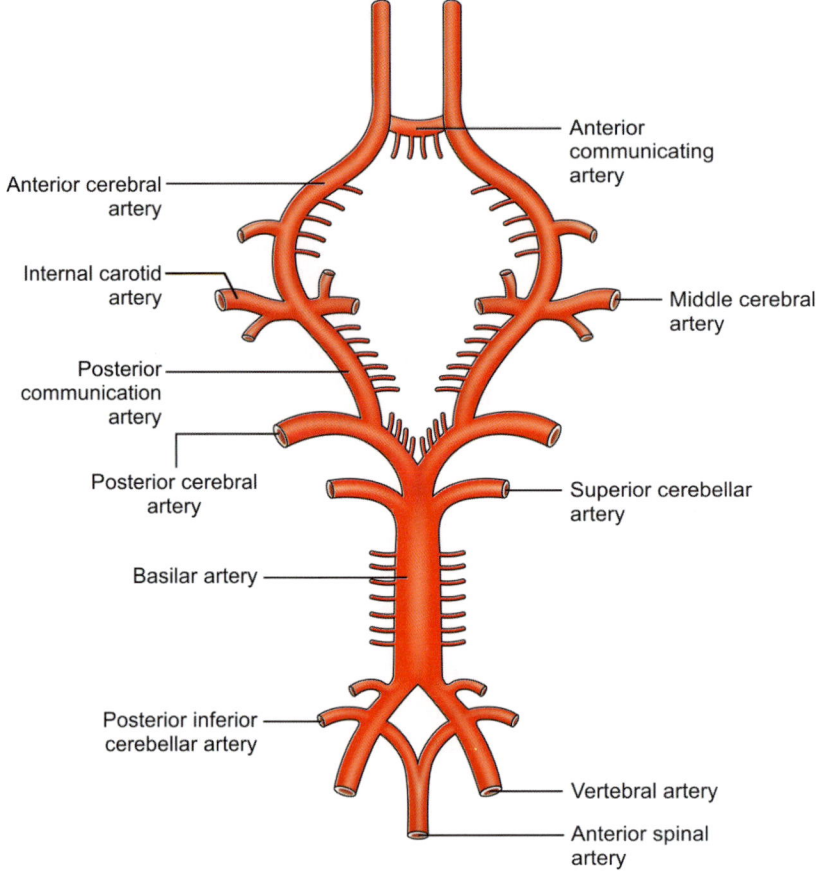

Fig. 4.2: Circle of Willis

Upper division of MCA supplies
- Broca's area
- Lower division supplies Wernicke's area

Lenticulostriate branch supplies: Upper half of internal capsule.

Areas which is not supplied by middle cerebral artery
- Occipital pole and lower temporal pole
- Frontal pole
- 2 cm of superolateral surface of cortex
- Medial half of orbital surface.

Anterior cerebral artery supplies
- Medial surface of cerebral hemisphere.
- Superior 2 cm of lateral surface of cerebral hemisphere.
- Orbital surface of frontal lobe and frontal pole.

Recurrent branch of anterior cerebral artery— Heubner's artery occlusion: Can result in facio-brachial monoplegia.

Posterior cerebral artery
- Division of basilar artery
- Supplies
  - Brainstem—midbrain
  - Pons
  - Medulla
  - Thalamus
  - Subthalamus
  - Cerebellum
- Part of temporal and occipital lobe—medial surface.

Basilar artery
- Supplies: Pons, cerebellum
- Divides into two posterior cerebral artery.

Blood Supply of Internal Capsule

Anterior limb

- *Superior part*: By anterior cerebral artery
- *Inferior part*: By middle cerebral artery
- *Genu*: By lenticulostriate branch of middle cerebral artery.

Posterior limb

- *Superior part*: By anterior choroidal artery.
- *Inferior part*: By posterior communicating artery.

CEREBRAL BLOOD FLOW

Normal cerebral blood flow

- 750 ml/minute (15% of cardiac output)
- 50–54 ml/100 gm of brain tissue/min.

Cerebral Venous System

Superficial venous system

- Dural venous sinuses
- Superior saggital sinus
- 2 transverse sinuses: They join to form 2 sigmoid sinuses
- 2 sigmoid sinuses continue as jugular veins and join SVC.

Deep venous system

- Deep veins of brain parenchyma join to form vein of Galen.
- Vein of Galen joins inferior sagittal sinus to form straight sinus which joins superficial venous system at confluence of sinuses.

Autoregulation of cerebral blood flow

- Normal cerebral blood flow is maintained by autoregulation of cerebral blood flow.
- Constriction of cerebral blood vessels occur whenever systolic blood pressure is very high and blood vessels dilate when systolic BP is very low.
- Cerebral blood vessels and blood flow is also influenced by CO_2 concentration of blood.
- High CO_2 content of blood dilates the cerebral blood vessels and low CO_2 content of blood constricts them.

Cerebral blood flow is influenced by

- Metabolic parameters
- Blood pressure in the cerebral vessels
- Chemical content of blood like CO_2 level and O_2 level
- Neural mechanisms.

LOCALISATION OF LESION IN NERVOUS SYSTEM DISORDER

Cortical Lesions

Features

- A—Agnosia, aphasia, apraxia
- B—Bladder involved
- C—Convulsions
- D—Disturbed consciousness

Other features

- Cortical sensory loss
- Primitive reflexes.
- Only monoparesis can occur

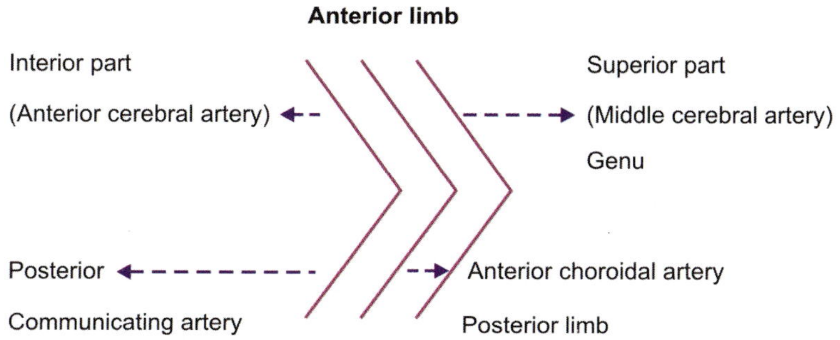

Fig. 4.3: Blood supply of internal capsule

Subcortical lesions

Corona radiata

- No central speech defect or convulsions
- Can have hemiparesis with disproportionate weakness.

Internal capsule

- No evidence of central speech defect or convulsions
- Presence of hemiplegia hemi-anesthesia, hemianopia
- UMN facial palsy on the hemiplegic side
- Equal involvement of upper and lower limbs

Basal ganglia: Different types of involuntary movement, presence of rigidity.

Thalamic lesions

- Opposite hemianesthesia
- Hyperpathia (increase threshold for pain stimuli with displeasing sensation with more severe and more lasting pain sensation)
- Basal ganglia and thalamic lesions can have rarely central speech defect.

Brainstem involvement

Common features

- Ipsilateral LMN cranial nerve palsy.
- Contralateral hemiplegia.
- Internuclear ophthalmoplegia.
- Horner's syndrome.
- May have hydrocephalus.
- Altered sensorium if ARAS involved.

Midbrain lesions

- 3rd and 4th cranial nerve palsy
- Opposite side hemiplegia
- Occasionally vertical gaze palsy.

Pontine lesions

- Horner's syndrome
- Pain and temperature loss—opposite side
- If PPRF-involved horizontal gaze palsy.
- Opposite pyramidal signs
- Involvement of 5th, 6th, 7th and 8th cranial nerves—same side.

- Can have cerebellar signs.
- If medial lemniscus involved—touch and proprioception can be affected

Medulla

- 9th, 10th, 11th and 12th cranial nerve palsy—same side.
- Evidence of Horner's syndrome
- Opposite side hemiplegia
- Involvement of centers like respiration.

Craniovertebral junction/high cervical cord

- Neck pain
- Down beat nystagmus
- Lower cranial nerves involvement
- Cerebellar signs
- Pyramidal signs in the limb

Craniovertebral anomaly

- Low hair line
- Short neck
- Down beat nystagmus
- Mirror movement
- Other features as lesion at high cervical cord.

Possible sites of lesions in a patient of hemiparesis without cranial nerve palsy.

1. Cortical lesions: Cranial nerve like facial may not be involved.
2. Medullary pyramid lesions
3. Cervical cord lesions
4. Subcortical lesions with minimal facial involvement which has resolved.

Cerebellar involvement

Cerebellar hemisphere involvement: Ataxia of limbs on the same side of lesion.

- Midline cerebellar lesion: Truncal ataxia with wide based gait.
- *Other features*
  - Nystagmus
  - Hypotonia
  - Dysarthria.

DISEASES OF CEREBRAL HEMISPHERE

Main Brodmann areas and their localisations
Motor cortex: Area no. 4: Precentral gyrus

Premotor cortex: Area no. 6

Primary sensory cortex: Area no. 1, 2.3—post-central gyrus

Frontal eye field: Area no. 8.

Broca's area: Area no. 44—inferior frontal gyrus—dominant side.

Wernicke's area: Area no. 22, 23—near auditory cortex—posterior 1/3 of superior temporal gyrus (dominant side).

Primary visual cortex: Area no. 17—occipital cortex.

Visual association areas: Area no. 18 and 19—occipital cortex.

Auditory cortex: Area no. 41, 42—superior temporal gyrus.

- Heschl's gyrus.

Frontal lobe

Parts of frontal lobe

- Primary motor area—area no. 4—precentral gyrus.
- Additional motor cortex: Premotor area—area no-6—rostral to area number 4.
- Supplementary motor area—medial surface of area number 6 (takes part in complex movements).

Other important parts of frontal lobe

- Motor speech area
- Area no 8: Frontal eye field—center for conjugate horizontal eye movement

Functions and clinical significance of frontal lobe

- Contralateral motor control
- Language and speech function
- Cortical control of bowel and bladder
- Conjugate movement of eyes
- Plans movements of the body and sequence of movements.

Lesion of frontal lobe produces

- Motor aphasia (dominant side)
- Micturition—impaired—cortical bladder.
- Loss of motor control—opposite side hemiparesis.

- Irritative lesion of frontal eye field—produces conjugate deviation of eyes to opposite side.
- Paralytic lesion of frontal eye field—conjugate deviation of eyes of the side of lesion.

Specific features of frontal lobe dysfunction

Clinical features	Site of lesion
• Pyramidal signs on one side	• Opposite frontal lobe
• Grasp reflex on one side	• Opposite frontal lobe
• Bilateral grasp reflex	• Bilateral frontal lobe
• Central speech abnormality	• Bilateral frontal lobe (mainly left side)
• Micturition abnormality	• Paracentral lobule
• Emotional and behavioral abnormality	• Prefrontal lobe with its connections

Prefrontal lobe: Area no. 8, 9, 10, 11, 12, 13, 14, 24, 25, 32, 44, 45, 46 and 47.

- Parts of prefrontal cortex
- Dorsolateral prefrontal cortex
- Medial prefrontal cortex
- Orbitofrontal prefrontal cortex

There is connection to caudate nucleus, thalamus and limbic system.

Functions of prefrontal lobe

- Decision making
- Integration of thoughts
- Behavioral changes
- Working memory
- Cognitive and executive functions
- Emotional behaviors.

Bilateral lesion of prefrontal lobe produces: Personality and behavioral changes.

Causes of prefrontal lobe dysfunction

- Deficiency B12
- Demyelination: Multiple sclerosis
- Trauma: Head injury
- Degenerative dementias.

Diffuse cerebrovascular disease and dementias can also cause frontal and prefrontal lobe dysfunction.

Clinical signs of prefrontal lobe dysfunction

- Decrease in the attention and concentration.
- Memory loss
- Abnormal behavior
- Defective cognitive and executive functions.
- Presence of frontal lobe release signs.

Parietal Lobe

Important parts of parietal lobe
- Postcentral gyrus—area no 3, 2, 1—sensory cortex.
- Posterior parietal lobule.

Functions of parietal lobe
- Localisation of touch and two-point discrimination
- Discrimination of primary sensations received from thalamus.
- Sensory aspects of speech
- Recognition of dimension of objects.
- Simple and complex calculations.
- Construction of 2 or 3 dimensional diagrams.
- Spatial orientation of different parts of the body and sensory motor representation of extra personal atmospheric events.

Effects of lesions of parietal lobe
Dominant side
- Central speech defect.
- Left angular gyrus: Gerstmann's syndrome.

Non-dominant
- Anosognosia
- Autotopognosia
- Sensory inattention.

Deep parietal lobe lesion
- Opposite: Lower quadrantanopia
- Apraxia agnosia

Other features
- Loss of optokinetic nystagmus—opposite parietal lobe lesion
- Cortical sensory loss.

Hemineglect in a Patient of Parietal Lesion

- Unilateral right hemispheric lesion causes left neglect.
- Unilateral left hemispheric lesion—may not produce significant hemineglect on the right side because right hemisphere controls both sides spatial orientation
- Bilateral lesions of parietal lobe can cause right hemispatial neglect.

Examination for Hemineglect

Features of hemineglect
- Usually on the left side: Person is unable to read the left half of the writing.
- Person is not eating the food which is kept on the left side.
- Person is not able to shave, dress on the left side.

Bedside Tests for Hemineglect

- Draw a circle and ask the patient to put dots or numbers inside the circle.
- Persons will put more dots on the right while keeping the left side of the circle blank.

Sensory in attention/extinction
- Person is able to identify the touch (stimuli) when it is given unilaterally on one side of the body.
- When person is given stimuli (touch) on both sides of the body on mirror image points (touch Acromion on both sides) simultaneously (patient closing the eyes) he fails to identify the stimulus on one side (usually left side).

Other features of parietal lobe dysfunction
- Anosognosia (person denies defect on one side).
- Autotopognosia: Person is unaware of body part on one side.

Deficit in bilateral parietal lobe dysfunction can occur due to
- Bilateral MCA and PCA water shed infarct.

- Superior sagittal sinus thrombosis.
- Hypoglycemia.

Parietal lobe atrophy (wasting): Parietal lesion can cause contralateral muscular atrophy and hypotonia.

Temporal Lobe

Functions of Temporal Lobe

Main function: Language and memory.

Other functions

- Auditory and vestibular information and upper visual pathway.
- Control of visceral motility, sexual function and respiratory function.
- Central representation of taste and smell.
- Connection with frontal lobe for behavior.
- Memory and learning—mainly represented in the Hippocampus.
- Hearing: Represented in bilateral temporal lobe.

LIMBIC SYSTEM

Parts

- Amygdaloid body
- Hippocampus
- Thalamic nucleus: Anterior and medial
- Parts of striatum
- Hypothalamus

Functions of limbic system

- Involved in endocrine function and autonomic function
- Recent memory, emotional aspects and motivation

Symptoms of temporal lobe dysfunction

- Seizures—complex partial seizures
- Déjàvu and jamaisvu phenomenon
- Abnormal and spontaneous lip smacking and facial grimaces
- Abnormalities of language memory and personality changes.

Signs: Dominant lobe

- Sensory aphasia

- Reading difficulty
- Verbal memory impaired
- Word deafness

Nondominant lobe

- *Impaired:* Nonverbal memory
- Impaired musical skills
- Sensory aphasia.

Signs

- Drowsiness
- Hemiparesis
- Upper quadrantic field defect.

Bilateral lesions of temporal lobe

- Deafness
- Behavioral abnormality
- Impaired memory and learning
- Korsakoff's psychosis
- Kluverbucy syndrome—due to bilateral lesion of medial temporal lobe and amygdaloid nucleus (visual agnosia, hypersexuality and excessive eating).

Occipital Lobe

- Contains primary visual cortex—area no. 17.
- Visual association area—18, 19
- Area no 17—primary visual cortex—receives fibers coming from geniculocalcarine fibers.
- *Unilateral lesion causes:* Homonymous hemianopia with macular sparing
- Area No 18, 19—visual association area
  - For recognition and identification of object.
  - For storage of visual memory
- Defect of area No 18, 19: Can cause visual inattention and visual agnosia.
- *Bilateral occipital damage:* Bilateral visual loss with macular involvement.
- Denial of blindness—cortical blindness—Anton's syndrome.

Prosopagnosia

- Person has got difficulty in recognizing familiar face including his own face in the mirror.

- Lesion—bilateral lesion of occipitotemporal cortex.

Object agnosia: Difficulty in recognizing object and its use can also occur in bilateral occipito-temporal cortex.

Causes of bilateral lesions of occipitotemporal cortex
- For example, bilateral PCA territory infarct.
- Degeneration of temporal cortex.

Limbic Network and Memory
- Memory function—requires intact limbic system
- Memory is also distributed throughout the cerebral cortex.

Types of memory loss
- *Anterograde amnesia*: Inability to learn new knowledge
- Retrograde amnesia: Loss of ability for the past memory.

Confabulation: Occurs in acute memory loss—person tries to explain which is not accurate to the situation.

Testing the memory function
- *Immediate memory*: Person is asked to repeat the words from 1 to 5 immediately.
- *Recent memory*: Person is asked to repeat three words after 3 to 5 minutes.
- *Remote memory*: Person is asked about the past events (or about the names of past prime ministers, etc.).
- Bilateral damage to limbic system: Global memory loss.

Causes of memory loss
- Werneck's encephalopathy
- Temporal lobe epilepsy
- Tumors of temporal lobe
- Dementias

Transient global amnesia (TGA)
- Sudden onset of memory loss, persisting for 24–48 hours for both past and new memories.

- Can occur in patients with posterior cerebral artery disease
- Occurs in temporal lobe epilepsy and migraine.

Examination of Handedness
Following factors will help in deciding handedness
- *Hand*: Which is used for writing and drawing.
- *Hand*: Which is kept uppermost while clapping
- *Ear*: Which is used for conversation through telephone
- *Eye*: Which is preferred for seeing though a key hole.
- Handedness is used for deciding the dominant hemisphere (left hemisphere containing speech center).

CEREBROVASCULAR DISEASE

Middle Central Artery Occlusion

Clinical signs	Lesions vessels involved (opposite side)
1. Hemiplegia, hemianesthesia and hemianopia + global aphasia	MCA stem occlusion on dominant side
2. Anosognosia, constructional apraxia Hemineglect	MCA stem occlusion, non-dominant side
3. Facial palsy + Broca's aphasia	MCA branch occlusion—dominant side
4. Hand ± ARM weakness	MCA branch occlusion (opposite)
5. Facial palsy + Broca's aphasia ± Arm weakness (frontal opercular syndrome)	MCA branch occlusion—dominant side
6. Hemiplegia + Broca's aphasia + Hemianaesthesia	MCA—upper division, occlusion dominant side
7. Sensory aphasia with or without weakness, superior quadrant—anopia	MCA—lower division—dominant side.

Lacunar Stroke

Occurs due to the occlusion of lenticular striate branches of middle cerebral artery.

Pathology

Fibrinoid necorsis or segmental lipohyalinosis of small arterioles.

Characteristics

Hypertension is present in 80–90% of patients.
- Diabetes mellitus is an important risk factor
- White matter is affected and grey matter is not affected
- Lacunes (little cavities are associated with infarcts (2–15 mm))
- Treatment of hypertension is associated with good prognosis
- Administration of antiplatelets is beneficial.

Types of Lacunar Syndrome

1. *Pure motor—most common*
   - Hemiparesis involving limbs + facial involvement
   - Site of lesion: Posterior limb of internal capsule or corona radiata
2. *Ataxic hemiparesis*
   - Hemiparesis with predominant cerebellar features on the same side
   - Usually site of lesion: Contralateral internal capsule—posterior limb due to involvement of corticospinal tract and fronto-ponto-cerebellar fibers
   - Contralateral basis pontis: Due to involvement of corticospinal tract and pontocerebellar fibers
   - Other rarer sites: Corona radiata, midbrain.
3. *Dysarthria—clumsy hand syndrome*
   - Weakness of hand, clumsiness of hand, facial weakness and dysarthria.
   - It is a variant of ataxic hemiparesis. Lesion is same as ataxic hemiparesis.
4. *Pure sensory*: Hemianesthesia on one side
   - Site of lesion: Contralateral thalamus, rarely internal capsule/corona radiata.

5. *Mixed sensory motor type*: Site of lesion: Posterior limb of internal capsule.

Anterior Cerebral (ACA) Occlusion

Clinical signs	Vessel involvement + site of involvement
1. Abulia Bilateral pyramidal signs para/quadriparesis	Single unpaired ACA
2. Opposite lower limb weakness and upper limb minimal weakness Cortical sensory loss—opposite side Cortical bladder	ACA occlusion

Hemiplegia, Hemi-anesthesia and Hemianopia

Possible sites of vascular occlusions (opposite side)
- MCA stem occlusion
- Anterior choroidal occlusion (branch of internal carotid artery).
- Possible site of lesion; contralateral internal capsule.

Internal Carotid Occlusion
(Carotid Hemiplegia)
- Usually behaves like MCA occlusion additionally person will have ipsilateral blindness due to ophthalmic artery occlusion.
- Rarely anterior cerebral and middle cerebral can get occluded due to top of carotid block causing abulia.

Common carotid occlusion: All signs of internal carotid occlusion. Person may have claudication of jaw.

Posterior Cerebral Artery Occlusion
- Causes all brainstem syndromes
- Can cause temporal and occipital lobe signs.

Clinical features	Vessel involvement
Contralateral sensory loss with hyperpathia	Thalamic syndrome Vessel-thalamic or thalamogeniculate artery.
Abulia, drowsiness + upward gaze palsy	Artery of Percheron

Anton's Syndrome

Due to: Bilateral distal PCA occlusion.

Features

- Person denies blindness
- Cortical blindness
- Can have gun barrel vision

Balint's Syndrome

Area involved: Parieto-occipital cortex (bilateral visual association areas due to infarct in the watershed area between MCA and distal PCA territory).

Features:

Optic ataxia: Visual targets are difficult to reach manually.

Oculomotor apraxia: Person is unable to visually scan the environment.

Simultanagnosia: Person has got difficulty in synthesizing whole image of the entire field of vision visually.

Dressing and constructional apraxia can also be the manifestations of bilateral parietal or right parietal lobe lesions.

Top of Basilar Syndrome

Vessel involved: Usually embolic occlusion of top of basilar artery.

Site involved: Bilateral thalamus, rostral midbrain, parts of temporal and occipital lobe.

Features

- Visual and oculomotor deficit (bilateral ptosis, lack of light reflex)
- Behavioral abnormality
- Drowsiness, hallucinations
- Motor involvement—rare.

COMA

Anatomy and Physiology of Coma

For maintenance of alertness requires intact-function of cerebral hemisphere and special thalamocortical projecting system called reticular activating system.

Ascending Reticular Activating System

- Present in the brainstem in the upper pons and midbrain and projects to thalamus and entire cerebral cortex.
- Posterior part of hypothalamus also participate in the maintenance of consciousness.

Structural Lesions Producing Coma

1. Cerebral hemispheric lesions
2. Brainstem lesions involving reticular activating system
3. Disorders affecting both hemispheres.

Cerebral Hemisphere Lesions

1. *Unilateral hemispheric lesions*: Can cause herniation, compression of the upper midbrain and reticular activating system. Increased intracranial pressure—causing herniation into the brainstem.
2. *Bilateral extensive lesions of hemisphere can cause loss of consciousness*: Metabolic disturbance, renal and hepatic dysfunction, drugs and toxins can alter the function of reticular activating system and cerebral hemisphere.

Localisation of Lesion in a Patient of Altered Consciousness

Pupillary reaction

- Upper brainstem lesion—pupils are fixed and dilated with loss of eyeball movement.
- If papillary reactions are normal, coma may be due to metabolic cause *or* diffuse bilateral hemispheric lesion.

Different Types of Cerebral Herniation

Cerebellar tonsillar herniation

- Herniation of cerebellar tonsils through foramen magnum.

- Causes respiratory arrest and death due to medullary compression.

Herniation of medial thalamic structures

- Can herniate through the tentorial opening.
- Result in compression of brainstem.

Herniation of uncus and medial part of temporal gyrus

Medial part of temporal gyrus (uncus) herniates through the tentorial opening: Can compress the 3rd nerve on the same side causing papillary enlargement.

Because the displaced parahippocampal gyrus presses the midbrain against the tentorial edge of the opposite side. Person will develop coma. Displaced midbrain can compress the opposite cerebral peduncle—causing opposite side hemiparesis (Kernohan-Woltman sign)—opposite to the side of hemiparesis already caused by the mass.

- Causes infarction of the brainstem due to compression of vascular structure.
- Hydrocephalus occurs due to compression of CSF flow.

Important clinical points

- Medullary lesion can cause apnea
- In acute hemiplegia—there may be transient loss of corneal and pharyngeal reflexes.
- Stupor is a condition wherein vigorous stimulus can make the patient wake up.

APRAXIA AGNOSIA APHASIA

Apraxia

Inability to perform voluntary movement correctly in the presence of normal sensory, motor and coordination function.

Types of Apraxia

Ideational: Forming the idea to carry out the complex act is defective.
Lesion: Dominant parietal lobe (sylvian gyrus).

Ideomotor apraxia: Inability to carry out the act on command (automatic acts may be performed normally).
Site of lesion: Dominant parieto temporal cortex, basal ganglia, corpus callosum.

Constructional: Loss of ability to copy figures or designs or make designs.
Lesion: Non-dominant parietal lobe lesion.

Dressing apraxia: Loss of ability to put dress and undress clothes.
Lesion: Non-dominant parietal lobe.

Bucco facial: Apraxic defect of face and lips and mouth.
Lesion: Either hemisphere/left hemisphere.

Patients with Broca's aphasia may also have Bucco facial apraxia.

AGNOSIA

Gnosis means presence of knowledge.
Agnosia: Failure to recognise objects.
Types of agnosia = visual, tactile, auditory

Visual agnosia: Inability to name or describe the use of the shown object (can identify by touch/smell).
Sites of lesion: Dominant occipital cortex and visual association area.

Tactile agnosia: Inability to recognise the details of the object by touch.
Lesion: Contralateral supramarginal gyrus (parietal lobe).

Auditory agnosia: Person will have normal hearing—there will be difficulty in recognising different types of sounds.
Lesion: Damage to the auditory cortex bilateral or left temporal lobe/superior temporal gyrus.

Autotopagnosia
Anosognosia   } See above
Prosopagnosia
Simultanognosia

Gerstmann's Syndrome

Lesion: Angular gyrus = left (inferior parietal lobule).

Defects
- Right to left confusion.
- Acalculia
- Agraphia
- Finger agnosia.

DISORDERS OF SPEECH AND LANGUAGE

Different Types of Speech Sounds Produced by Participation of Different Mouth Parts

- By participation of tongue: t, d, l
- By participation of lips: b, p, m
- Modified labials by lip contraction: o, u, i, e.
- Produced due to articulation between back of the tongue and soft palate are called gutturals: k, g, ng.
- Produced by articulation between dorsum of the tongue and hard palate: ch, g, gn.

Terminologies used While Approaching a Patient of Speech Defect

Aphasia (Dysphasia)
- Person has inability to express the meaningful words or
- Thoughts—articulation is normal.

Paraphasia: Wrong word or sound is substituted.

Dysarthria: Slurring/distortion of articulation or pronounciation of words/phrases.

Aphonia: Volume of sound produced is deficient.

Mutism: Consciousness is normal but without production of sound or attempt to speak.
Lesion: Bilateral posteromedial surface of frontal lobe.

Palilalia: Person's own speech/words are repeated.

Echolalia: Whatever sound heard is repeated meaningless.
Site of lesion: Diffuse cerebral dysfunction. Perisylvian region of dominant hemisphere.

Perseveration = person is asked various questions—one reply or idea is persisting (even after stopping of the stimulus, e.g. significant brain injury).

Neologism: Person is constructing a new meaningless word.

Important anatomical areas of brain concerned with speech and language function

Broca's area (motor speech area)	Left inferior frontal gyrus
Sensory speech area (Wernicke's area)	Left superior temporal gyrus
Connection between Wernicke's and Broca's area	Arcuate fasciculus
Concerned with reading	Left angular gyrus (inferior parietal lobule)
Concerned with writing	Wernicke's area

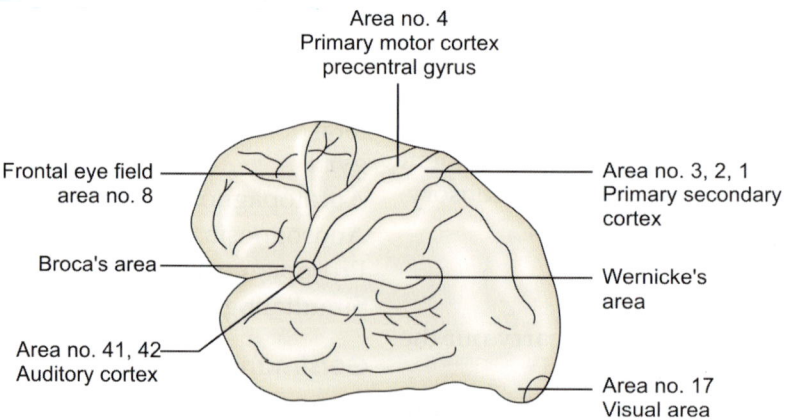

Fig. 4.4: Different cortical areas and areas of speech

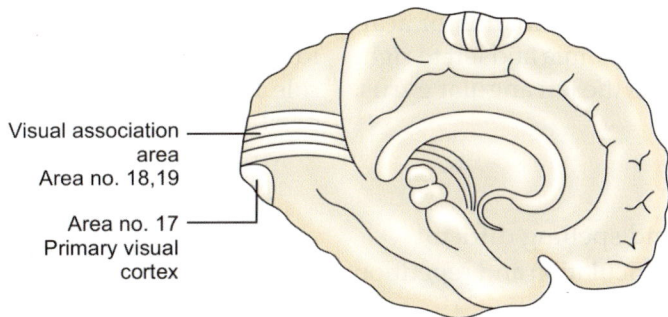

Visual association area
Area no. 18,19

Area no. 17
Primary visual cortex

Fig. 4.5: Different areas of visual cortex

Approach to a Patient of Aphasia

- Most of the persons: Right handed 90–95% with left hemisphere dominant (presence of speech center).
- Even in left-handed persons, left hemisphere dominant (60–70%).
- Some left-handed individuals—speech center is right-sided or both hemisphere dominant.
- Normal person: Person is able to express around 100–115 words/minute.
- Person is nonfluent—if he expresses less than seven words—usually less than 4 words/minute.

Test the following aspects of speech and language while examining the patient for aphasia

- Comprehension
- Naming
- Reading
- Repetition
- Word output
- Writing

Broca's aphasia

Features

- Decrease of word output
- Agrammatism.

Patients with Broca's aphasia can have dysarthria due to

- Associated UMN facial palsy
- Apraxia of muscles of articulation
- Apraxia of speech—cortical dysarthria— may be a form of "minor Broca's aphasia".

Wernicke's aphasia: Comprehension is usually lost. Can have difficulty only in understanding complicated grammatical words.

Alexia: Person has impaired ability to read or understand the written word.

- Vision is normal
- Lesion = dominant angular or supra-marginal gyrus.
- Disconnection between left occipital cortex, splenium of corpus callosum
- Left side language area and angular gyrus.

Word blindness: Same as alexia (difficulty in understanding the meaning of words seen).

Agraphia: Loss of ability to communicate through writing, motor power and coordination is normal.

Lesion: Between left angular gyrus and motor area.

Word deafness

- Difficulty in recognising the spoken word, but can appreciate other environmental nonverbal sounds.
- There is difficulty in writing from dictation.
- Spontaneous speech, reading, writing and hearing is normal.
- It is also called auditory verbal agnosia.

Lesion: There is loss of connection between bilateral auditory cortex with Wernicke's area on the left side.

Acalculia: Inability to perform simple mathematical calculations. Dominant parietal lobe pathology. Part of Gerstmann's syndrome.

Gerstmann's syndrome: Combination of acalculia, agraphia, finger anomia and left to right confusion. Lesion is in the left angular gyrus.

ANOMIA

Deficit: In naming
- Word findings and spelling difficult
- Understanding, articulation and repetition of speech are normal.

Causes: Metabolic encephalopathy
- Head injury
- Site of lesion—left temporal cortex.

APHEMIA

Deficit: Fluency of speech is lost
Lesion: Left hemisphere—lesion of supplementary motor area or partial lesion of Broca's area.

Aprosodia

Deficit: Stress and intonation of speech is lost.
Lesion: Right hemisphere—perisylvian area.

Subcortical aphasia

Features: Central speech defect.
Repetition intact, can be associated with hemiplegia
Lesion: Thalamus, caudate nucleus
Due to connection between cortical and subcortical structure is defective.

APPROACH TO A PATIENT OF DYSARTHRIA

Dysarthria

Difficulty in articulation occurs due to defective mechanism involving muscles supplied by cranial nerves, muscle disease, neuromuscular or cerebellar or extra pyramidal dysfunction.

Production of Sounds/Speech and Articulation

Peripheral

Following structures take part in the production of sounds, speech and voice.
Articulation: Tongue, lip, soft palate

Voice/sound production—larynx/pharynx: Respiratory muscles also play an important role in the mechanisms of sound and voice production.
- Muscles of the tongue—supplied by 12th nerve take part in the production of T, d, l, etc. (linguals).
- Labial (lip) muscles—supplied by 7th nerve
- Take part in the production of P, b, m (labials)
- Tongue and soft palate—together produce gutturals, e.g. ng, g

Causes and Types of Dysarthria

Due to cranial nerve palsy
- Lingual dysarthria—12th nerve palsy.
- Labial dysarthria—7th nerve palsy
- Nasal quality of speech—9th and 10th nerve palsy.

Due to lesion of basal ganglia and substantia nigra, e.g. Parkinsonism

Due to lesion of cerebellum—ataxic type (staccato and scanning)

Due to bilateral UMN lesions involving lower cranial nerves—spastic dysarthria (hot potato speech).

Due to LMN lesion involving lower cranial nerves, e.g. bulbar palsy—flaccid dysarthria.

Due to involvement of muscles and neuromuscular junction, e.g. myopathy and myasthenia gravis (muscle fatigue and slow decrease of voice).

Key Points in Dysarthria

- LMN facial palsy is more likely to produce dysarthria compared to UMN 7th nerve palsy.
- *Bulbar palsy*
  - Speech is indistinct
  - Speech is slow and hesitation to articulate
- *UMN lesion*—pseudobulbar palsy
  - Spastic (pseudobulbar): Hot potato speech
  - Thick bulbar speech
  - Takes strain to speak.

HEADACHE

Primary Pain Producing Structures in the Head

- Structures of scalp
- Pial arteries and their proximal segments
- Sinuses in the duramater
- Middle meningeal artery
- Falx cerebri

Structures Which do not Produce Pain

- Parenchyma of the brain
- Choroid plexus.

Approach to a Patient of Headache

Causes of Acute Onset of Headache

Infective disorder: Meningitis

Intracranial bleeding

- Subdural hematoma
- Epidural hematoma
- Subarachnoid hemorrhage.
- Intracranial space occupying tumors
- *Raised intraocular pressure*: Glaucoma
- *Disorder related to sinus*: Acute sinusitis

Headache which are clinically significant

- Acute—very severe headache.
- Associated with projectile vomiting.
- Progressive worsening of headache
- Headache disturbing the sleep and worse on morning.
- Headache associated with fever and neurological deficit.

Look for following signs in a patient of headache

- Signs of meningeal irritation
- Intraocular pressure
- Sinus tenderness
- Measurement of blood pressure
- Look for refractory error
- Palpate the temporal artery
- Oral and dental examination
- Optic fundus

Different Types of Headache

Due to intracranial space occupying lesion

- Early morning headache
- Severe throbbing

- Projectile vomiting*
- Disturbs sleep

*Projectile vomiting

- Sudden forceful vomiting
- No preceding nausea
- Vomitus will be thrown into a distance

Headache of temporal arteritis

- Tenderness over the temporal artery—unilateral/intermittent headache
- Can present with blindness due to occlusion of ophthalmic artery.

Acute congestive glaucoma

- Severe headache
- Red eye
- Pain in and around the eye
- Vomiting

Meningitis

- High grade fever
- Photophobia
- Neck stiffness
- Headache and vomiting.

Subarachnoid hemorrhage

- Sudden onset severe headache
- Neck stiffness

Headache which is due to previous trauma (post-traumatic): History of previous trauma to the head.

Previous infective illness: There can be persisting headache for longer duration—postviral illness.

MIGRAINE

Features

- Unilateral severe pulsating headache
- Associated with nausea and vomiting
- Photophobia/phonophobia

Cluster headache

- Usually starts in the retro-orbital region
- Unilateral
- Patient is awakened from sleep

- Comes in attacks of clusters
- Associated with autonomic symptoms.

Tension headache
- Tight band like sensation
- Can fluctuate
- Other features of migraine are absent like vomiting, photophobia and phonophobia.

CRANIAL NERVES

Clinically Significant Anatomical Aspects of Brainstem

General Description of Terms

1. *Nucleus of the nerve*: Indicates cranial nerve nuclei
   Cranial nerve nuclei in the brainstem
   - Midbrain: 3rd and 4th cranial nerve nuclei
   - Pons: 6th, 7th, 8th (parts of 8th) cranial nerve nuclei
   - Medulla—parts of 8th and 9th, 10th and 11th and 12th cranial nerve nuclei.
2. *Tectum of midbrain* (literally means roof of midbrain.)
3. Tegmentum refers to mid-portion.
4. *Fascicle of the nerve*: Intraparenchymal part of the cranial nerve.

Superior colliculus and lateral geniculate body: Has got important role in visual reflexes.

Inferior colliculus and medial geniculate body: Relay station for auditory pathway.

Red nucleus: Takes important part in maintaining flexor tone—facilitates flexor tone.

Crus Cerebri
- Anatomically internal capsule continues as crus cerebri.
- It contains corticospinal and corticobulbar fibers.

Pons: Contains nucleus of cranial nerves and trigeminal sensory pathways.

Medulla
- 90% of corticospinal tract decussate at pyramid level.

- 10% of fibers continues as anterior corticospinal tract and decussate at spinal level.
- Corticospinal fibers supplying arm lie medial to leg fibers and upper limb fibers cross first and then the lower limb fibers.

Reticular activating system
- Present in the brainstem.
- Made up of cells and fibers—network with connections.
- They are important in maintaining consciousness.
- They terminate in the intralaminar nucleus of thalamus.

3 main nucleus of reticular activating system
Raphe nucleus—connect with brainstem, cerebral hemisphere, cerebellum, and spinal cord.

Lateral reticular nucleus: Predominantly afferent—receiving fibers from long.

Tracts: Connects with medial reticular nucleus.

Medial reticular nucleus—take part in reticulospinal tract.

CRANIAL NERVES

Olfactory Nerve

Anatomical aspect
- Sensory cells in the upper part of nose
- They are bipolar cells
- They form the first order neurons.

Olfactory nerve: Unmyelinated neurons of sensory cells unite to form olfactory nerve on each side.

Olfactory bulb: Olfactory nerve pierces the cribriform plate of ethmoid bone, reach the olfactory bulb—from this 2nd order neurons arise.

Olfactory tract: 2nd order neurons from the olfactory bulb arise to form olfactory tract. They occupy inferior surface of the frontal lobe.

Course of olfactory tract
- Olfactory tract divides into medial and lateral striae

- Medial striae ends in cingulate cortex.
- Lateral striae ends in the temporal lobe (uncus, pyriform area, amygdala and hippocampus).

Entorhinal cortex
- Important part of smell localization. Uncus and orbitofrontal cortex constitute entorhinal cortex.
- Fibers concerned with smell also connect with thalamus, hypothalamus and reticular activating system.

Foster Kennedy syndrome: Due to meningioma of the olfactory groove.

Features

On the side of tumor: Optic atrophy on the side of the tumor—due to direct compression of the optic nerve.

Papilledema on the opposite side: Due to increased intracranial pressure.

OPTIC NERVE

Key Points While Testing Acuity and Field of Vision

- Snellen's charts is held at 20 feet distance from the patient
- For near vision—Jaeger type card—held at a distance of 30 cm.
- Goldmann perimetry is used for detecting scotomas.
- In the center of the visual field—a circle of around 5° is macular vision.
- While testing visual field—an object like red or white pin can be used.

Field defect—important clinical points
- Retrobulbar neuritis and optic nerve compression produces central scotomas.
- If the defect in the field of vision is similar shaped in each eye, it is called congruous hemianopia and lesion is more likely to be posterior.
- If the field defect is not similar shaped in each eye, it is called incongruous hemianopia and lesion is more likely to be anterior.

Macular sparing hemianopia: Macular vision is usually spared in unilateral occipital lobe lesion.

Reason for macular sparing in unilateral lesion
- Macula is supplied by both middle and posterior cerebral arteries.
- Possibly double macular representation in each occipital cortex.

Toxic damage to the optic nerve
Causes
- Drugs
  - Ethambutol
  - INH
  - Iodoquinol
- Toxins
  - Alcohol
  - Tobacco
  - Deficiency: B12 deficiency

Consecutive optic atrophy: Secondary to extensive disease of the retina and choroid, e.g. retinitis pigmentosa.

Causes of Visual Loss
Transient Loss of Vision

Transient unilateral loss of vision
- Episode of migraine
- Vasculitis
- Embolization (amaurosis fugax)
- Psychogenic

Transient bilateral loss of vision
- Migraine episode
- ↓Blood supply to occipital lobe—both
- An attack of seizure.

Permanent and sudden loss of vision one eye
- Vitreous hemorrhage
- Retinal detachment
- Central retinal artery or venous occlusion
- Ischemia to the optic nerve

Sudden loss of vision—both eyes
- Bilateral occipital lobe infarction
- Trauma to the head
- Pituitary apoplexy
- Functional disorder

Localisation of Lesion along the Visual Pathway

Lesion of retina and optic nerve

- Unilateral—usually total loss of vision
- Optic disc may be normal or abnormal
- Light reflex affected.

Optic chiasma

If crossing fibers involved, e.g. pituitary tumor.
- Bitemporal hemianopia
- Optic disc—usually normal
- Light reflex may be affected

Lateral chiasma lesion—nasal field is affected

Optic tract

- Homonymous hemianopia
- Light reflex affected.

Visual radiation

- Light reflex not affected.
- Temporal lobe pathology: Involvement of Mayer's loop
- Contralateral upper quadrantanopia
- Parietal cortex affected—contralateral lower quadrantanopia.

Lesion of unilateral occipital cortex

- Homonymous hemianopia
- Macular sparing
- Light reflex not affected.

Bilateral occipital cortex (visual cortex involving occipital pole): Produces Anton's syndrome.

Anton's syndrome

- Loss of vision with denial of blindness (cortical blindness)
- Macula involved.

 Note

Macular cortex has double blood supply from middle cerebral artery and posterior cerebral artery independent of each other.

EXAMINATION OF OPTIC FUNDUS

Key Points

- Macula is about 2 disc diameter from temporal border of the optic disc.

- Normally nasal border of the disc is less clear.
- Temporal half of the retina is less vascular and may be pale.
- Drusen of the optic nerve (developmental abnormality in the optic nerve head) can cause visual loss (due to collection of protein and calcium in the optic nerve can cause pseudopapilledema).

Papilledema

- Swelling of the optic nerve head due to raised intracranial tension as a result of intracranial mass lesion.
- Other conditions which cause swelling of optic nerve head is called edema of optic nerve head.

Conditions Which can Mimic Papilledema

- Myelinated fibers
- High myopia
- Deep optic cusp

Pathogenesis of Papilledema

- Increased in the CSF pressure—causes edema of the axons causing decreased axoplasmic flow.
- Venous congestion occurs due to swelling of axons causing disturbance in the retinal venous return. This increases the swelling of axons further causing edema of the optic nerve head.

Effect of Long Standing Papilledema

Results in visual field defect and optic atrophy (secondary).

Effect of Papilledema on the Retina and Optic Nerve Head

- Edema of cells of retina
- Exudates and hemorrhage in the retina
- Causes blind spot enlargement
- Gliotic changes in the optic nerve head.
- Other abnormalities like structural lesion of the nervous system which causes papilledema can also cause visual defect.

Different Types of Visual Field Defects

Incongruous hemianopia: Occurs due to lesion of optic tract and chiasma—outline of visual field loss in both eyes is different.

Congruous hemianopia

Lesion—optic radiation: Outline of visual field loss in both eyes are similar.

Lesion of lateral geniculate body causes congruous homonymous field defect.

Parietal lobe lesion

- Results in visual inattention.
- Failure to perceive an object in one-half of the visual field when presented
- Bilaterally
- Can cause opposite lower quadrantanopia.

Monoocular visual loss

Occurs due to

- Optic neuritis
- Multiple sclerosis
- Orbital tumor

Binocular visual loss

- Chiasma compression
- Increased intracranial pressure
- Toxins like alcohol.

Pseudopapilledema

- There will be optic disc appearing filled
- No congestion of veins
- There will be apparent swelling of the optic disc.

Causes

- Myelinated nerve fibers
- Drusen of the optic nerve
- Hypermetropia.

3rd, 4th and 6th Cranial Nerves

Important Clinical Points

3rd cranial nerve: There is single unpaired nucleus for both-sided levator palpabrae superioris.

4th cranial nerve

- Passes posteriorly emerges from dorsum of the midbrain.

- Left 4th nerve nucleus supplies opposite superior oblique.

Movement of eyes

- Upward direction: 30°–40°
- Downward direction: 50°–60°
- Medial direction: 50°
- Lateral direction: 60° to 70°

Action of extraocular muscles

Recti-act in the direction according to their names and act when the eye is in abducted position.

Oblique

- Act in the direction opposite to their names.
- Act when the eye is in adducted position.

Superior recti—elevate
Inferior recti—depress
Superior oblique—depress
Inferior oblique—elevate
Internal rotation

- Superior oblique
- Superior rectus

External rotation

- Inferior oblique
- Inferior rectus.

Bilateral Ptosis

Causes

- Myasthenia gravis
- Myopathy
- Bilateral Horner's syndrome
- Snakebite
- Botulism.

Differences between paralytic squint and concomitant squint

Paralytic squint	Concomitant squint
• Occurs in adults	Occurs as congenital defect
• Diplopia is present	Diplopia is absent
• No visual defect	Vision affected
• Eye movement affected	Eye movements not affected

Oculomotor (3rd) Nerve

Clinical Aspects

- Superior rectus is supplied by contralateral 3rd nerve nucleus
- Single nucleus supplies both levator palpabrae superioris
- Pupillo-constrictor fibers—parasympathetic fibers lie superficially in the 3rd nerve.
- Recti muscles which vertically act are most active when the eye is abducted
- Oblique muscles are active when the eye is adducted.

Extraocular Muscle Testing

Direction of action of muscles

- Medial rectus—inwards and horizontal
- Lateral rectus—outwards and horizontal
- Interior rectus—eye is down and out
- Superior rectus—eye is up and out.
- Inferior oblique—eye is up and inwards.
- Superior oblique—eye is down and inwards
- Levator palpabrae superioris—elevation of upper eyelid.
- When testing for extraocular muscles—test the individual eye separately and hold the object at a distance of one foot.

3rd Nerve Palsy

Features

- Complete ptosis (diplopia is usually absent due to complete ptosis)
- Pupil fixed and dilated.
- Eye down and out.

Outward position: Due to action of lateral rectus.

Downward position: Due to superior oblique secondary depressive action.

Ptosis of 3rd nerve palsy

- Ptosis complete (inability to lift the upper lid even with effort).
- Wrinkling of forehead occurs due to compensatory action of frontalis in an attempt to lift the upper eyelid.

 Note

In myogenic ptosis it is usually unilateral and pupil is not involved.

Testing for 4th nerve in the presence of 3rd nerve palsy

- Patient is asked to look downwards and towards the nose (medially)
- If intact 4th nerve eyeball movement does not occur but blood vessels of the conjunctiva appear to intort.

Marcus Gunn Phenomenon

- Winking movement of upper eyelid occurs whenever there is lower jaw movement.
- Due to motor branch of trigeminal nerve supplying lateral pterygoid becomes aberrantly connected with fibers of 3rd cranial nerve supplying levator palpabrae superioris.
- May be a genetic disorder.

PUPIL

- Normal pupil size 2–5 mm
- Miosis—pupil less than 2 mm
- Midriasis—pupil more than 6 mm

Clinical Aspects

- In compressive pathology of 3rd nerve pupil is involved early, e.g. uncal herniation: Hutchison's pupil.
- Diabetic can have abnormal pupil due to autonomic neuropathy.
- Diphtheria can cause paralysis of accommodation.
- In Wernicke's hemianopic pupil: Light reflex response is better when the light is shown to intact half of retina.
- Diabetics develop pupil sparing ophthalmoplegia.

Light Near Dissociation

- Accommodation reflex preserved
- Light reflex is affected

- Can occur in neurosyphilis
- Dorsal (rostral midbrain lesion—pinealoma, Parinaud's syndrome).

Argyll Robertson Pupil (ARP)

Features

- Light reflex is lost or very poor. Accommodation reflex is intact—light near dissociation.
- Light reflex pathways are damaged.
- Pupil is irregular and small and atropine cannot dilate it.
- Local lesion of the iris may be present.

Lesion: Rostral midbrain/pre-tectal area

Causes

- Neurosyphilis
- Diabetes mellitus

Marcus Gunn Pupil

- Occurs in patient with retrobulbar neuritis.
- Afferent pupillary reflex pathway is defective.
- When the affected eye is directly stimulated
- There will be short duration of slow incomplete constriction of pupil
- Direct light reflex is weaker compared to consensual reflex.

Swinging Torch Test for Demonstration of Marcus Gunn Pupil

Throw the light and swing it from one eye to the other

- Light is thrown to the normal eye—both pupils constrict.
- This is due to intact light reflex of normal eye and normal consensual reflex of the affected side eye.
- Swing back to the light to the affected eye—observe for dilatation of pupil due to weaker light reflex due to afferent pathway defect on the affected side and more effective consensual reflex on the affected side.

- Swinging of light from one eye to the other normal eye constricts, affected eye dilates.

Wernicke's Hemianopic Pupil

- Present in patients with the lesion of the optic tract.
- There will be absent of light reflex and pupillary constriction when light is shown on the temporal half of the retina on the affected side and nasal half on the opposite side.
- Light reflex is present when the light is thrown on the nasal half of the retina on the affected side and temporal half on the opposite side.

Diplopia

Clinical Aspects

- Separation of image is greatest in the direction of action of weak muscle.
- False image is more peripheral.
- Cataract and macular disease can cause uniocular diplopia.
- Binocular diplopia occurs due to extra ocular muscle paralysis.
- Horizontal diplopia occurs due to recti (medial and lateral recti) muscle weakness.
- Vertical diplopia occurs due to oblique muscle weakness.

TROCHLEAR (4th Cranial Nerve)

Clinical Aspects

- Has got longest intracranial course
- Get injured in a patient of head injury
- Diplopia—maximal with downward gaze
- Head tilt will be away from the affected side.

Head tilt in 4th nerve palsy: Head tilt in 4th nerve palsy will be to the opposite side of the side affected to avoid diplopia. By this there will be better alignment of eyes.

TRIGEMINAL NERVE

Trigeminal nerve has got both motor and sensory components.

Motor component—mandibular division supplies: Muscles of mastication.

Sensory components

- Ophthalmic ⎤
- Maxillary   ⎬ Facial
- Mandibular ⎦ sensation
- Motor-nucleus-midpons

Muscles of Mastication

Masseter

- Temporalis
- Medial pterygoid
- Lateral pterygoid
- Other muscles supplied
  - Anterior belly of digastric
  - Mylohyoid
  - Tensor veli palatini
  - Tensor tympani.

Sensory Part of Trigeminal Nerve

Sensory ganglion: Gasserian ganglion lies in the apex of the Petrous part of temporal bone (Meckel's cave).

3 sensory divisions

Ophthalmic branch

- Upper part of face up to vertex
- Orbital structures
- Upper part of nose tentorium cerebelli, dura mater. Falx cerebri
- Maxillary division—middle part of facial structures. Middle cranial fossa
- Sphenopalatine ganglion and lacrimal gland.
- Mandibular nerve: Lower part of facial structures up to the angle of the mandible.

Note

Angle of the mandible is supplied by C2/C3 segment.

Key Points Regarding Sensory Supply of Face

- There is onion skin like representation of facial sensations.
- Fibers from central part of face synapse— most rostrally in the nucleus of spinal tract of trigeminal nerve in the brainstem.

- Fibers from outer part of face synapse at the level of C2–C3 in the nucleus of spinal tract of trigeminal nerve.
- Corneal reflex is lost early in the initial lesion of Vth nerve.
- Motor nucleus of the trigeminal nerve lies in the pons and supplies muscles of mastication

Sensory nuclei of trigeminal nerve

1. Fibers carrying proprioception predominantly of muscles of mastication after entering the pons travel up to the midbrain (mesencephalon) and terminate in the mesencephalic nucleus.
2. Fibers carrying touch, pressure and vibration sensation of face enter the pons and terminate in the principal sensory nucleus in the pons itself.
3. Fibers carrying pain and temperature of face travel down to the cervical cord and terminate in the nucleus of spinal tract of trigeminal nerve.

Clinical Examination of Vth Nerve

Clinical Aspects

- Wasting of temporalis produces hollowing of temple part of face.
- Wasting of masseter produces flattening of jaw on one side

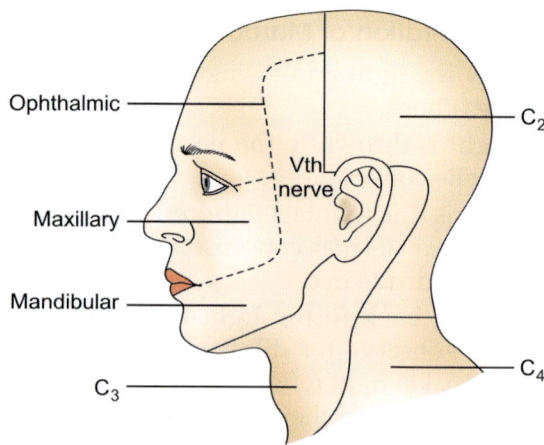

Fig. 4.6: Sensory supply of trigeminal nerve

Flowchart 4.1: Sensory pathway of trigeminal nerve

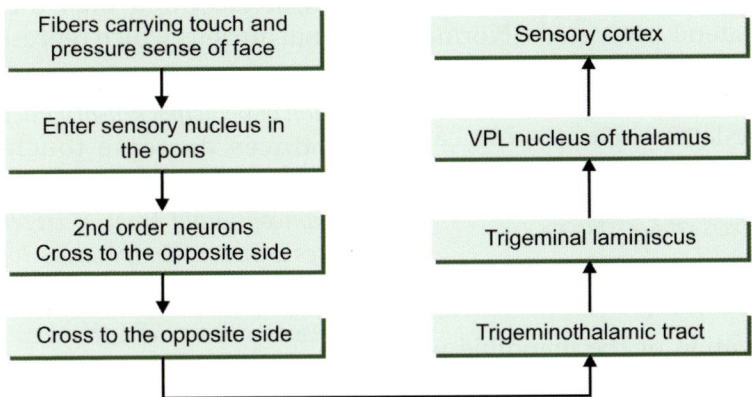

Flowchart 4.2

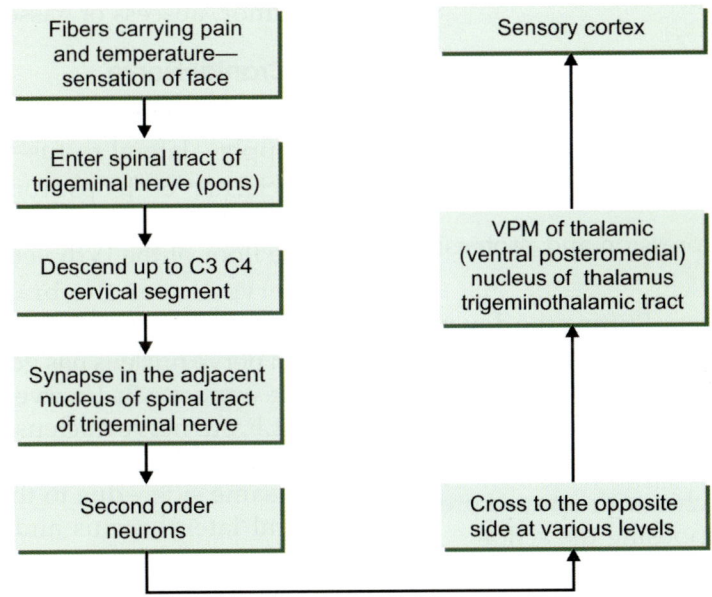

Flowchart 4.3

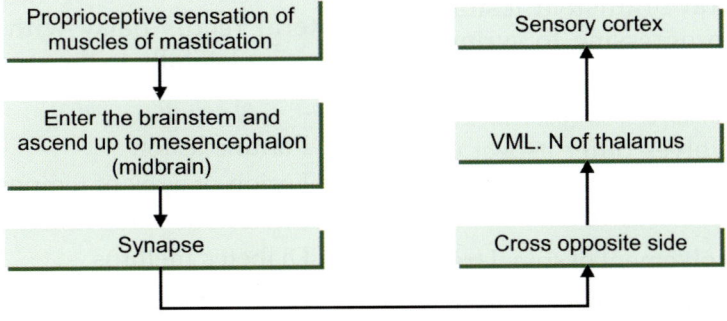

- Vth nerve lesion on one side—jaw deviates to the same side due to unopposed action of opposite lateral pterygoid. (Normally incisor teeth, philtrum of lip and tip of nose should be in the same line).
- Amyotrophic lateral sclerosis can cause dropping of the jaw.

Actions of Muscles of Mastication

Masseter: Elevation of mandible and closing the mouth. Can help in protrusion of the jaw.

Temporalis: Elevation of the mandible with closing the jaw. Can retract the jaw with pulling the posteriorly.

Medial pterygoid: Elevation of the mandible and closure of the jaw. Can cause protrusion of the jaw.

Lateral pterygoid
- *Acting bilaterally*: Forward movement of the jaw.
- *Unilateral action*: Side to side movement of the jaw.
- Can help in depression and protrusion of the jaw.

Testing for jaw closure: Putting the downward pressure with the examiner's thumb kept over the bony prominence of the patient's chin with patient opposing the action.

Testing for jaw opening: Putting the finger or thumb under the chin with upward pressure and the patient opposing the action.

Sensory Aspects of 5th Nerve

Balaclava helmet distribution of sensory loss (onion skin or onion peel sensory loss): Occurs in central brainstem lesion, e.g. syringomyelia progressing to syringobulbia.

Distribution of sensory loss (balaclava helmet distribution): Involves outer aspect of face sparing central part like mouth and nose resemble balaclava helmet.

Due to initial involvement of spinal tract and nucleus of trigeminal nerve (lower part at cervical level first representing the outer part of face) and then the upper part of spinal nucleus which represents central part of face.

Lesion of principal sensory nucleus in the pons— produces decrease touch and pressure sensation over the facial structures.

Lesion of spinal tract of trigeminal nerve produces pain and temperature loss of facial structures.

Causes for lesion of Vth nerve
- Tumors of Vth nerve
- Demyelination.
- Vascular lesion of brainstem
- Syringomyelia
- Tumor/abscess of gasserian ganglion

6th Cranial Nerve

- Nuclear position: Pons
- Supply—lateral rectus—same side
- Facial nerve—loops around the sixth nerve nucleus forms facial colliculus visible in the floor of the IVth ventricle.
- Nerve leaves the brainstem at ponto medullary junction.
- 6th nerve nucleus has got connection with the opposite 3rd nerve nucleus through MLF. 6th nerve nucleus is responsible for horizontal gaze (movement of both eyes to same side—due to the action of ipsilateral lateral rectus and opposite medial rectus).

Nuclear lesion of 6th nerve Results in horizontal gaze palsy to the same side.

Nerve lesion of 6th nerve: Results in ipsilateral lateral rectus palsy with diplopia while looking laterally to the same side.

Causes of 6th nerve palsy
- Pontine lesion
- Lesion of apex of temporal bone.
- Cavernous sinus lesion
- Diabetes mellitus
- Vasculitis.

False localising lesion of 6th nerve

False localising lesion: Neurological abnormality results due to the pathology at a site which is away from the actual site of anatomical abnormality.

False localising sign 6th nerve: Due to raised intracranial tension. There will be downward displacement of brainstem with compression of 6th nerve.

Pseudoabducens palsy

Features:
- Abducens nerve normal
- Abduction is affected.

Lesion: Due to involvement of inhibitory convergent pathways which inhibit convergence which descend from temporo-occipital cortex to the upper midbrain.

Site of lesion: Thalamus, upper midbrain.

CLINICAL EXAMINATION OF FACIAL NERVE

Anatomical Aspects

Facial nucleus
- Motor nucleus: Pons
- Lacrimal nucleus and superior salivatory nucleus: Pons: For lacrimal and salivary glands.

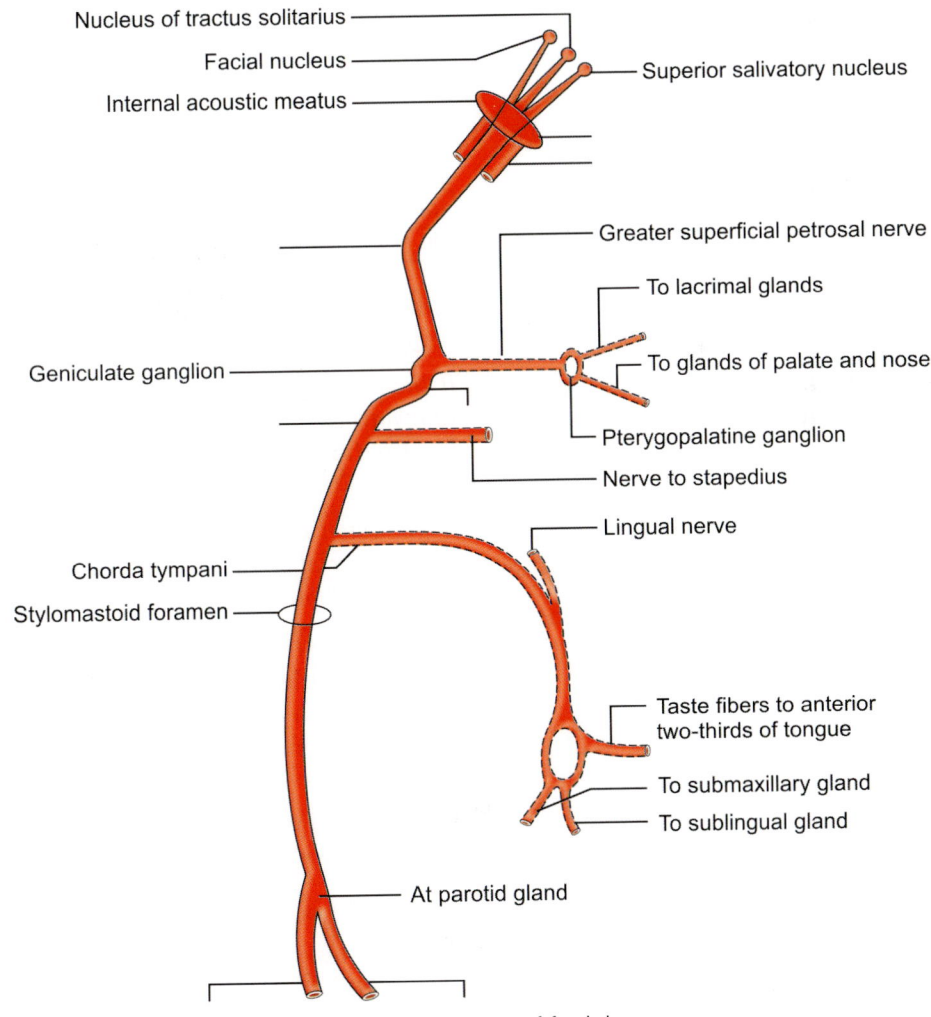

Fig. 4.7: LMN course of facial nerve

Nucleus of solitarius: For taste fibers of anterior two-thirds of tongue.

Nervous intermedius: Joins the motor component as it exists from the pons.

Nervous intermedius has got following connections

Superior salivatory nucleus (pons)

- Via greater superficial petrosal nerve supply fibers to lacrimal glands
- Via chorda tympani nerve to submandibular and salivary glands

Nucleus solitarius (medulla)

Via chorda tympani nerve: Taste fibers for anterior two-thirds of tongue.

Types of Facial Palsy

Upper motor neuron facial palsy

- Volitional
- Mimitic

Lower motor neuron facial palsy

Mimitic (emotional) facial palsy

- Facial palsy is present only on emotional movement like laughing.
- Voluntary movement does not show any abnormality.
- Can have masked-like face.

Lesion

- Frontal lobe.
- Fibers of emotional movement travel separately from corticobulbar fibers of facial nerves. Occurs usually in bilateral lesion.

Unilateral LMN facial palsy: Whole of face is affected on the side of the lesion with the presence of Bell's phenomenon.

Bilateral LMN facial palsy

Features

- All voluntary movements not possible.
- Normal facial folds are lost. Verify
- Sagging of corners of mouth
- When patient is trying to close the eyes sclera is seen.

Bilateral UMN facial palsy: Occurs in pseudobulbar palsy.

Causes

- Multi-infarct state
- Amyotrophic lateral sclerosis

Features

- UMN facial on both sides (may behave like bilateral LMN facial palsy)
- May have involuntary crying and laughing
- Brisk jaw jerk
- Bilateral pyramidal tract signs
- Blinking—not affected
- Bell's phenomenon absent.

Minimal facial palsy

- Ask the patient to close the eye tightly
- If orbicularis oculi is weak—it can be easily opened with the thumb—indicates minimal weakness of orbicularis oculi.

 Note

Normally when the person is asked to close the eye tightly vibrations of the eyelid can be felt. This may be lost in early facial palsy.

Other Important Clinical Aspects of LMN Facial Palsy

If the lesion lies between brainstem and chorda tympani origin: There will be loss of salivation, lacrimation, taste and there will be hyperacusis with same side facial palsy.

If the lesion is before chorda tympani and after the superficial petrosal nerve: Taste and salivation is lost but lacrimation is normal.

Melkersson syndrome

- Combination: LMN 7th nerve paralysis (recurrent) and facial swelling especially upper lip and fissuring of tongue (Table 4.1).
- May have genetic origin.
- It can be a manifestation of Crohn's disease or sarcoidosis.

Aberrant Innervation of Facial Nerve

Crocodile tears

1. Activity of facial muscles such as eating causes tearing.

Table 4.1: Difference between bilateral UMN 7th versus bilateral LMN 7th nerve palsy

Bilateral UMN 7th nerve palsy	*Bilateral LMN 7th nerve palsy*
Long tract signs +	No long tract signs
Brisk jaw jerk	Jaw jerk not involved
Emotional fibers spared	Involved
Bell's phenomenon absent	Present
Corneal reflex preserved	Absent

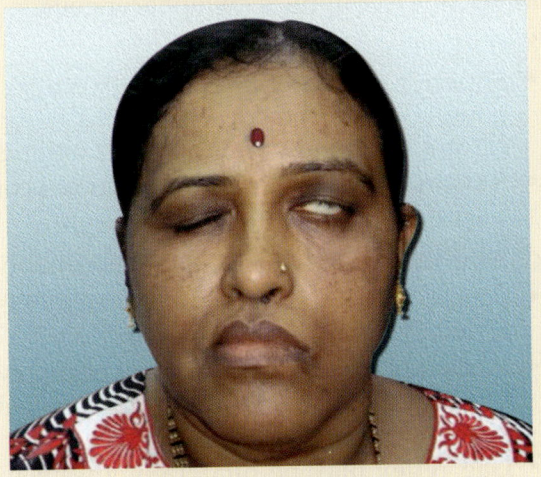

Unilateral LMN facial palsy (left)

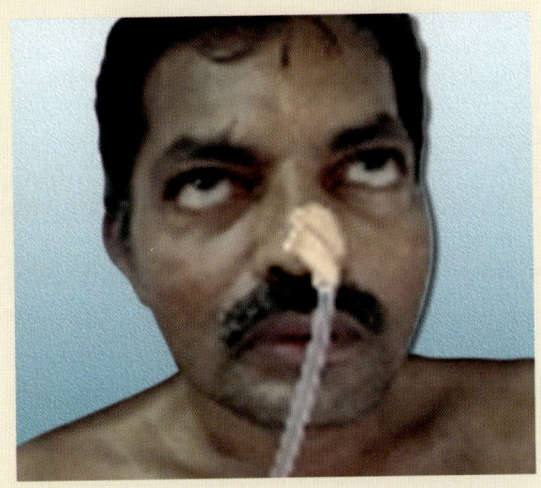

Bilateral LMN facial palsy in a patient of GB syndrome (note the Bell's phenomenon)

Due to nerve fibers which are originally innervating facial muscles become innervating lacrimal gland.

2. Closure of eyelid due to facial movement. Aberrant innervations of orbicularis oculi by the fibers which were innervating orbicularis oris.

8th Cranial Nerve (Vestibulocochlear Nerve)

Vestibular component and pathway

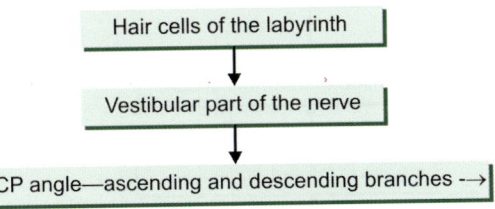

End in vestibular nuclei of pons and medulla (medial, lateral, superior and inferior vestibular nuclei).

Vestibular nuclei connect with
- Spinal cord
- Cerebellum
- Thalamus
- Sensory and motor cortex
- Temporal lobe.

Clinical aspects of vestibular nerve
- Each vestibular system on one side tries to push the body, extremities and eye to the opposite side.
- There is a tendency to fall to the side of lesion.
- Direction of nystagmus (fast component) opposite to the side of lesion.
- Normal doll's eye phenomenon indicates intact brainstem connection between vestibular nuclei and cranial nuclei in pons and midbrain.
- For positional nystagmus Hallpike or Nylen-Bárány maneuver—*refer to Manipal Manual of Clinical Medicine.*

Auditory pathway (Flowchart 4.4)
Cochlear component.

📝 *Note*

- *Cochlear nerve in the brainstem joins ventral and dorsal cochlear nucleus. From the ventral cochlear nucleus fibers cross to the opposite side and joins lateral leminiscus.*
- *Fibers from the dorsal cochlear nucleus cross to the opposite side and joins the superior olivary nucleus and then joins the lateral lemniscus.*

Cochlear component (Clinical aspects)

- Air conduction occurs through pinna, tympanic membrane and ossicles of the ear.
- Bone conduction occurs from skull bones directly to the inner ear of the same side and also to the opposite side.

Weber's test: In sensory neural hearing loss both bone conduction and air conduction is decreased on the affected side.

During Weber's test: Lateralised to normal ear in neuronal deafness (affected ear hearing is decreased both by air and bone conduction because of nerve pathology).

Lateralised to affected ear in conductive deafness (better bone conduction on the affected side through skull bones and external noise is masked because of conductive deafness).

Rinne's test in conductive deafness: Bone conduction is better than air conduction because there is inhibition of conduction through ear passage and middle ear.

GLOSSOPHARYNGEAL NERVE

Location of the nucleus—medulla: Passes through jugular foramen, reaches the carotid sheath and reaches lateral pharyngeal wall.

Motor supply: Supplies stylopharyngeus.

Sensory and autonomic supply

- Superior and inferior glossopharyngeal ganglia—connected with carotid body, carotid sinus and posterior 1/3 of tongue.
- Sensory fibers terminate in the nucleus of tractus solitarius.

Clinical aspects of glossopharyngeal nerve

- Posterior 1/3 of tongue taste sensation is tested by galavanic stimulation.
- While testing gag reflex afferent pathway is mainly contributed by glossopharyngeal nerve.
- Gag reflex may be bilaterally absent in some normal individuals.
- Lowering of palatal arch may occur on the affected side due to 9th nerve palsy.

Vagus nerve

Dorsal motor nucleus of vagus: Supplies all visceral structures.

Nucleus ambiguous

- Supplies pharyngeal and laryngeal muscles.

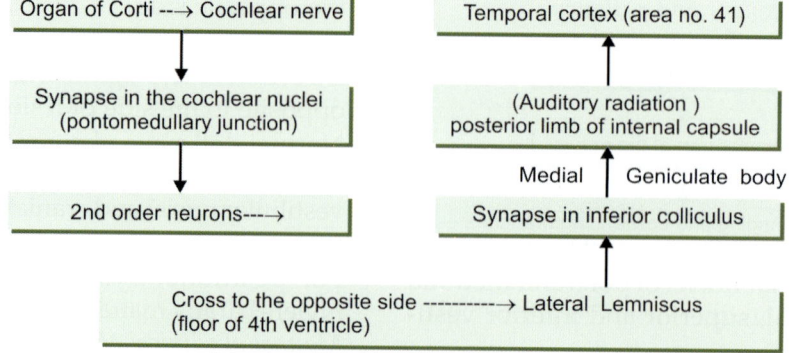

Flowchart 4.4: Auditory pathway

- Taste fibers from epiglottis reach nucleus of tractus solitarius.
- Sensory from oropharynx, viscera and upper bowel reach the vagus.

ACCESSORY NERVE

Cranial Part

Cranial part of the accessory nerve joins the vagus nerve and supplies muscles of soft palate.

Spinal part: Arise from C1–C5 segments of cervical spinal cord and joins the cranial part.

Spinal part supplies: Sternomastoid and trapezius and cervical muscles.

Supranuclear control of sternomastoid
- Control is ipsilateral
- In hemiplegia due to vascular lesion, e.g. internal capsular lesion. There will be sternomastoid weakness on the side of the lesion.

Clinical aspects of 11th cranial nerve
- Atrophy of trapezius causes depression of the shoulder with loss of contour of the shoulder.
- Dropped head can occur in patients with myasthenia gravis, amyotrophic lateral sclerosis and polymyositis.

12th Cranial Nerve (Hypoglossal Nerve)

Motor nucleus: Medial medulla

Supply: Muscles of tongue

Clinical aspects
- Ipsilateral involvement of hypoglossal nerve causes deviation of tongue to the same side (because of action of opposite genioglossus) of the lesion.
- In long standing atrophy of tongue— becomes curved to the ipsilateral side.
- In LMN paralysis of 12th cranial nerve there will be fasciculations on the affected side of the tongue which can appear like bag of worms.

OCULAR MOVEMENTS AND GAZE PALSY

Types of Eyeball Movements

Saccadic Eyeball Movements
- There is rapid movement of eyes
- Rapid changing of point of fixation occurs
- There is rapid jump from one eye position to the other.
- Usually occurs while scanning a visual scene.

Smooth Pursuit Movement

Occurs whenever smooth tracking of the object in the visual field occurs.

Centre of pursuit movement: Junction of occipito-parietal and temporal cortex.

Vergence movement
- Both eyes may move in a different direction so that nearer or further away object in the visual field is seen.
- It may be convergence or divergence of eye movement.

Vestibulo-ocular movement
- This is the eye movement which occurs in response to the position of the head/neck.
- This movement helps for focusing of the eye on the target whenever there is movement of head.
- This movement takes place with the participation of vestibular nucleus and its connections with the cerebellum, nuclei of 3rd, 4th, 6th nerves, parapontine reticular formation and MLF.

Conjugate movement of eyes: Both eyes move in the same direction and angular relationship of these eyes is maintained.

Gaze Palsy
- Inability of the conjugate movement or difficulty to move both eyes in the same direction is called gaze palsy.
- Gaze palsies may be vertical or horizontal. Vertical gaze palsy may be for upward or downward gaze.
- Patients with gaze palsy do not complain of diplopia

Vertical Gaze

Supranuclear Control and Connections

Cortical center: No single cortical center.

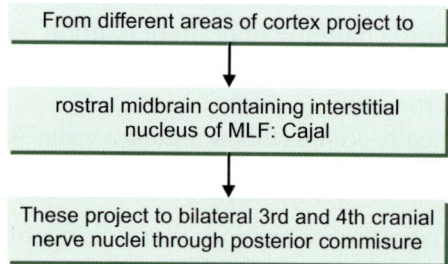

From different areas of cortex project to
↓
rostral midbrain containing interstitial nucleus of MLF: Cajal
↓
These project to bilateral 3rd and 4th cranial nerve nuclei through posterior commisure

Vertical gaze palsy: Inability of both eyes to move either upward or downward.
Upward gaze center: Rostral midbrain
Downward gaze center: Rostral midbrain

Vertical gaze palsy

Causes

- Progressive supranuclear palsy.
- Huntington's chorea.
- Wernicke's encephalopathy
- Parkinson's disease.
- In progressive supranuclear palsy there is initial difficulty of downward gaze and then of upward gaze.

Horizontal gaze: Ability of the two eyes to move in the same direction in a horizontal plane.

Cortical center and connections

- *Frontal eye field (area no. 8)* is the cortical center for horizontal gaze.
- Activation of frontal eye field, there will be horizontal movement of eyes to the opposite side.

Frontal eye field (area no. 8) is connected to

- Corona radiata, and internal capsule
- Project to the opposite parapontine reticular formation (PPRF) and also abducens.
- Nucleus

↓

- Connect to opposite 3rd nerve nucleus through MLF

- Stimulation of PPRF and abducens nucleus move the eye to the same side.

Median longitudinal fasciculus (MLF)

- Present in the brainstem
- Arises from abducens nucleus in the pons and connects the contralateral 3rd nerve nucleus in the midbrain.

Gaze Preference in a Hemiplegic

Cortical lesion (frontal eye field—area no. 8)
Irritative lesion of area no. 8: Eyes are horizontally deviated to the opposite side (eyes look towards the hemiplegic side).
Paralytic (destructive lesion of area no. 8): Eyes are horizontally deviated to the side of lesion (person looks away from hemiplegic side).

Brainstem lesion

Destructive lesion of pons: Eye is deviated to the hemiplegic side (opposite PPRF pulls the eye towards the hemiplegic side)—away from the site of lesion.

Pursuit Movement Pathway

Occipital eye field → Pontine nuclei → Ponto cerebellar fibers → Floccules of the cerebellum → Vestibular complex → Nuclei of extra ocular muscles

Basal ganglia disease and gaze palsy

- Over action of basal ganglia causes occulogyric crises.
- Underactivity of basal ganglia causes impaired vertical gaze.

In progressive supranuclear palsy: Impairment of downward gaze initially and then upward gaze.

Internuclear ophthalmoplegia: Occurs due to the lesion of MLF. There is disconnection between one side ipsilateral 3rd nerve nucleus and opposite side 6th nerve nucleus.

Anterior internuclear ophthalmoplegia

Features: Defective convergence on the ipsilateral side with abducting eye showing nystagmus (adducting eye fails to adduct and abducting eye shows nystagmus).

Lesion: Midbrain

Cause of nystagmus in internuclear ophthalmoplegia:

Possible attempt by the brain to compensate for the adduction weakness.

Posterior internuclear ophthalmoplegia

• Convergence—not affected
• Lesion—near midbrain.

One and half syndrome: Occurs in lesion of pons midline lesion due to the lesion of VIth nerve nucleus or parapontine reticular formation and MLF on one side.

Results in: Horizontal gaze palsy.

One and half syndrome occurs due to (if on right side)

• Right VI nerve nuclear palsy—failure to abduction to right
• Right MLF lesion—failure of adduction of right eye
• Right MLF lesion—failure of adduction of left eye
• Only movement possible—left eye abduction.

Bilateral internuclear ophthalmoplegia

Lesion: Midbrain

Involves bilateral MLF and 3rd nerve nucleus.

Features

• Affects convergence
• There will be bilateral divergence of eyes
• It is called walled eye bilateral INO (WEBINO)

PSEUDOBULBAR PALSY

What is Pseudobulbar Palsy?

Features of involvement of lower cranial nerves but lesion is above the brainstem.

Site of lesion: Bilateral frontal cortex

Causes

• Motor neuron disease
• Multiple infarcts.
• Multiple brain trauma
• Osmotic demyelination
• Multiple sclerosis.

Structures involved: Bilateral descending corticobulbar, pyramidal tract including emotional control fibers.

Features

• Emotional incontinence
• Lower cranial nerve involvement of UMN type
• Brisk jaw jerk
• Bilateral pyramidal tract involvement

Speech in (due to small and stiff tongue) pseudobulbar palsy

• Called hot potato speech
• Due to inadequate movement of tongue
• Inadequate movement of muscles of speech production causes spastic dysarthria (strainful speech).

Bulbar Palsy

Due to lesion in the medulla causing LMN cranial nerve palsy—lower 9th, 10th and 11th and 12th nerves (either the nuclear lesion or lesion of the fascicle of the nerves).

Table 4.2: Differences between bulbar and pseudobulbar palsy		
	Bulbar palsy	*Pseudobulbar palsy*
• Type of lesion	LMN	UMN
• Facial muscles	Uni/bilateral (weak)	Bilateral (stiff)
• Gag reflex	Absent	Brisk
• Tongue involvement	Flabby with fasciculations	Small and stiff
• Emotional upsets	No involuntary laughing/crying	Involuntary laughing/crying
• Jaw jerk	Not involved/absent	Brisk
• Pyramidal signs	Absent	Bilaterally present with extensor plantar
• Speech	Nasal	Thick-spastic

Causes
- Vascular medullary infarction
- MND—progressive bulbar palsy
- Glioma of the medulla.

Features: LMN involvement of lower cranial nerves 9th, 10th, 11th and 12th.

Speech in bulbar palsy
- Nasal quality of speech
- Speech is slow and slurred.

Nystagmus
- Jerky oscillations—usually unequal
- Slow drift in one direction
- Fast drift—correcting movement

Type of Nystagmus and Site of Lesion

Type of nystagmus	*Site of lesion*
- Horizontal	Cerebellar
- Vertical	Brainstem
- Rotating	Labyrinthine

Convergence retraction nystagmus
- Occurs in Parinaud's syndrome
- Fast phase in convergent direction

See-saw nystagmus
- Movement of one eye will be raising and intorting.
- Movement of other will be falling downwards and extorting.
- *Site of lesion*: Midbrain tegmentum

Down beat nystagmus: Site of lesion CV junction anomaly.

CEREBELLOPONTINE ANGLE

Cerebellopontine angle (CP angle) is the triangle formed by
- Medially cerebellum and lateral part of pons
- Laterally by inner part of petrous part of temporal bone

Vertical extent of CP angle
- Upper part Vth nerve
- Lower part 9th cranial nerve
- 6th cranial nerve runs upwards and over the medial edge of the triangle

Structures traversing through the triangle: Facial and vestibulocochlear nerves traverse through the angle from internal auditory meatus.

Causes of CP angle mass lesions
- Acoustic neuroma (schwannoma of vestibulocochlear nerve)
- Tumor of the facial nerve
- Meningioma
- Arachnoid cyst

Features
- Can present as slowly progressive lesions (may grow up to 20–30 years)
- Can start as decrease of hearing
- Vertigo, ataxia, numbness over the face and hemifacial spasm can be the manifestations at presentation and can cause hydrocephalus.

Signs
- Corneal reflex can be early host.
- CP angle mass can lift and distort the afferent fibers of corneal reflex.
- LMN facial palsy—may be late
- Can have 8th nerve lesions, cerebellar ataxia and pyramidal tract involvement.

HORNER'S SYNDROME

Horner's syndrome occurs due to: Interruption of sympathetic supply to the eye.

Triad of Horner's syndrome: Partial ptosis, miosis and anhydrosis of ipsilateral face.

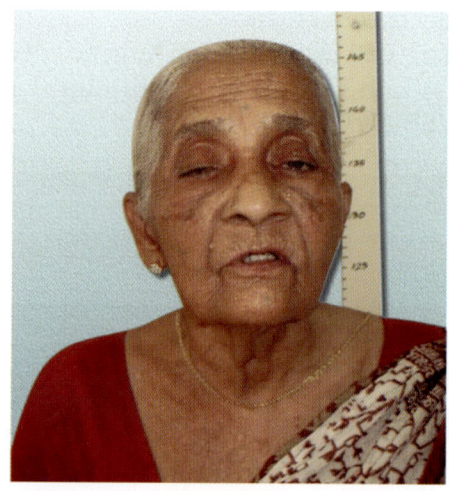

Fig. 4.8: Right ptosis in a patient of Horner's syndrome

Sympathetic supply to the eye
(Flowchart 4.5).

Causes of Horner's syndrome

1. *Due to lesion of higher centres (1st order neurons)*
   - Hypothalamic/cortical lesion
   - Brainstem lesion
   - Lateral medullary syndrome
   - Syringobulbia

- Multiple sclerosis
- Vertebral artery dissection

2. *At the level of cervical sympathetic chain and superior cervical ganglion*
   - Cervical rib
   - Pancoast's tumor
   - Lesion of common carotid
   - Injury to brachial plexus

Flowchart 4.5

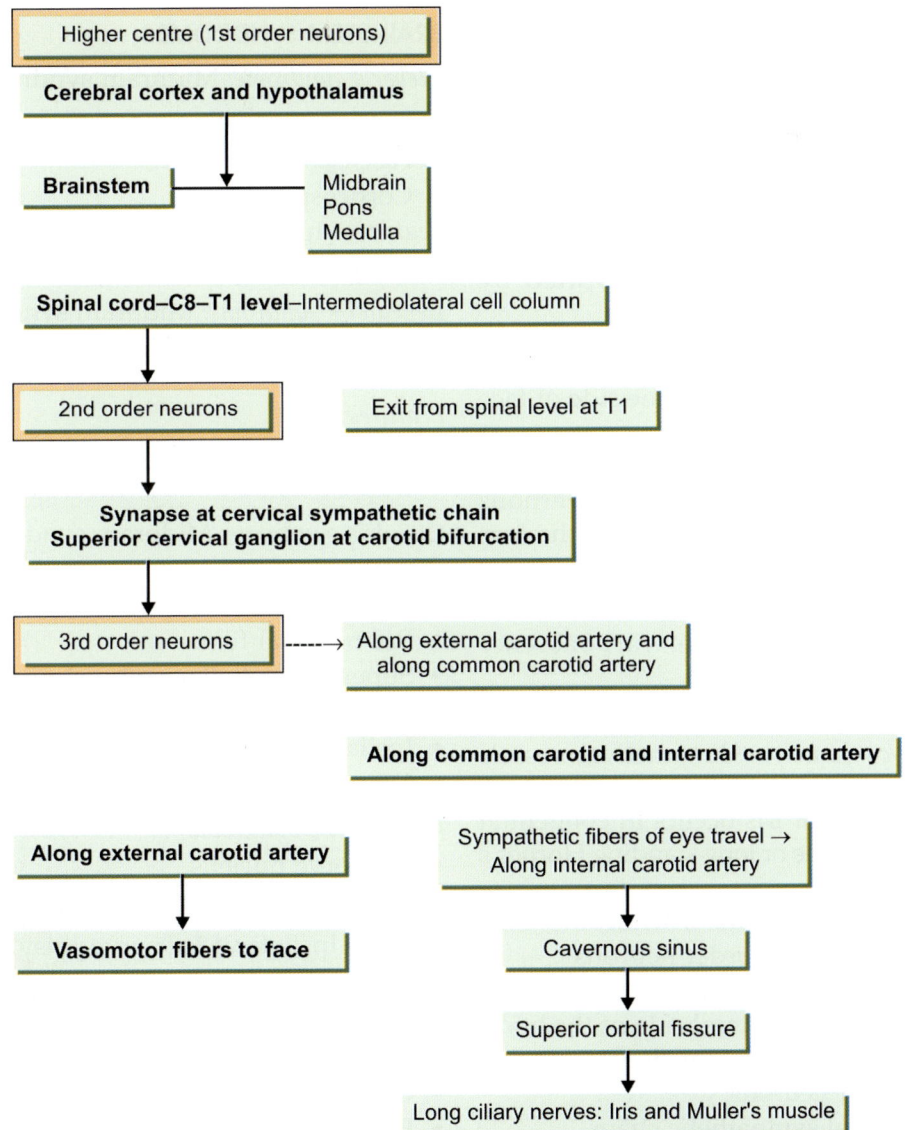

3. *After carotid bifurcation*
   • Dissection of internal carotid
   • Cavernous sinus lesions.

Clinical Features

1. *Ptosis*—partial ptosis due to Muller's muscle involvement.

 Note

Slight elevation of lower eyelid can occur due to involvement of lower eyelid muscle.

2. *Miosis* due to paralysis of sympathetic supply to iris.
3. *Enophthalmos*
   • Actual enophthalmos does not occur.
   • It appears due to narrow palpebral fissure.

Narrow palpebral fissure occurs due to
1. Ptosis of upper eyelid.
2. Elevation of lower eye due to involvement of lower eyelid muscle (supplied by sympathetic).

Anihidrosis
• Loss of sweating on the same side of face of the side of lesion.
• If sympathetic fibers of eye get affected after carotid bifurcation, e.g. cavernous sinus thrombosis—anhidrosis of the face will be absent.

Loss of ciliospinal reflex: If the skin on the back of the neck is pinched—there will be absence of dilatation of the pupil.

Other features
Blood shot conjunctiva: Conjunctival vessels dilate due to absence of vasoconstriction. (Heterochromia of iris occurs in congenital Horner's syndrome or long standing Horner's syndrome).
• Site of lesion in Horner's syndrome
• Higher centers: 1st order neurons
Features
• Anhidrosis of ipsilateral side of the body
• Other cortical/brainstem signs.
  – 2nd order neurons
  – At cervical sympathetic chain

• Signs depending on the cause of lesion
• Ipsilateral face will have anhidrosis

After carotid bifurcation and at the level of cavernous sinus
• Associated with 5th, 6th cranial nerve palsy
• No anhidrosis of face.

 Note

Massive infarct of one hemisphere, or thalamic hemorrhage can cause Horner's syndrome on the side of the lesion.

BRAINSTEM SYNDROMES

Weber's syndrome: Midbrain syndrome.

Structures involved
• Fascicles of 3rd nerve
• Corticospinal fibers.
Features: Ipsilateral 3rd nerve palsy with opposite side hemiplegia.

Benedict's syndrome: Midbrain syndrome.
Structures involved: Fascicles of 3rd nerve and red nucleus.
Features
• Ipsilateral 3rd nerve palsy
• Opposite side tremor/choreoathetosis.

Claude's syndrome: Midbrain syndrome.
Structures
• 3rd nerve involved; Red nucleus
• Rubrodental fibers
• Superior cerebellar peduncle
Features
• Ipsilateral 3rd nerve palsy
• Opposite side: Ataxia and tremor.

Nothnagel's syndrome
• 3rd nerve nucleus
• Superior cerebellar peduncle.

Features: Ipsilateral 3rd nerve palsy, opposite side ataxia.

Millard-Gubler syndrome: Lesion: Ventral pons
Structures involved
• Cranial nerves VI and VII nerve
• Pyramidal tract.

Features
- Ipsilateral 7th nerve palsy
- Ipsilateral lateral rectus palsy
- Contralateral hemiplegia.

Foville's syndrome: *Lesion:* Dorsal pons
Structures involved
- Cranial nerve nuclei: VI and VII
- Corticospinal tract

Other structures can be involved
- Medial longitudinal fasciculus
- Medial lemniscus
Features: Same side
- LMN 7th nerve palsy
- Lateral gaze weakness
Opposite side: Hemiplegia.

Involvement of artery of Percheron
Structures involved
- Infarct in the posterior circulation.
- Infarct of the paramedian thalamus-bilaterally
Features
- Altered sensorium
- Vertical gaze palsy
- Loss of memory

Raymond's syndrome
Site of lesion—ventral median pons
Structures involved (on the side of lesion)
- Fascicle of the VI nerve (on the side of lesion)
- Corticospinal tract
Features
- Ipsilateral 6th nerve palsy
- Contralateral hemiplegia
Top of basilar syndrome
- Embolic occlusion of top of basilar artery
- Causes ischemia of bilateral thalamus.
Features
- Drowsiness
- Abnormal behavior
- Vertical gaze palsy
- Visual and oculomotor defect
- Defective reaction of the pupil
- Motor deficit is usually absent.

Collet-Sicard syndrome: Lesion at jugular foramen and hypoglossal canal: Resulting in cranial nerve palsy: IX, X, XI, and XII.
Causes: Tumor, vascular lesions, metastasis.

Vernet syndrome (jugular foramen syndrome)
Due to glomus jugular tumor, Schwannoma.
Features: Cranial nerve palsies: IX, X and XI nerves.

Villaret syndrome
Lesion: At retroparotid space.
Features: Ipsilateral paralysis of 9th, 10th, 11th and 12th nerve with Horner's syndrome.

Medial medullary syndrome
- Site of involvement: Medial medulla
- Artery involved: Vertebral artery/anterior spinal artery/basilar artery.
Features
- On the side of lesion: 12th nerve palsy (involvement of 12th nerve nucleus)
- Opposite side: Hemiplegia (pyramid tract involvement)
- Opposite side: Hemisensory loss (medial leminiscus).

Lateral medullary syndrome (Wallenberg syndrome)
Site of lesion: Lateral part of medulla.
Artery involved: usually: Vertebral artery
Posterior inferior cerebellar artery (PICA)
Structures involved

On the side of lesion	Deficit
• Spinal tract of Vth nerve	Pain and temperature: Loss on same side of face
• Inferior cerebellar peduncle	Ataxia on the side of lesion
• Vestibular nucleus	Vertigo and nystagmus
• Nucleus ambiguus— 9, 10, 11th nucleus	Dysphagia, hoarseness (9, 10, 11th cranial nerve palsy).
• Descending sympathetic chain	Horner's syndrome

On the opposite side of lesion
- There will be pain and temperature loss of the upper limb and lower limb.

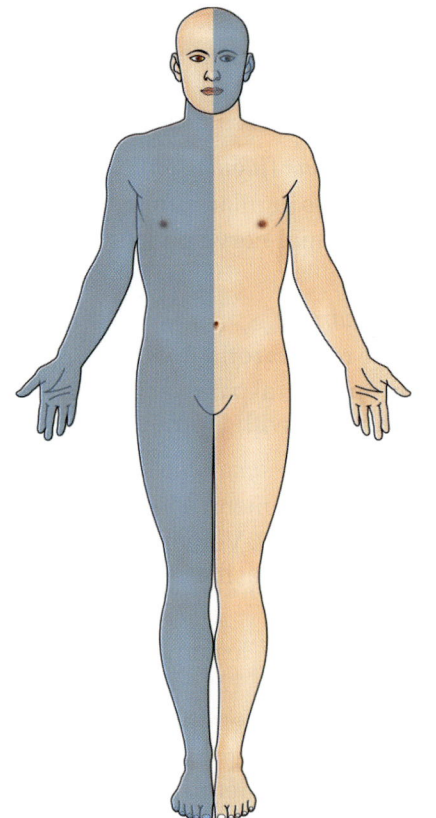

Fig. 4.9: Distribution of pain and temperature loss in lateral medullary syndrome—lesion left side

- Due to involvement of spinothalamic tract on the side of lesion.

Other structures which can be involved in lateral medullary syndrome
1. Due to involvement of nucleus and tractus solitarius—taste loss on the side of lesion.
2. Due to involvement of UMN fibers of 7th nerve which is descending down to medulla and deflected upwards to supply—ipsilateral 7th nucleus—UMN facial palsy on the side of lesion.
3. Due to involvement of cuneate and gracilis nucleus—numbness of ipsilateral arm, leg and body.

Variants of lateral medullary syndrome
Opalski's variant
- *Additional feature*: Hemiplegia on the side of lesion.

- Due to infarct extending into the caudal part of medulla.
Results in: Involvement of pyramidal tract after crossing over.

Babinski-Nageotte variant:
Additional feature: Hemiplegia on the opposite side.
Due to infarct extending downwards.
Results in: Involvement of pyramid tract before crossing over.

📝 *Note*

There can be occasionally partial lateral medullary syndrome or there can be combination of lateral and medial medullary syndrome.

Parinaud's syndrome: Dorsal midbrain syndrome.
Causes
- Infarction of the midbrain
- Tumor of pineal gland and encephalitis.
Signs: Vertical gaze palsy: Usually upward gaze palsy
- Light near dissociation (loss of papillary light reflex)
- Pseudoabducens palsy (loss of convergence)
- Convergence retraction nystagmus
- Convergent down gaze (setting sun sign)
- Upper eyelid retraction.

MOTOR SYSTEM

Pyramidal tract—arising from precentral gyrus.
Arrangement of fibers in the internal capsule
Anterior limb
- Frontopontine tract
- Anterior thalamic radiation
- Fibers from cortex to corpus callosum
Genu-corticobulbar tract
Posterior limb
- Corticospinal
- Corticostriatal
- Corticorubral

- Corticoreticular
- Cortico-olivary
- Post-thalamic radiations: Optic, auditory, sensory, occipitopontine temporopontine.

Corticospinal tract

Controls

- Continuous, discrete, isolated motor response.
- Fine voluntary movement.
- Controls speed of distal extremity movement.

Primary motor cortex

- Area no. 4—precentral gyrus.
- Large coordinated response with more stereotyped movement.

Premotor area no. 6

- Lies anterior to the primary motor cortex
- Controls sensory guidance of movement
- Lesion can cause apraxia

Supplementary motor area

- Lies anterior to the leg area of the primary motor cortex on the medial surface of the frontal lobe.
- Takes part in the planning of complex movement of contralateral extremities.

MOTOR SYSTEM EXAMINATION

Nutrition

Causes of Muscle Hypertrophy

- *Physiological*: Work hypertrophy.
- *Pathological conditions*:
  - Localized muscle enlargement
    - Tumors
    - Abscess
    - Cysticercosis
    - Muscle rupture

True hypertrophy: Can occur in myotonia congenita due to constant activation of muscle.

Pseudohypertrophy

- Muscle appears enlarged due to accumulation of fat and fibrous tissue.

- Muscle power is decreased with fatigue, e.g. Duchenne muscular dystrophy.

Usual muscles involved

- Calf muscles
- Deltoid
- Infraspinatus.

Hoffmann's syndrome

- Occurs in a patient of hypothyroidism
- Muscles appear enlarged (calf muscle) with fatigue and decreased strength.
- Muscle enlargement appears to be due to connective tissue deposition
- There will be delayed relaxation of ankle jerk
- Associated with proximal muscle weakness.

MUSCLE TONE

Muscle tone is defined as degree of tension developed in the muscle at rest.

Regulation of muscle tone: Regulated predominantly by muscle spindles and also by Golgi tendon with the participation of gamma motor neurons.

Muscles spindle

- Specialised type of muscle fibers
- Sensitive to stretch
- Helps in regulating muscle tone.

Golgi tendon organs

- Present in the tendon
- Sensitive to muscle stretch
- Senses the amount of force being applied to the muscle
- Prevent over stretching of muscle.

   If the muscle is overstretched—stimulation of Golgi tendon organ inhibits contraction of agonists and causes contraction of antagonists resulting in decreased muscle stretch.

Spasticity

Characteristics

- Increase tone in anti-gravity muscles
- Tone increase is not uniform throughout the range of movement.

- Tone varies with speed of movement
- Associated features
  - ↑Deep tendon reflexes
  - Plantar↑
  - Presence of clonus

Clasp-knife phenomenon
- Increase resistance to initial movement followed by sudden decrease of tone.
- Due to inverse stretch reflex mediated by Golgi tendon organs causing stimulation of inhibitory interneurons.

Extrapyramidal rigidity
- Site of lesion—basal ganglia
- Type of hypertonia—rigidity

Rigidity
- Constant level of increase of tone
- Affects both agonists and antagonists
- Increase tone occurs throughout the range of movement
- No change with speed of movement.

Types of rigidity
Lead pipe
- Involved muscles become rigid throughout the range of movement/movement may not be possible.
- Patient offers smooth resistance throughout the range of movement.

Paratonia—variable resistance to movement.

Paratonic rigidity of Gegenhalten
- Resistance to passive movement varies as the examiner varies the resistance.
- Resistance to passive movement increases as the examiner's efforts to move the part.
- For example, Parkinsonism—arteriosclerotic
  - Anterior cerebral artery occlusion
  - Diffuse cerebral dysfunction.

Cog wheeling
- Rigidity is interrupted by tremor.
- There will be regular, repeated and alternate contraction of agonists and antagonists.

For example, idiopathic parkinsonism.

Catatonia
- Resistance offered to passive movement is of lead pipe type.
- If the extremity is held in one particular position—it will be kept in that position for a prolonged duration.
- Can be associated with psychosis.

Decortication: Flexion of elbow and wrist with extension of legs and feet.

Decerebration: Limbs are kept in extended position—increased contraction of extensor muscles of extremities.

Rigidity	Spasticity
Extrapyramidal	Pyramidal
Tone is increased throughout the range of movement	Tone is increased initially
Tone is increased in both agonists and antagonists	Tone is increased in antigravity muscles
Not velocity dependent	Velocity dependent
Other features of extrapyramidal involvement	Features of pyramidal involvement

Muscle Weakness

Distribution of pyramidal weakness
- Upper limb: Extensors and abductors
- Lower limb: Flexors
- Loss of power is interpreted as weakness by the patient which is different from fatigability.

Easy fatigability
Patient is not making an attempt to move the limb and not able to sustain the movement.

Bradykinesia
Patient is taking more time for movement and movement is slow.

Different groups of muscles and their nerve root supply
Muscles of neck
- Neck flexors: Strap muscles of neck (C1 to C3)
- Neck extensors: Splenius capitus (C1 to C3)

Muscles of upper limb and their nerve supply

Shoulder		
Flexors	Pectoralis major	C5 and C6
	Anterior deltoid	C5 and C6
Extensors	Posterior deltoid	
	Infraspinatus	C5 and C6
	Teres major	
	Teres minor	
	L. dorsi	C5 and C6
Adduction	Pectoralis major	C5 and C6
	L. dorsi	C5 and C6
Abduction	Supraspinatus	C5 and C6
	Deltoid	C5 and C6
Elbow		
Flexors	Biceps	C5 and C6
Extensor	Triceps	C6 and C7
Pronation	Pronator teres and pronator quadratus	C6, C7 and T1
Supination	Supinator and biceps brachii	
Wrist		
Flexion	Flexor carpi ulnaris	C8 and T1
Extensor	Extensor carpi ulnaris	C6, C7 and C8

Hand muscles—*see* under peripheral neuropathy.
Lower limb muscles—*see* under paraplegia.

Causes of Muscle Weakness

Proximal muscle weakness
Upper limb
- Inflammatory myopathy
- Muscular dystrophy
- Syringomyelia
- C5–C6 lesion
- MND/spinal muscular atrophy
Lower limb
- Inflammatory myopathy
- Endocrine myopathy
- Guillain-Barré syndrome
- Lumbar root involvement
- Osteomalacia
- Diabetic amyotrophy
- Muscular dystrophy.

Distal weakness
Upper limb
- Syringomyelia
- Pancoast's tumor
- C8-T1 lesions
- MND
- Distal muscular dystrophy
- Pyramid tract disease
Lower limb
- Peripheral neuropathy
- Pyramidal weakness
- MND
- Myotonic dystrophy

Muscle disorders causing distal weakness
- Myotonic dystrophy
- Inclusion body myositis
- Mitochondrial myopathy
- Distal type of muscular dystrophy

Causes of anterior horn cell disease
Infective
- Poliomyelitis
- Tick paralysis.

Compression: Syringomyelia
Vascular: Anterior spinal artery occlusion
Degenerative
- MND
- Spinal muscular atrophy

Toxin induced: Triorthocresyl phosphate exposure.

Causes of weakness of both upper limbs
- Syringomyelia
- MND
- Bilateral upper cervical radiculopathy
- Bilateral brachial plexopathy
- Rarely lesion at cervicomedullary junction

Muscle weakness
Minimal weakness upper limb—test for pronator drift.

Testing for pronator drift
- Keep the palm upwards with eyes closed
- Hold the palms up for 20–30 seconds

Observe for

Corticospinal lesions: Minimum pronation of hand with slight flexion of the elbow on the affected side.

Severe drift: Significant pronation of entire arm with downward drift, due to overaction of pronators compared to supinator.

Cerebellar disease: Drifting of hand occurs in outward and slightly upward direction towards the site of lesion.

Parietal drift: Raising of the involved arm with drifting upwards. And outwards indicates lesion in the contralateral parietal cortex. (due to loss of position sense).

Minimal weakness of lower limb

Patient is asked to walk on heels: Sensitive way for foot dorsiflexor weakness.

Patient is asked to walk on toes: Sensitive way for testing plantar flexor weakness.

Testing minimal weakness of lower limb

Leg or knee drifting test

- Patient is in supine position.
- Hip and knee are flexed with the knee forming an angle of around 45 degrees with the heel resting on the table.

In corticospinal lesion

- Observe for sliding downwards of heel gradually and slow extension of knee.
- Hip extends with external rotation and abduction.

SENSORY EXAMINATION

Different Types of Sensations

Exteroceptive sensation

- Source of sensation is from outside of the body.
- For example, pain, light touch and temperature.

Proprioceptive sensation

- Source of sensation is body part itself, e.g. joint sense
- Position and pressure sense
- Deep pain
- Vibration

Cortical sensation: Finer discrimination of sensation with participation of sensory cortex.

Interoceptive sensation: Visceral sensation.

Sensory Receptors

For pain: Cutaneous receptors.

For vibration: Pacinian corpuscle.

For temperature: Cutaneous sensory receptors for hot and cold.

For touch: Cutaneous mechanoreceptors/ naked nerve endings.

For joint sense: Joint capsules/tendon endings/ muscle spindles.

Sensory Pathways

Flowcharts 4.6 and 4.7.

Flowchart 4.6: Spinothalamic pathway

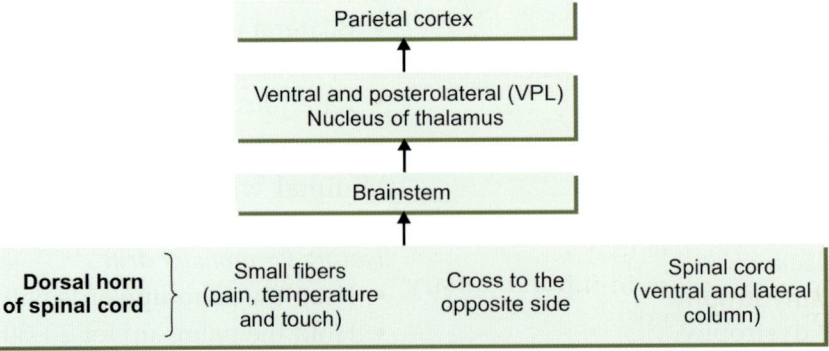

Flowchart 4.7: Posterior column pathway

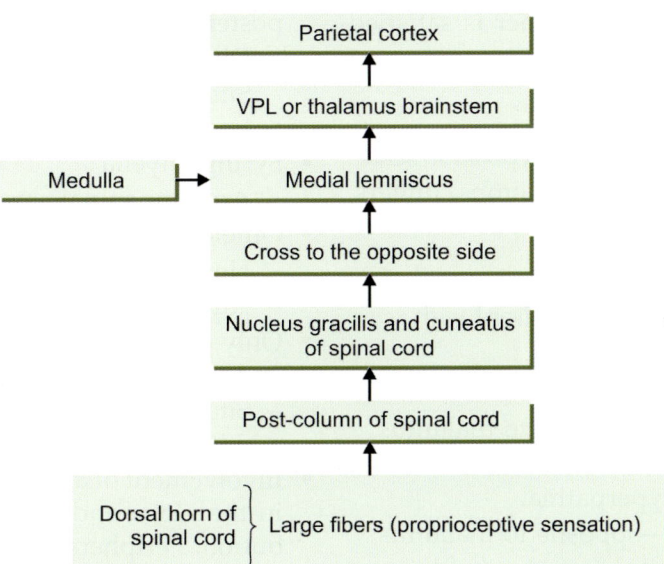

CORTICAL SENSORY LOSS

Key Points

- Patients with cortical sensory loss will have intact primary modalities of sensation.
- Contralateral parietal cortex is the site of lesion if there is cortical sensory loss on one side.
- While testing two-point discrimination 3 mm of discrimination is detected over the pulp of fingers.
- Back of the body, dorsum of hand and foot-less sensitive compared to other parts.
- Tip of tongue, lips—most sensitive parts of the body.
- While testing for graphesthesia letter/figure of 1 cm are written over the skin in the form of figures of 4, 8, 5, etc.

Key Points While Examining Sensory System

- Vibration sense is lost early in diabetes mellitus and also in elderly.
- Sacral sparing occurs in intramedullary lesions of cervical cord.

- Subacute combined degeneration of spinal cord produces more of vibration sense loss compared to position sense loss.
- Tabes dorsalis produces more of position sense loss.
- Central cord lesions produce funicular type of pain.
- Lateral spinothalamic tract by convention is called spinothalamic tract.
- Band like hyperaesthesia around the body is a manifestation of posterior column pathology.

Joint Sense

Key Points

- Hold the joint on sides and hold parallel to the plane of movement.
- Hold the joint lightly to avoid pressure sensation.
- Avoid up and down movement alternatively—may give indirect information of movement to the patient.
- Touch applied to the anterior and posterior aspects of the joint may give indication to the movement of the joint and to be avoided.

- Perform the test till successive response is obtained/till the examiner is satisfied with the response.

Pseudoathetosis

- Occurs in patients with loss of position sense.
- Involuntary movement of limbs/fingers, occurs when the hand is out stretched while closing the eyes.

Localisation of Lesions in Patient with Sensory Abnormality

- Unilateral loss of sensation of all modalities:
  - Site of lesion—opposite to thalamus.
- Unilateral loss of sensation with increased threshold and hyperpathia.
  - Site of lesion—opposite to thalamus
- Unilateral cortical sensory loss with intact primary sensations:
  - Site of lesion—contralateral parietal cortex.
- Loss of pain and temperature on one side of face and opposite side limbs:
  - Site of lesion—lateral medullary syndrome.
- Bilateral loss of all forms of sensation below a horizontal level:
  - Site of lesion: Gross lesion of spinal cord.
- Contralateral loss of pain and temperature below a certain level with ipsilateral loss of touch sensation below the level.
  - Site of lesion: Brown-Séquard syndrome.
- Impairment of pain and temperature over several segments with normal sensation above and below—"suspended jacket".
  - Site of lesion: Intrinsic lesion of spinal cord, e.g. syringomyelia
- Crossing sensory fibers are damaged.
- Sacral sparing of sensation.
  - Site of lesion: Intramedullary lesion of cervical cord.
- Saddle anesthesia:
  - Site of lesion: Conus/cauda equina lesion.
- Loss of all forms of sensation over a clearly defined part of the body on one side.
  - For example, nerve root/lesion.

- Pain and temperature loss with preserved posterior column sensation:
  - Dissociated anesthesia.
  - Site of lesion: Crossing spinothalamic tract
- Syringomyelia
  - Anterior spinal artery occlusion.
- Other causes: Leprosy
  - Hereditary sensory motor neuropathy
  - Amyloidosis.
- Only proprioceptive loss with intact pain and temperature:
  - Site of lesion—posterior cord syndrome with involvement of posterior column.
- Involvement of all modalities of sensation in the glove and stocking type of distribution: Peripheral neuropathy.

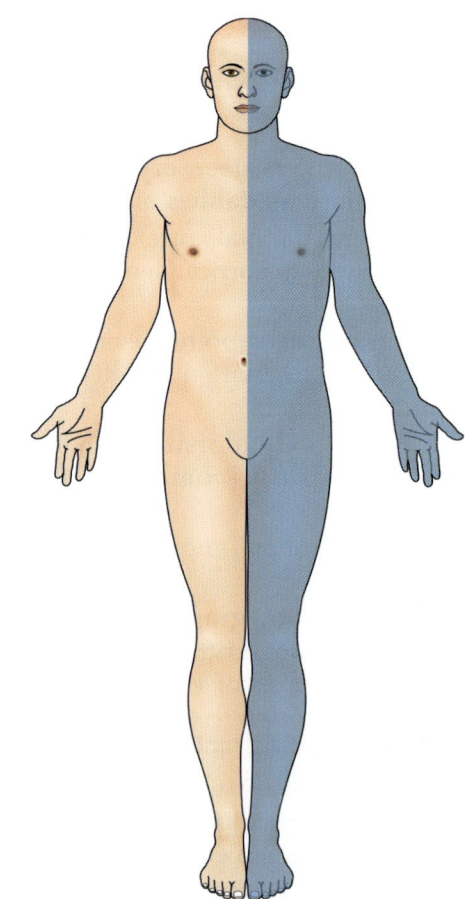

Fig. 4.10: Thalamic lesion

Important Clinical Points

Barber's chair sign (Lhermitte's sign): Occurs in:

- Multiple sclerosis
- Cervical spondylosis

Phantom limb: Pseudoperception of the part of the body which is not present (amputated limb)

Causalgia (complex regional pain syndrome type II): Chronic burning type of pain associated with hyperaesthesia in the distribution of the nerve when the nerve is cut/injured.

REFLEXES

Superficial Reflexes

Plantar Reflex

- Extensor plantar is the hardest sign of pyramidal lesion.
- Can be reinforced by movement of head/neck to the opposite side.

Different Methods of Plantar Reflex Elicitation Apart from Babinski Method

Chaddock's sign: Stroke the area below the lateral malleolus and observe for the response.

Oppenheim's sign: Apply pressure firmly from below the knee with the fingers up to the ankle.

Gordon's sign: Squeeze the calf muscles.

Schaeffer's sign: Squeeze the Achilles tendon

Minimal Babinski

- Elicit for plantar response.
- Palpate the thigh for contraction of hamstrings and tensor faciae latae.

Crossed plantar extensor

Stimulation of one side of foot results in bilateral extensor plantar.

Lesion: Bilateral cerebral cortex or spinal cord.

Physiological basis for plantar reflex

- Physiologically plantar extension is shortening of limb (flexor response) with the maturation of corticospinal system—there

will be suppression of primitive flexion response for maintaining normal posture.

- Pyramidal lesion—plantar becomes extensor.

Deep Tendon Reflexes

Key Points

- After a stage of neuronal shock extensor plantar appears earlier than deep reflexes.
- Hoffman's and Wartenberg's sign is more important if present unilaterally.
- Abdominal reflex can be brisk in patient with anxiety and psychoneurosis.
- Clonus elicitation results in alternate contraction of agonists and antagonists—alternate stretch reflex.
- Elicit triceps jerk by tapping the knee hammer 1 inch above olecranon and for supinator jerk 4 inches above base of the thumb.

Reinforcement of Deep Tendon Reflexes

- For upper limb reflexes—clenching the teeth.
- For lower limb reflexes—Jendrassik's maneuver.

Inverted Jerks

Inverted supinator jerk suggests C5 lesion.

Inverted biceps: Striking the biceps tendon—there will be extension of elbow.

Inverted triceps: Flexion of elbow while eliciting triceps jerk—suggests lesion of C6, C7.

Physiological basis for inverted jerks: Underlying hyperreflexia due to UMN lesion (below the level of spinal cord lesion)—lowers the threshold for elicitation of lower segmental reflex and reflex becomes excitable due to transmission of vibrations when the higher segmental reflex is elicited—which is as such is absent due to the spinal cord lesion (LMN lesion at the level of lesion).

Pendular knee jerk: Present if 3 or more full to and fro oscillations occur while eliciting knee jerk due to impaired check reflex and hypotonia.

Hung up reflex: Delayed relaxing ankle jerk (Woltman's sign) occurs in hypothyroidism.

Pectoral jerk: Place the finger as nearly as possible on the tendon of pectoralis major muscle near its insertion on the greater tuberosity of humerus.

Elicitation: Tap the finger.

Response: Adduction and slight internal rotation of arm at the shoulder.

Root value: C3–C4.

Adductor reflex: **Keep the finger on the adductor tendon** at its insertion on the medial condyle of the femur. Tap the finger and observe for adduction of the hip.

Root value: L2 to L4.

PRIMITIVE REFLEXES

Snout, suckling and palmomental reflex: Occurs in patients with diffuse frontal lobe disease.

Groping reflex: Person follows the objects moving in front of them and attempts to move their hand forward. May be accompanied by grasp reflex. Present in patient with frontal lobe disease.

Lesion: Contralateral frontal lobe.

Mirror movement: With the movement of one hand—the other hand also performs the similar movement, e.g. Parkinsonism, craniovertebral anomalies.

Explanation
- May be due to defect in the inhibition of contralateral cortex.
- Defect in the decussation of pyramidal fibers at lower medullary level.

Grasp reflex

Method of elicitation: Keep an object over the palm or keep the examiners finger between the thumb and forefinger of the patient. It will be grasped with the palmar grasp.

Significance: Lesion of contralateral frontal lobe.

Forced grasping—similar to above: Flexor response of fingers and hand occur when skin of palmar surface of hand is stimulated.

Lesion: Contralateral frontal lobe.

Suckling reflex: Movement of lips occurs in a suckling manner whenever lips are stimulated.

Rooting: Turning the head forwards and towards the object whenever the cheek is strolled or stimulated till the object is found.

Snout
- *Elicitation*: Tapping the upper lips lightly.
- *Observe*: Protrusion of the lips—muscles around the mouth and base of the nose—contracts.

Palmomental
- *Elicitation*: Thenar eminence is stroked briskly with a thin stick: Proximal to distal (edge of the wrist to the base of the thumb).
- *Positive response*: Twich of chin muscle—contraction of mentalis, orbicularis oris with wrinkling skin of chin, elevation of angle of the mouth.
- Suckling, rooting, snout and palmomental reflex positivity suggest diffuse frontal lobe disease.
- *Avoiding response*: Lesion—contralateral parietal lobe.

Other Reflexes

Bulbocavernosus Reflex

Detects intact S2, S3 and S4.

Technique: Squeezing the glans penis/tagging the catheter if the patient is on Foley's catheter—look for anal sphincter contraction.

Can be absent in spinal shock and lesion of S3, S4 and S5.

Anal reflex
- *Root value*: S3, S4 and S5
- Absent in S3, S4 and S5 lesions

- Stimulate the skin/mucosa of the perianal region by scratching it. Feel for the contraction of the external anal sphincter by introducing the finger into the anal canal.

INVOLUNTARY MOVEMENTS

Different Types of Movement Disorders

Hyperkinetic movement disorders
- Athetosis
- Ballism
- Chorea
- Dystonia
- Myoclonus
- Tics
- Tremors

Hypokinetic movement disorder: Parkinsonism

Athetosis
- Slow sinuous/writhing movement.
- Can affect fingers, hands and feet.
- Absent during sleep
- Not altered by eye closure
- Can occur at rest and can increase by anxiety and interferes with voluntary movement.

Lesion: Basal ganglia
- Pseudoathetosis—*see* under sensory system.

Ballism
- Wide flinging movement of limb on one side of the body.
- Affects proximal muscles
- Can occur in resting state.
- Interferes with voluntary movement.

Lesion: Opposite subthalamic nucleus

Chorea
- Irregular nonrepetitive movement.
- Occurs at rest, appears to mimic semi-purposeful activity.
- Involves extremities, trunk and face.
- Increases by anxiety and absent during sleep.
- Tone is increased except in patients with rheumatic chorea (tone is decreased).

Causes
- Rheumatic: Sydenham's chorea (Saint Vitus dance)
- Huntington's chorea
- Chorea gravidarum
- Senile/atherosclerotic

Site of lesion: Basal ganglia

Myoclonus: Sudden jerk-like movement of the part of the body.

Causes
- Myoclonic epilepsy
- Metabolic/toxic encephalopathy

Types
- Epileptic/non-epileptic
- *Positive myoclonus:* Occurs due to contraction of muscle.
- *Negative myoclonus:* If the interruption occurs in a contracting muscle.
- It may be focal, segmental or generalised.
- Action myoclonus—myoclonus precipitated by action.
- Reflex myoclonus—stimulated by light/sound/touch.
- **Asterixis** is an example for negative myoclonus.

TICS (Habit spasm)
- Repetitive stereotyped movement occurs at rest.
- Can be suppressed by the person and can be precipitated when observed.
- Increases during anxiety and can be associated with depression/personality disorder.
- Decreases during sleep and when distracted.

Types: Motor, vocal and sensory.

Tremors
- Involuntary rhythmic oscillations of part of the body
- Can occur at rest: Parkinsonism
- Action tremor—during voluntary movement
  - For example, benign essential
- Postural: When the hand is outstretched
  - For example, anxiety

- Thyrotoxicosis
- Alcohol
- Benign essential
- Flapping tremor: Metabolic encephalopathies.
- Intention tremor: Cerebellar disturbances.

Titubation: Occurs in cerebellar disease/benign essential tremor.

Rubral tremor (red nucleus tremor): Due to the lesion of red nucleus.
- Coarse and slow tremor which is increased by postural adjustment.

Wing beating tremor: Present in patients with Wilson's disease.

Characteristics: Sustained abduction of proximal arm with flexion of elbow and downward facing palm. Low frequency high amplitude tremor.

Hemifacial spasm and blepharospasm: Facial muscle contraction on one side. Rapid, brief and repetitive spasm of facial muscles. Can become sustained tonic spasm.
Causes: Compression of facial nerve by a vessel, by a tumor, CVA, demyelination, idiopathic.

Akathesia movements
- Person is not able to sit still.
- Person feels an inner feeling of restlessness which is decreased by moving about.
- Can have focal/generalised stereotyped movements.

Dystonia: Characterised by abnormal positioning, twisting movement of part of body.
Types
- Most common: Focal dystonia
- For example, torticollis, writer's cramp, blepharospasm
- Drug induced due to L-Dopa/neuroleptics
- Due to lesion of: Basal ganglia, thalamus, brainstem.
- Dystonia may be a part of Wilson's disease or parkinsonism.
- Dystonia increases by fatigue and stress and can decrease by relaxation.

INVOLUNTARY MOVEMENTS

Extrapyramidal System

Consists of striatum with following structures
- Caudate nucleus
- Putamen
- Substantia nigra
- Subthalamic nucleus.

Above structures connect with
- Circuits connecting voluntary movements
- Limbic connections
- Oculomotor system

Parts of extrapyramidal system connect with
- Brainstem reticular formation
- Inferior olivary nucleus
- Vestibular nucleus

Vestibulospinal tract—influences extensor muscle tone of trunk and extremities.

Rubrospinal—facilitate flexor muscle tone of upper limb.

Tectospinal arises from superior colliculus: Influences muscles of neck and upper trunk (maintain the position of head to the body position).

Pontine reticulospinal—facilitate extensor muscle tone of the trunk and proximal muscles.

Medullary reticulospinal inhibits antigravity muscle tone and is involved in autonomic function.

Disorders of extrapyramidal system
- Increase inhibitory effect on basal ganglia—causes bradykinesia, e.g. Parkinsonism.
- Reduction in normal inhibition on movements results in hyperkinetic movement disorder, e.g.
  - Chorea
  - Athetosis
  - Dystonia
  - Tremors
  - Tics

Approach to a Patient of Movement Disorder

Importance of history in a patient of movement disorder

Ask for the following details to the patient or the bystander regarding the movement disorder

- What part of the body is affected
- Whether the involuntary movement is constant/episodic
- Whether it occurs at rest or on voluntary movement
- Does voluntary movement increase or decrease the involuntary movement
- What is the type of involuntary movement
- What is the effect of sleep on involuntary movement
- Does involuntary movement is interfering with voluntary activity
- Does the involuntary movement is associated with fever and other systemic symptoms
- Are there any precipitating factors like drugs/toxins
- Whether there is any positive family history

What part of the body affected?

- Tremors—distal part
- Myoclonus—whole limb.
- Spasms
  - Focal dystonia
  - Hemifacial spasm
  - Blepharospam
- Focal involuntary movements: Focal seizures.
- Involuntary movements—constant/episodic
- Constant movements; Resting tremors of Parkinsonism
  - Benign essential tremors
  - Epilepsia partialis continua
- Episodic attacks
  - Myoclonic jerks
  - Generalised epilepsy

Only at rest or only on movement

At rest

- Resting tremor of parkinsonism
- Chorea
- Myoclonus

On movement: Action tremor.

Does voluntary movement increase or decrease the involuntary movement

Increase on voluntary movement

- Anxiety/action tremor
- Intention tremor

Decrease on voluntary movement: For example, tremor of parkinsonism.

What is the type of involuntary movement?

- Rapid rhythmic oscillations of part of the body: *Tremors*
- Slow writhing movement: *Athetosis*
- Sudden jerky movement: *Myoclonus*
- Wide flinging movements of proximal part of the limb: *Ballism*
- Non-repetitive, semi-purposive movement: *Chorea*
- Abnormal posturing of part of the body: *Dystonia*
- Sudden jerky movement—occurring during sleep: *Myoclonus*

What is the effect of sleep on involuntary movement

Involuntary movements which disappear during sleep

- Dystonia
- Tremors
- Chorea
- Hemiballism

Involuntary movement which persists during sleep

- Hemifacial spasm
- Restless leg syndrome
- Myoclonus

Does the involuntary movement interfere with voluntary activity

Involuntary movement interfering with voluntary activity

- Choreoathetosis

- Myoclonus
- Ballism
- Essential tremors/action tremors.

Involuntary movements which do not interfere with voluntary activity
- Tics
- Resting tremors

Involuntary movements which increase with anxiety
- Tremors
- Tics
- Chorea
- Dystonia
- Athetosis.

Involuntary movements which are relieved by alcohol: Benign essential tremors.

Involuntary movements which occur on mechanical stimulation: Fasciculations.

Relationship between eyeball movement and eyeball closure with involuntary movements:
- Pseudoseizure—patient will be closing the eye during an attack of seizure.
- During an attack of true seizure—eyes are kept opened with deviation of eyes.

 Note

- *Hysterical/pseudoinvoluntary movements occur— may be only on being watched.*
- *True involuntary movements occur even when the person is not being watched.*

Features which are not favoring epileptic seizure
- No postictal phenomenon
- Waxing and waning type of movement during seizure episode
- No eyeball movements/eyes are closed during seizure
- No evidence of injury to the body parts, no frothing or incontinence.

Factors precipitating seizure
- Consumption of alcohol
- Sleep deprivation
- Flickering light
- Drugs: Ciprofloxacin, theophylline

- Metabolic: Hypoglycemia
- Hypocalcemia
- Hypomagnesemia
- Hyponatremia.

Factors which relieve involuntary movement: Alcohol relieves benign essential tremors.

Focal involuntary movements which disturb the conscious level: For example, complex partial seizure.

Palatal nystagmus: Involuntary movement of soft palate and pharyngeal muscles due to defect in the Guillain-Mollaret triangle (consists of dentate nucleus, red nucleus and inferior olivary nucleus).

PARKINSONISM

Parkinson's Disease
(Idiopathic parkinsonism/paralysis agitans)
Disease Description
- Degenerative disorder of the nervous system.
- Age group involved: 7th to 8th decade.

Classical features
- Combination of: Rigidity, bradykinesia, resting tremor
- Associated with abnormality of gait.

Pathogenesis and pathology: Mutation in the LRRK2 and Parkin gene.
Site of lesion
- Substantia nigra
- Decrease of dopaminergic neurons
- Formation of inclusion bodies (Lewy body)
- Lewy body contains: Alpha-synuclein (protein substance)
- Can also have involvement of nondopa-minergic neurons containing noradrenaline. There is involvement of cerebral cortex, spinal cord, autonomous nervous system, brainstem and effector neurons.

Clinical Features
- Bradykinesia—slowness of movement
- Rigidity—can have cog wheeling

- Tremor—resting tremor
- Tremor of parkinsonism
  - Resting tremor
  - Increases with anxiety
  - Decreases with voluntary/purposeful movement
  - Pill rolling (due to biplanar movement: flexion and extension and adduction and abduction of thumb).

 Note

Cog wheeling is due to rigidity interrupted by tremor.

Other features
- Masked like—expressionless face
- Glabellar tap sign positive
- Monotonus speech
- Micrographia
- *Brainstem involvement*
  - Dysphagia
  - Hypophonia
  - Sleep disturbance, mood disorder and dementia
  - Motor power—normal
  - Reflexes normal

Autonomic dysfunction
Orthostatic dysfunction:
- GIT/genitourinary dysfunction
- Sexual dysfunction

Differential diagnosis
1. Idiopathic parkinsonism
2. Secondary parkinsonism
3. Atypical parkinsonism
4. Parkinsonism dementia disease
5. Systemic disease like hepatic failure.

Factors favoring idiopathic parkinsonism (Parkinson's disease)
- Usually starts unilaterally
- Initially gait disturbance and difficulty in walking is not a feature.
- There is no evidence of pyramidal involvement/dementia less common
- Classically associated with tremor
- Response to L-dopa present.

Causes of secondary parkinsonism
- Occurs due to a secondary cause resulting in parkinsonism
- For example, drugs: Reserpine, amiadarone, neuroleptics, lithium
- Vascular: Arteriosclerotic parkinsonism (usually hemiplegic parkinsonism) features of pyramidal involvement/multi-infarct state.
- Trauma—due to repeated head injury.
- Postencephalitic parkinsonism.
- Exposure to toxins like carbon monoxide, manganese, MPTP.
- Chronic hepatic failure including Wilson's disease.

Atypical Parkinsonism
- Widespread degeneration of nervous system:
  - For example, multisystem atrophy (C and P type), progressive supranuclear palsy, corticobasal ganglion degeneration.

Features of atypical parkinsonism
- Resting tremor is usually absent
- Impairment of speech and abnormality of gait occurs early.
- Does not respond to L-dopa when compared to idiopathic parkinsonism
- Disease—usually runs an aggressive course.

Multisystem atrophy (MSA)
- Combination of parkinsonism with cerebellar feature; C-type
- Combination of parkinsonism with postural hypotension (autonomic involvement: P-type)
- MRI shows typical hot cross bun appearance (due to atrophy of pons).

Progressive supranuclear palsy
Features
- Early disturbance of gait
- History of falling backwards (due to extensor hypertonia)
- Hyperextension of neck
- Vertical gaze palsy (initially for downward gaze)

- Associated with disorder of speech and cognition.
- MRI shows hummingbird sign (due to atrophy of midbrain with preservation of PNS).

Corticobasal ganglion disorder: Rare disorder.
- Associated with apraxia, agnosia, clumsiness of hand and dementia

Disorders of parkinsonism + dementia
1. Long standing idiopathic parkinsonism later may develop dementia.
2. Early dementia with parkinsonism—dementia with Lewy bodies.

Other disorders which are associated with rigidity/gait disturbance/higher mental function abnormality

Huntington's chorea
- Presence of chorea
- Abnormal behavior
- Impairement of judgement/self awareness

Normal pressure hydrocephalus (NPH)
Features
- Urinary incontinence
- Gait abnormality
- Memory impairment

 Note

Multiple cortical infarct state also have gait abnormality, pseudobulbar features with urinary incontinence.

DISORDERS OF THE SPINAL CORD

Anatomy of the Spinal Cord

Total spinal cord segments: 31
- Cervical: 8
- Thoracic: 12
- Lumbar: 5
- Sacral: 5
- Coccygeal: 1

Extent of spinal cord
Starts from foramen magnum and extends up to L1 vertebra.

Spinal cord segments and corresponding vertebral positions

At cervical vertebral level
- Add one to the lower cervical vertebral level
- C7 vertebra corresponds to C8 cervical spinal cord segment

At thoracic level
- Add 2 spinal cord segments to the upper thoracic vertebra (T1–T6)
- Add 3 to the lower thoracic vertebra (T7, T8, T9)
- T10 vertebral arch—corresponds to L1 and L2 lumbar segment.

At lumbar level
- T11 vertebral arch corresponds to L3 and L4 lumbar segment
- T12 vertebral arch—corresponds to L5 segment
- L1 vertebral arch—corresponds to sacral and coccygeal segments.

CLINICAL ASPECTS OF SPINAL CORD AND EXAMINATION OF SPINE

Blood supply of spinal cord
- Spinal cord is supplied by a single anterior spinal artery and 2 posterior spinal arteries.
- Anterior spinal artery supplies anterior 2/3 of spinal cord and posterior spinal artery supplies posterior column and posterior horn of spinal cord.

Anterior spinal artery: Originates at the level of foramen magnum. It is formed by joining of single branches from each vertebral artery and runs down anteromedially.

Anterior spinal artery is supplemented by following arterial branches
- Branches from thyrocervical trunk.
- Intercostal arteries
- Lumbar: Ileo lumbar and lateral sacral arteries.
- Artery of Adamkiewicz: Arteria magna.

Artery of Adamkiewicz (*Arteria Magna*)

- Largest supplementary artery to the anterior spinal artery.
- Usually found on the left side
- Arises from posterior intercostal arteries at the level of T8 to L1
- Supplies lumbar and sacral cord. Joins Anterior spinal artery.

Posterior spinal arteries

- Paired arteries: 2 in number.
- They may be in the form of plexiform channels rather than distinct arteries.
- Anterior spinal artery also gives branches to join posterior spinal arteries.
- Supply posterior column and posterior horn of spinal cord.

Susceptible levels of spinal cord to ischemia

- At thoracic T3–T4 level
- Watershed zone between connections of anterior and posterior spinal arteries.

Causes of anterior/posterior spinal artery occlusion

- Severe hypotension
- Vasculitis
- Cardioembolism
- *Aortic disease*
  - Aortic dissection
  - Aortic aneurysm
  - Atherosclerosis
  - Vertebral artery disease

Other vascular disease of spinal cord

- Spinal cord hematoma
- Hematomyelia
- Arteriovenous malformation.

Veins of spinal cord

- Form venous plexus corresponding to spinal arteries
- They join the veins of thoracic, abdominal and pelvic cavities.

Batson plexus of veins

- Part of cerebrospinal venous system

- Connect deep pelvic veins and thoracic venous channels to the internal venous plexus of vertebra and veins of CNS.
- *Special features*: Valveless.

Significance

- Transmit tumor cells from pelvis like rectal/prostatic malignancy to vertebra and brain.
- Transmit infection from urinary tract like pyelonephritis to vertebra.
- Occlusion of anterior spinal artery and artery of Adamkiewicz (*see* later).

Arrangement of Fibers in the Spinal Cord (at Cervical Level)

Motor fibers—pyramidal tract at cervical level
From medial to lateral: Cervical, thoracic, lumbar, sacral (C, T, L, S).
Cervical—medial most
Sacral—lateral most

Posterior Column Fibers (at Cervical Level)

From medial to lateral: Sacral, lumbar, thoracic, cervical (S, L, T, C).

Spinothalamic fibers (*at cervical level*): From medial to lateral: Cervical, thoracic, lumbar, sacral (C, T, L, S).

SPINAL CORD COMPRESSION

Causes of Spinal Cord Compression

Bony (vertebral) causes
- Intervertebral disc prolapse
- Fracture vertebrae
- Tuberculosis of the spine
- *Secondary metastasis from*
  - Prostate
  - Breast
  - Bronchogenic carcinoma
  - Myeloma

Meningeal causes
- Spinal epidural abscess
- Meningioma
- Neurofibroma
- Metastatic compression.

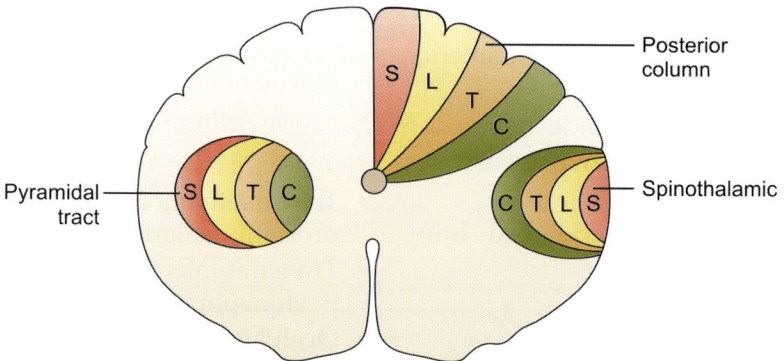

Fig. 4.11: Distribution of fibers in the spinal cord at cervical level

Spinal cord disorders

- Cervical spondylosis
- Craniovertebral anomalies
- Syringomyelia
- Bleeding into the cord
- Glioma and ependymoma
- Metastasis

Approach to a Patient of Spinal Cord Compression

Mode of Onset

Sudden

- Traumatic lesions
- Intervertebral disc prolapse

Rapid: Carcinomatous lesions

Gradually progressive: Benign spinal cord tumors like—meningioma/neurofibroma.

Pain Associated with Spinal Cord Compression

Types of Pain in Spinal Cord Lesions

Back pain—bony pain: In compressive lesions—present in both extradural/intradural lesions.

Root pain: Due to compression of nerve roots—in extradural/intradural lesions.

Funicular pain

- Burning type of pain
- Poorly localized
- Due to irritation of spinothalamic tract
- Can be present in intramedullary tumors or spinal cord injury

Pain due to spinal cord compression can be unilateral or bilateral.

Band of hyperaesthesia can be present in spinal cord lesions at the level of compression indicating posterior column involvement.

Types of Cord Compression Depending on the Site of Involvement

Extradural

Causes

- Trauma—intervertebral disc prolapse/vertebral fracture
- Spondylotic myelopathy
- TB spine
- Tumors—secondary metastasis

Features

- Presence of pain in the back (bony pain)
- Root pain may or may not be significant
- May be symmetrical in onset.
- Involvement of pyramidal tract first, then posterior column and then the bladder and bowel.
- There will be a horizontal level of lesion with radicular involvement with or without myelopathy.

Intradural

- For example, meningioma
- Neurofibroma

Features

- Duration of symptoms—prolonged due to benign nature of the disease.

- Root pain and paraesthesia—common as the lesion arises near the nerve root.
- Initially there may be posterior column involvement.
- Usually asymmetrical in onset.

Intramedullary compression

Causes
- Syringomyelia.
- Intramedullary tumors like gliomas

Features
- Not associated with root pain and back pain.
- There can be funicular pain—poorly localizing burning pain.
- Early involvement of bladder and bowel (except syringomyelia)
- Dissociated anesthesia
- Sacral sparing (cervical lesion)
- May be symmetrical in onset

Order of compression of structures in extradural compressions: There will be initial involvement of pyramidal tract followed by posterior column and then the spinothalamic tract.

Reasons for early involvement of pyramidal tract in extradural compression

- Pyramidal tract lies close to denticulate ligament and vulnerable to get damaged as the ligament will be subjected to traction because of compression.
- Terminal branches of spinal arteries supply pyramidal tract and is vulnerable to ischemia because of compression.

Mechanisms of neurological involvement in spinal cord compression

- Direct compression of nerve root and spinal cord.
- Ischemia of the cord due to interference in the blood flow of the longitudinal and radicular arteries caused by the lesion.
- Edema of the cord below the level of compression due to pressure effect on the ascending and longitudinal veins.

- Compression causes obstruction to the CSF flow and can cause changes in the CSF.

Clinical evidence of spinal cord involvement
- Definite level of lesion.
- Involvement of motor, sensory and autonomic functions and sphincters bilaterally below the level of lesion.
- No involvement of intracranial structure.

Features which suggest level of lesion
- Site of pain in the back and radicular pain—vertebral level.
- Band of hyperaesthesia
- Level of motor, sensory and reflex level.
- If the motor, sensory and reflex levels do not coincide—highest of the 3 levels to be taken as the level of involvement.

  Because the higher cord level can explain the lower cord lesions.

Nerve root involvement in spinal cord lesions
Due to
- Direct injury to the root and compression of the root
- Inflammation of the root
- Axonal loss/demyelination.

Motor features
Muscle wasting
- At the level of lesion and due to LMN involvement.
- Stiffness of limbs due to hypertonia below the level of lesion.

Extensor spasm
- Sudden extension and spasm of limbs
- Due to pyramidal lesion
- Causes paraplegia in extension.

Flexor spasm
- Due to progressive lesion of spinal cord
- There will be flexion of limbs
- Indicates bad prognosis
- Causes paraplegia in flexion.

Flexor spasm: Whenever a mechanical stimulus is given to a patient of progressive paraplegia, there will be immediate dorsiflexion of ankle, flexion of knee and hip. It is a flexor withdrawal reflex and is normally inhibited by vestibulo-spinal and reticulospinal pathways. In pro-gressive lesion of spinal cord, these pathways are damaged causing flexor spasm.

Features which affect prognosis in a paraplegia
- Presence of bedsore
- Urinary tract infection
- Malnutrition.

Sensory features
At the level of lesion:
- Root pain
- Girdle pain
- Band of hyperesthesia
- Dissociated anesthesia.

Involvement of posterior column
- Occurs early in posterior cord compression.
- Can be pressed against the ligamentum flavum.

Cervical cord: Intramedullary lesions can cause sacral sparing.

In spinothalamic lesions
- Final upper level of anesthesia lies several segments below the level of lesion.
- Due to crossing of fibers several segments above after entering the spinal cord.

Saddle anesthesia: Occurs in conus medullaris and cauda equina lesions.

Reflex involvement
- Superficial and deep reflexes are lost at the level of lesions.
- Deep reflexes are exaggerated below the level of lesion.
- Plantar extensor in UMN lesions.

Sphincter involvement: Symptoms like hesi-tancy, precipitancy and retention of urine and automatic emptying can occur.

Sexual function: Involved in cauda and conus lesions.

Mass reflex
- Occurs in severe myelopathy after the stage of spinal shock.

- Stimulation of the body part below the level of lesion;
  - Results in leg flexion, contraction of abdominal muscles, sphincter evacua-tion and sweating.
- Due to exaggerated autonomic res-ponse.

Remember
- In spinal cord lesions—at the level of lesion there will be LMN involvement and below the level of lesion there will be UMN signs.
- Flexor spasm suggests progressive lesion of the spinal cord and carries bad progno-sis.

Cervical Cord Involvement

Clinical Anatomy of Cervical Cord
- Spinal segments—C_1–C_8 and correspon-ding vertebra—C_1–C_7.
- At cervical level—spinal canal sagittal dia-meter is 15–20 mm.
- If the saggital diameter of the canal is less than 13 mm at the cervical level, it is suggestive of compression and narrowing of the cervical canal called cervical canal stenosis—can present as cervical cord compression.

Key Points Regarding Cervical Cord Lesions
- At the level of foramen magnum/higher cervical cord lesions—cause downbeat nystagmus.
- Even in higher cervical cord lesions maxi-mum deficit can occur at C_8–T_1 level
- At C_5 lesions: There will be loss of biceps jerk—with inverted supinator jerk.
- High cervical cord lesions cause sensory loss over the face due to involvement of spinal tract of trigeminal nerve.
- Sacral sparing occurs in intramedullary lesions of cervical cord.

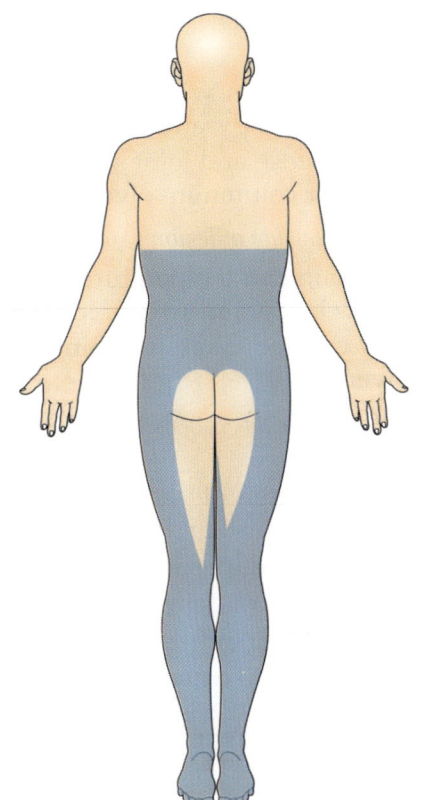

Fig. 4.12: Sacral sparing in intramedullary cervical spinal cord lesion

DIFFERENT SPINAL CORD SYNDROMES

Central Cord Syndrome

Occurs due to
- Selective damage to central gray matter nerve cells (softening of spinal cord).
- Damage to the crossing spinothalamic tract surrounding spinal canal.
- Common site involved—cervical spinal cord due to
  - Injury
  - Syringomyelia
  - Intrinsic cord tumors

Features
- Motor weakness more in the upper limb compared to the lower limb
- Dissociated sensory loss over the shoulder. lower neck and upper trunk (suspended jacket—cape distribution)

- Posterior column—normal
- Minor long tract signs
- Bladder distention with urinary retention.

Anterior cord syndrome
- Due to anterior spinal artery occlusion
- Results in para or quadriplegia (flaccid)
- Pain and temperature sensation are lost
- Posterior column sensation is preserved
- Sensory, motor and autonomic function are lost below the level of lesion.

Posterior cord syndrome
- Signs and symptoms of posterior column dysfunction.
- Lesion of posterior column of the spinal cord
- Unilateral/bilateral

Causes
- Trauma to the cord
- Posterior spinal artery occlusion
- Disc protrusion
- B12 deficiency
- Syphilis
- Multiple sclerosis
- Tumor compression
- Tabes dorsalis

Arteria Magna Occlusion

- Level of lesion can be at T_4–T_6—significant involvement of lumbar and sacral cord
- Produces central cord syndrome
- Acute flaccid paraplegia
- Urinary retention
- Spinothalamic sensory loss
- Posterior column—not involved.

Tuberculosis of Spine (TB Spine)

Common site of involvement—thoracolumbar spine.

Possible reasons for thoracolumbar cord involvement in tuberculosis
- Hematogenus spread of TB focus from lungs via intercostal arteries.
- Involvement of lymph node—like para-aortic nodes—vertebrae are contiguous

with the lymph nodes which can have TB foci

- Vertebrae are rich in arterial supply—can easily become affected.

Different types of spinal cord involvement in TB

- Due to mechanical compression of the spinal cord by
  - diseased vertebra and disc
  - adhesive arachnoiditis
  - Psoas abscess.
- End arteritis causing vascular lesions.
- Tuberculoma of the spinal cord.

Brown-Séquard Syndrome

Occurs due to hemisection of the cord

Features—at the level of lesion

- Presence of root pain on the side of the lesion
- Motor weakness and wasting at the level
- Presence of fasciculations
- Absence of deep tendon reflexes

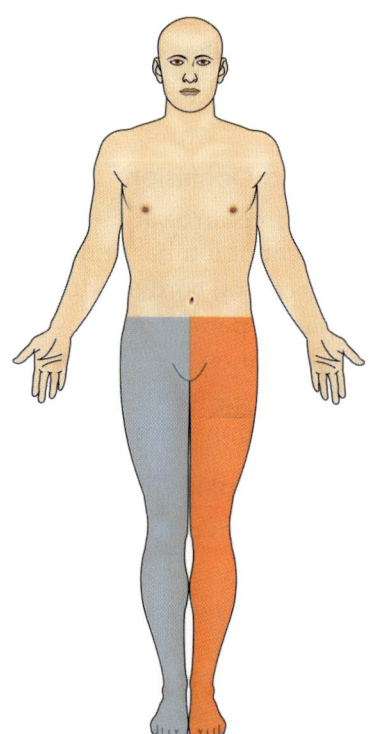

Fig. 4.13: Sensory loss in Brown-Séquard syndrome

Below the level of lesion

On the side of lesion

- Motor weakness with increased deep reflexes (due to pyramidal involvement).
- Vibration sense and joint sense loss (due to posterior column involvement).

On the opposite side of lesion

- Loss of pain and temperature one or two segments below the level of lesion.
- Due to crossed fibers of spinothalamic involvement

Causes of multiple levels of compression of spinal cord

- Multiple fracture of vertebra or multiple intervertebral disc prolapse
- Multiple secondaries in the spine
- Multiple levels of demyelination
- Adhesive arachnoiditis.
- Benign lesions like neurofibromatosis.

Compression of Spinal Cord from Metastatic Lesions

Source of Metastasis

- Neoplasm of lung, breast, prostate, kidney.
- Lymphoma and plasma cell dyscrasias.
- Due to the presence of higher content of bone marrow in the vertebral column, there is a tendency for solid tumors to metastasize into the vertebral column.

Most common site of involvement

- Thoracic spine
- Lumbar and sacral spine are usually involved by ovarian and prostatic malignancy.
- Root pain—may be caused by retroperitoneal mass entering through intervertebral foramina.

Features of metastatic spine disorders

- Severe pain in the back
- May be radiating pain over the trunk
- Pain increases on coughing/sneezing
- Severe pain at night.

Note

As thoracic spine is not usually involved in spondylosis, recent onset of back pain in the thoracic region—rule out metastasis to the spine.

Noncompressive Myelopathy

Causes

Acute onset
- Acute transverse myelitis
- Vascular involvement of spinal cord
- Demyelinating disorder
  - Chronic onset
- Infective
  - HIV involvement of spinal cord
  - HTLV myelopathy—tropical spastic paraplegia
  - Tabes dorsalis.
- Vascular
  - Vascular malformation of cord
  - AV fistula of the cord
- Demyelinating: Multiple sclerosis
- Deficiency: Subacute combined degeneration of spinal cord.

Degenerative
- MND
- Hereditary spastic paraplegia.

Vascular malformation of spinal cord and AV malformation of the cord
- Presents as progressive myelopathy
- Can have bruit over the spine and presents as vascular nevus.

HTLV Myelopathy
- Also called tropical spastic paraplegia
- Aetiological agent
- HTLV-I virus
- Human T cell lymphotropic virus type I

Features
- Insidious onset slowly progressive weakness of lower limb.
- Spastic paraplegia
- Sensory loss
- Bladder involvement.

Familial Spastic Paraplegia
- Presents as progressive weakness and spasticity of lower limb.
- Genetically mediated
- Sensory is usually not involved
- Bladder is involved
- Can also have ataxia, optic atrophy and nystagmus

DIFFERENT LEVELS OF SPINAL CORD LESIONS

High cervical cord lesions
Features
- Causes suboccipital pain which is radiating to the neck and shoulder.
- If C_2 segment is involved—it can cause sensory loss over the occipital area.
- Involvement of descending sensory tract of trigeminal nerve.
- Involvement of IX, X and XI and XII cranial nerves.
- Short neck and low hair line (associated with craniovertebral anomalies).

Short neck
- Hold the neck in neutral position
- Measure from external occipital protruberance to spine of C7 vertebra.
- Measure also the total body height.
- If the measurement of neck is less than 1/13 of the measurement of total body height, it is suggestive of short neck.

Low hair line: Posterior hair line is receding below C4 spine.

Lesion at the level of foramen magnum
- Results in cruciate hemiplegia
- Due to involvement of pyramidal tract after fibers decussate to upper limb have crossed but those of lower limb have not crossed.

Signs: Weakness of ipsilateral upper limb and weakness of contralateral lower limb.

Lhermitte's sign (Barber's chair sign)
- Electrical shock like sensation or sensation of tingling which is felt from neck above

down to the back when the person flexes the neck.

- Indicates distortion or inflammation of the cervical cord.
- Can occur in patients with
  - Multiple sclerosis
  - Cervical spondylosis

Elsberg's phenomenon

- Occurs in patients with cervical myelopathy.
- There will be U-shaped distribution of motor symptoms.
- Weakness starts with weakness of ipsilateral upper limb. Then involves ipsilateral lower limb, then contralateral lower limb and then contralateral upper limb.

Possible explanations

Compression on one side of the spinal cord and then being pushed to the opposite side causing contralateral side symptoms. Venous edema may also contribute to the clinical manifestations.

Lesions above C3 level

- Quadriparesis
- Diaphragm paralysis.

Below C3 level

- Quadriparesis
- Horner's syndrome
- Features also depend on the cervical segment involved.

C8, T1 involvement in high cervical cord lesions:
Higher cervical cord lesions cause ischemia and hypoxia at the level of C8–T1 due to venous congestion and ischemia occurs as a result of watershed territory of blood supply.

Sacral sparing in cervical cord lesions

- Occurs in patients with intrinsic lesions of cervical spinal cord
- Features—sparing of sacral sensation
- Due to longest sensory fibers from sacral segments come to lie most superficial and fibers from more rostral level occupy deeper levels.

Summary of Features of Cervical Cord Lesions

- Lower cranial nerve involvement (high cervical cord)
- Cerebellar involvement (high cervical cord)
- Downbeat nystagmus (high cervical cord)
- Diaphragm involvement (up to C3 level)
- Spinal tract of trigeminal nerve involvement (up to C5 level)
- Horner's syndrome
- Elsberg phenomenon
- Lhermitte's symptom
- Significant involvement of C8 and T1
- Sacral sparing (intramedullary lesions)

Cervical Spine Disease

Different Types of Neurological Involvement in Cervical Spine Disease

Compression of nerve roots
Due to

- Osteophytes
- Disc protrusion
- Hypertrophic facets of vertebra and joints.
- Common roots compressed—C6 and C7 roots.

Compression of spinal cord in cervical spondylosis occurs due to

- Ischemia occurring due to compression of vertebral artery.
- Osteophytes cause narrowing of spinal canal.
- Herniation of intervertebral disc (central or lateral).
- Posterior longitudinal ligament becomes ossified and can cause compression.

Spondylotic myelopathy: Occurs in patients with cervical spondylosis.

Clinical features
Presents with

- Neck pain and stiffness of neck.
- Root pain—referred to the upper limb.
- Weakness of upper limb and lower limb and involvement of small muscles of hand.

- Elsberg phenomenon—in the distribution of symptoms and signs.
- Stiffness of lower limb.
- Lhermitte's symptoms.
- Bladder and bowel—later or may not be involved.

Signs
- Lower motor neuron signs in the upper limb with upper motor signs in the lower limb.
- Sensory signs in the distribution of root involved.

Other causes of LMN signs in the upper limb and UMN signs in the lower limb.
- Syringomyelia
- Amyotrophic lateral sclerosis.

Involvement of Thoracic Spinal Cord

Compression—causes—TB spine
- Secondary metastasis
- Spinal cord benign tumors.

Features
Site of pain
- Well localized to the back
- Weakness of lower limb with spastic paraparesis.
- Involvement of bowel and bladder.
- Sensory level over the trunk.
- Abdominal reflexes—may be absent (T6–T12 level)

Lesion at T10: Sensory level at T10 (at umbilicus) and presence of Beevor's sign.

Lumbar Cord

Causes of compression of lumbar cord
- Trauma to the spine
- Lumbar disc prolapse
- Secondary deposits
- Spinal epidural abscess.

Features of lumbar cord compression
- Low back pain
- Root pain—mainly radiate to the lower limb.

If the lesion is at L2, L3 and L4
- Weakness of extensors of knee.
- Loss of knee jerk

If the lesion is at L5–S1
- Weakness of foot and ankle.
- Loss of ankle jerk.

Lumbar Canal Stenosis
- Characterised by narrowed lumbar spinal canal.
- Usually asymptomatic
- When becomes symptomatic, presents with neurogenic claudication.

Causes of lumbar canal stenosis
- Common cause: Congenital
- Less common: Acquired
- Congenital: Spinal canal narrowing occurs due to short and thick pedicle of the vertebra.
- Acquired: Trauma to the lumbar spine.
  - Lumbar spondylosis
  - Sclerosis of lumbar spine
  - Paget's disease of bone
  - Spondylolisthesis of lumbar spine.
- Significant narrowing of neural foramina results in sensory loss across the lower limb with focal weakness and loss of tendon jerk.

Characteristic features of neurogenic claudication
Site of pain
- Posterior aspect of buttocks, legs and back.
- Bilateral
- May be associated with neurological symptoms.
- Precipitating factors immediately on standing.
- Relieving factors—sitting, leaning forwards, pain relief takes minutes.

Clinical examination: Peripheral pulses normally felt.
- Can have motor weakness and reflex changes in the lower limb.
- Pain relief in flexed position in lumbar canal stenosis:

- Flexion causes increase of anteroposterior diameter of spinal canal and decreases intraspinal venous hypertension and pain.

Features of vascular claudication

Site of pain—usually calf and unilateral.

Precipitating factors—climbing/walking

Co-morbidities—smoking, diabetes mellitus

Relieved by stopping the exercise, relieves within seconds.

Examination: Peripheral pulses are absent. No neurological deficit.

CAUDA EQUINA AND CONUS MEDULLARIS

Cauda Equina

Anatomy

- Bunch of nerve roots arise from conus medullaris
- Resembles horsetail
- Consists of 10 pairs of nerve roots
  - From L2–L5
  - S1–S5
  - One pair of coccygeal root

Blood supply: Anterior and posterior spinal arteries.

Function

- Receive and send signals between pelvic organs, lower limb, genital organs and rectal organs.
- Also contain preganglionic parasympathetic fibers from S2 to S4 to innervate detrusor muscle of urinary bladder.
- Somatic LMN fibers from S2 to S4 for voluntary muscle of external sphincter of anus and rectum.

Causes of Cauda Equina Lesion

- Trauma to the back
- Spinal tumors in the low back region
- Spinal epidural abscess
- Degenerative disease of spine
- Lumbar canal stenosis.

Symptoms of Cauda Equina Lesion

Back pain: Less compared to root pain.

Root pain

- Severe in the distribution of nerve root
- Usually sciatic nerve

Symptoms

- Predominantly unilateral.
- Gradually progressive

Sensory features

- Symptoms in the distribution of dermatome involved
- Numbness of pelvic area, glans and clitoris, saddle area can be involved.

Symptoms: Symmetrical and may be unilateral.

Motor features

- LMN type of involvement
- Muscle involved—hypotonic
- Thinning of muscles—atrophy
- Deep reflexes—absent
- Motor involvement—usually asymmetrical
- In higher up lesions of cauda equina there will be involvement of spinal cord causing UMN signs. There can be brisk reflexes and extensor plantar (cauda + conus involvement).

Sphincters and sexual function

Presents as

- Difficulty in initiating micturition with hesitancy
- Urinary retention with overflow incontinence
- Sphincter tone—lost.

S_1 and S_2 lesions

- Weakness of flexors of knee
- Intrinsic muscles of foot—paralysed and wasted
- Knee jerk is preserved
- Ankle jerk is lost
- Anal and bulbocavernous—not lost

S_3, S_4 and S_5 lesions

- Lower limb weakness—may not be present
- Deep reflexes—not lost
- Saddle anesthesia
- Urinary and fecal retention
- Bowel and bladder paralysed
- Paralysis of external sphincter
- Anal and bulbocavernous reflexes lost.

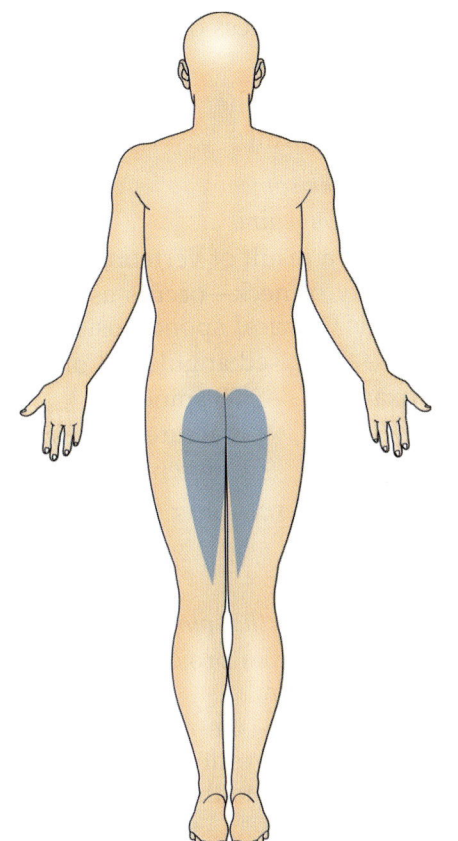

Fig. 4.14: Saddle anesthesia in conus medullaris lesion

Conus Medullaris

Terminal Part of Spinal Cord

- Corresponds to T_{12} to L_1 vertebra
- Rarely L_1–L_2 vertebra
- Epiconus—cord segments—L_4–L_5 and S_1 rarely S_2.
- Conus medullaris at T_{12}–L_1 vertebra. It is the tapered end of the spinal cord involving.
- Segments: S_2, S_3, S_4, S_5 and coccygeal 1.
- At the end of conus medullaris pia mater continues as filum terminale as a slender filament attached to the coccyx.

Periconus: Epiconus + conus medullaris.

Blood supply: Anterior and posterior spinal arteries.

Causes of conus medullaris involvement

- Trauma to the back
- Spinal tumors: Dermoid/lipoma
- Degenerative disease of spine

Features of Conus Medullaris Involvement

Symptoms

- Low back pain—severe
- Radicular pain—less severe
- Bilaterally symmetrical
- May be of sudden in onset.

Table 4.3: Differential features between conus medullaris and cauda equina lesions

	Conus medullaris	Cauda equina
Onset of pain	Bilaterally symmetrical and usually sudden	Unilateral and gradual
Back pain	Bilaterally symmetrical Pain less severe, felt in the Thigh and perineum	Symmetrical root pain severe
Motor system	Symmetrical weakness Of lower limb—fasciculation May be present	Severe weakness asymmetrical No fasciculation
Sensory	Bilaterally symmetrical—saddle anesthesia Dissociated anesthesia— may be present	Unilateral and asymmetrical have saddle anesthesia
Sphincter and sexual function **Segments involved**	Severe and early involvement Epiconus L_4, L_5, S_1 and S_2 Conus S_3, S_4, S_5, and coccygeal	Late and less severe Roots: L_2, L_3, L_4, L_5 S_1–S_5 and coccygeal

Sensory
- Dissociated anesthesia
- Bilaterally symmetrical
- Saddle anesthesia (S_3–S_5)

Motor
- Spasticity
- Bilaterally symmetrical distal paralysis of lower limb
- Brisk ankle jerks
- If the lesion is above S1—plantar is extensor.

Sphincters and sexual function
- Early and severely involved
- Impotence
- Urinary retention with overflow incontinence
- Early fecal incontinence with atonic sphincter.
- Loss of anal and bulbocavernous reflex.

EXAMINATION OF SPINE

Important Anatomical Landmarks While Examining the Spine and Back

- Cervical—C7 spine: Most prominent spine over the back
- T7 spine—at the level of inferior angle of scapula
- L2—spine at the level of lower rib
- L3/L4 spine—at the level of iliac crest
- S2—corresponds to dimple at posterior superior iliac spine.

Inspection of Spine

Look for Following Abnormalities

- Deformity
- Gibbus
- Asymmetry
- Kyphoscoliosis
- Lumbar lordosis

Examination of Spine

Palpation of Spine

- Tenderness
- Step deformity over the spine
- Movement of spine.

Percussion: Tenderness over the spine.

Auscultation
- Bruit over the spine
- Renal angle bruit

Inspection of the spine
Deformity—congenital
- Occurs as a result of vertebral disease.
- Deformity of neck—occurs as a result of torticollis/cervical spondylosis
- Gibbus—localised angulation of spine
- For example: – TB spine
                 – Fracture vertebra
                 – Congenital.

Also look for tenderness over the spine
- Renal angle
- Sacroiliac joint.

Step deformity over the spine
- Palpable step-like projection at the level of L_5–S_1 junction.
- Palpating finger is moved down over the spine from above downwards over the lumbar spine up to the sacrum.
- Indicates spondylolisthesis.

Percussion = For tenderness over the spine.

Auscultation

Bruit over the spine: Occurs in patients with AV malformation of spinal cord.
Bruit over the renal angle: Renal artery stenosis.

Flattening of lumbar lordosis
Causes
- Infection of the vertebra
- Osteoarthritis
- Prolapsed disc
- Ankylosing spondylitis

Asymmetry of paraspinal area: Look for asymmetry in the prominence of paraspinal muscles: Indicates muscle spasm.

Kyphoscoliosis
- Normal spine: Lordosis is present at cervical and lumbar levels.
- Kyphosis—occurs at thoracic level.
- Scoliosis—lateral bending of spine.

Postural scoliosis: Due to defective posturing of body and spine—disappears with forward flexion of spine.

Structural scoliosis: Persists with forward flexion of spine and there will be persistence of rib hump.

Tenderness over the spine
- Occurs due to infection
- Fracture
- Neoplastic disorders.

Tenderness can also occur due to
- Soft tissue tenderness
- Paravertebral muscles spasm.

Inspection of the skin over the spine
- Look for previous scar of surgery
- Presence of sinus: Indicates pilonidal sinus

Tuft of hair/pad of fat/dimple of skin = at the lower spinal level suggests spina bifida occulta/meningocoele/meningomyelocoele.

Color changes
- Pigmentation/café-au-lait spot:
- Suggests neurofibromatosis.

Look for maculoanesthetic patch over the back and buttocks—patch of leprosy: Decubitus ulcers— common in bed-ridden patients.

Spina bifida occulta
- Presence of gap in the vertebra due to defective closure.
- Can have meningocele/meningomyelocele.
- Produces urinary incontinence and neurological involvement in the lower back (L_4, L_5 and S_1 involvement).

Other system examinations along with examination of spine
- Movement of spine, shoulder, and hip
- Examination of nervous system
- Per abdominal examination
- Per rectal examination
- Examination of prostate and anal sphincter.

Important Clinical Signs While Examining Spine

Straight leg raising (SLR) sign
- Keep the patient in supine position
- Flex the patient's lower limb at the hip which is kept in extended position.
- Normal person—can flex the hip up to 80°.
- Further dorsiflexion of foot after maximum flexion of hip = further stretch produces pain.
- *Conclusion*: Causes stretch of L5–S1 root and sciatic root.

Crossed SLR
- Specific test for herniation of intervertebral disc.
- Flexion of one leg on one side results in pain on the other side.
- *Conclusion*: Nerve root involved—damage to the nerve root on the side of the pain.

Reversed SLR
- Ask the patient to stand.
- Extend the lower limb with the knee fully extended: Patient will have pain.

Conclusion: Stretch of L_2, L_3, and L_4 nerve roots, lumbosacral plexus and femoral nerve.

GUILLAIN-BARRÉ SYNDROME

Type of Disease

It is an acute inflammatory demyelinating polyneuropathy.

Pathogenesis
- Autoimmune disorder
- Antibodies against gangliosides of nerve tissues
- Compliment activation with damage to myelin and axons
- Predominantly of motor nerve roots and extraocular motor nerves.

Pathology
- Predominantly demyelinating form produces conduction block
- Rapid demyelination can occur
- Axonal form—slow recovery.

Precipitating Factors

- Preceding (1–3 weeks before): Gastro-intestinal/respiratory infection.
- Most common infection: *Campylobacter jejuni* infection.

 Note

Surface glycoproteins of C. jejuni can cross react with gangliosides of nerves.

Clinical Features

- *Rapid progression of motor weakness*
  - Proximal > distal
  - Lower limb > upper limb
  - Ascending type
- Sensory symptoms—very minimal
- Deep tendon reflexes—absent
- Urinary bladder: Not involved or very minimal
- Pain in the limbs
- *Rapidly can progress to*
  - Bulbar muscle involvement
  - Bilateral facial involvement
  - Respiratory difficulty requiring ventilatory support
- *There can be autonomic involvement can result in*
  - Postural hypotension
  - Hypertension
  - Cardiac arrhythmias

Different Types

Common type—AIDP: Acute inflammatory demyelinating neuropathy.

Other precipitating factors

- *Infection with*
  - CMV virus
  - HIV virus
  - Epstein-Barr virus
  - Hepatitis E
  - Mycoplasma infection
- *Types*
  - AMAN: Acute motor axonal neuropathy

- AMSAN: Acute motor sensory axonal neuropathy
- Acute autonomic neuropathy—pandysautonomia
- Ophthalmoplegia
- Pure sensory form

Miller-Fisher Variant

- No motor weakness
- Ataxia
- Loss of deep tendon reflexes
- Ophthalmoplegia
- Paralysis of papillary function.

Other conditions which may cause AIDP like presentation

- Lymphoma
- SLE
- Retroviral infection
- *Consider alternate diagnosis in a patient of suspected GB syndrome if following features are present*
  - Presence of fever at starting of illness
  - Intact/brisk deep tendon reflexes
  - Early and severe bladder involvement
  - Horizontal level of sensory loss
  - CSF cell count high (>50 cells/cmm)

Antibodies associated with different types of GB syndrome

- Anti-GM_1 antibody: AIDP.
- Anti-GD1 antibody: Acute Motor axonal neuropathy.
- Anti-GM_2 antibody: Bulbar and facial involvement.
- Anti-GQ1D antibody: Miller-Fisher variant.

Differential Diagnosis

- Poliomyelitis
- Myelopathy
- Diphtheria
- Porphyria
- Tick paralysis
- Vasculitis: Neuropathy/mononeuropathy multiplex
- Botulism
- Myasthenia gravis

Differentiating Features

- *Poliomyelitis*
  - Fever, asymmetrical weakness
  - Fasciculation
- *Myelopathy*: Horizontal level, motor, sensory and bladder involvement.
- *Diphtheria*: Diphtheritic membrane over the tonsil/pharynx, pupil involvement, myocarditis.
- *Porphyria*: Pain abdomen, precipitating drugs.
- *Vasculitis*: Other features of vasculitis.
- *Myasthenia gravis*: Fatigue, progressive weakness fluctuating.

Lab Features

- Demyelinating neuropathy—conduction block on nerve conduction velocity.
- Axonal neuropathy—reduced amplitude of conduction.
- CSF after 1 week—albumino cytological dissociation (raised protein—may raise up to 1 Gr without raise in the CSF cell count).

Conditions which mimic GB syndrome with raised CSF cell count
- Sarcoidosis with neurological involvement
- HIV infection
- Viral myelitis
- Hematological malignancy with neuronal involvement, e.g. lymphoma/leukemia.

Features which require early intervention in GB syndrome
1. Rapidly progressive weakness
2. Severe muscular weakness
3. Bulbar and respiratory involvement
Course of illness
- Usually slowly progressive
- Can slowly recover within 4–8 weeks
- 30% of patients—may require respiratory support

Spinal Epidural Abscess

- Abscess in the spinal epidural space.
- Results in progressive compressive myelopathy

- Organisms responsible
  - *Streptococcus pyogenes*
  - *Staphylococcus aureus*
  - Gram-negative bacilli
  - Anaerobic infection
  - Tuberculosis

Pathology
- Formation of an abscess
- Compression of spinal cord
- Venous stasis.

Predisposing factors
- Uncontrolled diabetes mellitus
- Chronic renal failure
- Malignancy
- Other immune compromised state

Possible source of infection
- Endocarditis
- Skin and dental infection

Duration of symptoms
- Usually 1–2 weeks
- Occasionally longer

Presenting features
- Back pain with or without radicular pain.
- Fever, lower limb weakness.

Investigation: MRI spine.

Tethered Cord Syndrome

- Developmental disorder of lower spinal cord.
- Results in involvement of lower spinal cord and nerve roots.
- Can cause back pain
- Can have tuft of hair, dimple over the skin over the lower back.

MRI: Thickening of filum terminale on the low lying conus medullaris.

Neuromyelitis Optica (NMO)

Demyelinating disorder causing severe spinal cord involvement.
Features:
- Bilateral optic neuritis, longitudinal spinal cord involvement for 2–3 segments.

- Occasionally brainstem is involved.
- CSF—mononuclear pleocytosis, oligoclonal band present

Characteristic antibody

- Autoantibody against aquaporin-4 channel
- Can be associated with SLE, APLA syndrome.

ACUTE TRANSVERSE MYELITIS

Inflammatory Lesion of Spinal Cord

Characteristics

- Inflammation of spinal cord
- Horizontal level of lesion
- Neurological involvement below the horizontal level on both sides of spinal cord.

Meaning of transverse myelitis

- Across the spinal cord—pathology occurs at a transverse level.
- Complete transverse lesion may not occur.

Clinical Features

Onset

- Sudden or gradual over 1–4 weeks
- Starts as vague back pain or sudden sharp shooting pain.

Motor features: Weakness of arms and legs below a horizontal level.

Sensory features: Sensory loss below a horizontal level of all modalities of sensation.

Sphincters and sexual function: Bowel, bladder and sexual function are lost.

Most common spinal cord level involved—thoracic cord level.

Course of events: Initially behaves like LMN lesion with hypotonia, and loss of reflexes, below a horizontal level due to spinal shock and later develops spasticity and exaggerated deep reflexes and plantar extensor bilaterally.

Exclude following disorders in a patient of acute transverse myelitis

- Compressive pathology of spinal cord
- Vascular occlusion

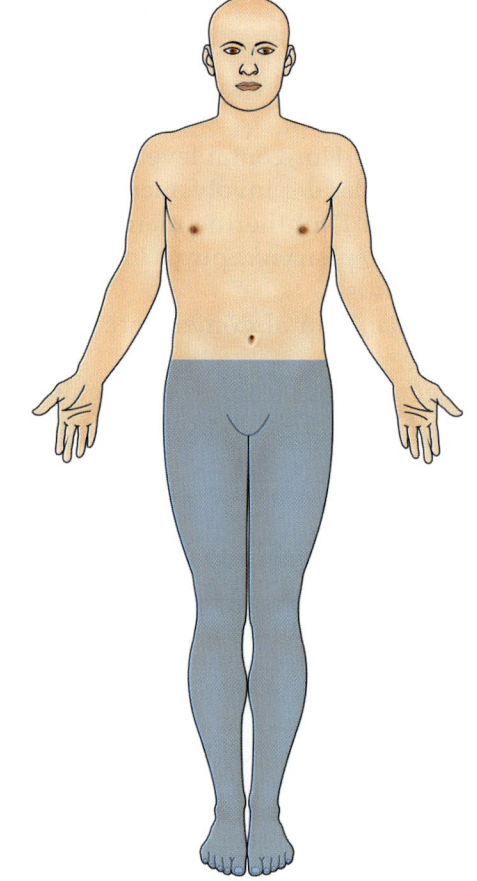

Fig. 4.15: Sensory loss in acute transverse myelitis

- AV malformation of the cord
- Radiation-induced myelitis
- ADEM.

Causes of acute transverse myelitis

Infective—viral

- Herpes zoster
- Herpes simplex
- HIV infection.

Bacterial

- Mycoplasma infection
- Lyme disease
- Syphilis.

Postvaccinal

- MMR vaccine
- Diphtheria, tetanus vaccine

- Anti-rabies vaccine
- Hepatitis B vaccine.

Systemic disease
- SLE
- Sjögren's syndrome

Demyelination
- Multiple sclerosis
- Neuromyelitis optica

Occasionally idiopathic
Investigations
- CSF—for pleocytosis
- MRI spine—evidence of cord involvement
- Serology for infective etiology.

Brown-Sèquard Syndrome

- Occurs due to pathology in one-half of the spinal cord.
- Usual site involved: Cervical cord.

Features

- Ipsilateral hemiplegia
- Ipsilateral proprioceptive loss
- Contralateral pain and temperature loss (a few segments below the level of lesion).

Causes

- Trauma
- Spinal tumor
- Multiple sclerosis
- Disc lesions
- Rare: Hemorrhage/ischemia of the cord
- Loss of pain and temperature several segments below the level of lesion as pain and temperature fibers ascend a few segments before crossing to the opposite side.

Endemic fluorosis

- Disease caused by drinking water with high fluoride content over a prolonged period of time.
- Increased incidence in India (Andhra Pradesh), Africa, etc.
- Safe content of fluoride in the water: 0.8 ppm.

Clinical Manifestations
Dental
- Mottled enamel, chalky white opacities and brownish discoloration.
- Mottled enamel is indicative of excessive ingestion of fluorine since childhood.

Skeletal fluorosis: Pain and stiffness of joints specially spine. Formation of exostosis.

Spine
- There will be calcification of ligaments
- Fusion of vertebrae
- Marked kyphosis
- Compressive myelopathy

Characteristic feature: Ossification of interosseus membrane of leg and forearm.

Advanced cases
- Renal involvement
- Thyroid and parathyroid involvement
- Severe anemia

LATHYRISM

- Due to excessive consumption of *Lathyrus sativus* caused by the neurotoxic substance beta-N-oxalyl-amino-alanine (BOAA).
- Irreversible nonprogressive spastic paraparesis.
- Due to degenerative changes in the spinal cord.

NEUROGENIC BLADDER
Micturition Centers
- Cortical center—frontal lobe (2nd frontal gyrus)

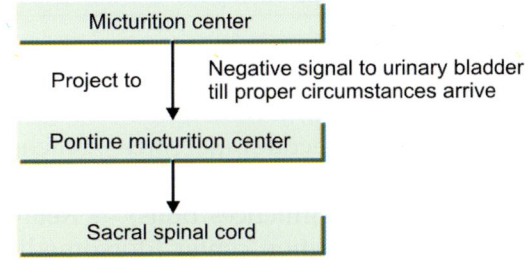

- Cortical center—sends negative signal to the lower centers until proper circumstances arrive to urinate.
- Pontine center—excitatory center—facilitates detrusor contraction and sphincter relaxation—act of micturition.
- Cortical center is taken control over by the pons by 3–4 years of age.

Nerve Supply of Urinary Bladder

Parasympathetic supply
- From S2, S3, S4 intermediolateral column (segment) of the spinal cord.
- Causes detrusor contraction
- Relaxes internal sphincter
- Inhibits pudendal nerve—causes external sphincter to relax and emptying of the bladder
- So parasympathetic supply is called nerve of bladder emptying.

Sympathetic supply
- From T12-L1 level of spinal cord
- Innervate the bladder through inferior hypogastric plexus
- Results in increase in the bladder capacity and contraction of internal sphincter.
- They are called nerve of bladder filling.
- Somatic supply: S2, S3, S4—motor nucleus—via pudendal nerve—innervate external sphincter.

Nucleus of Onuf: Additional motor nucleus located in nearby anterior horn cell near the sacral region. Innervate the external sphincter via pudendal nerve.

 Note

Nucleus of Onuf is spared in patients with MND.

Micturition Reflex

Stretch of the urinary bladder →
Impulse reaches sacral spinal cord → reaches cortical center
Cortical center (influences pons) → Relays to pontine micturition center (dorsomedial pontine segment) → Descending fibers to parasympathetic centre in sacral cord → Detrusor contraction and relaxation of internal Sphincter → Micturition

Features of Neurogenic Bladder

Different Levels of Lesion at Nervous System

Cortical bladder (uninhibited bladder)
Lesion of frontal micturition center
Features
- Sudden emptying of bladder which is uncontrollable.
- There will be detrusor hyperreflexia causing urgency at lower bladder volumes.
- Residual urine is usually absent
- Social inhibition for urination is lost
- May be associated with other cortical abnormalities.

Pontine lesions: Can cause retention of urine due to damage to pontine facilitatory center.
Lesion of the spinal cord
Lesion of spinal cord above the sacral cord produces UMN bladder (spastic bladder—automatic bladder)
- External sphincter and bladder are spastic.
- If the lesion is above T6 segment, there will be associated mass reflex.
- If the lesion is below T6, mass reflex is absent.

Features of automatic bladder
- Reflex emptying of bladder without filling
- Evacuation may be incomplete
- Frequency and urgency of micturition is present.

Other associated features
- Bilateral pyramidal signs in the lower limb
- Flexor spasms
- Mass reflex

 Note

In the initial stage of spinal cord lesion there is a stage of spinal shock. Person will have urinary retention with constipation.

Sacral cord lesion along with involvement of nerve roots

Due to

- Tumors
- Herniated intervertebral disc
- Trauma
- Tethered cord
- There will be interruption of sacral reflex arc controlling the bladder.
- There may be damage to the motor and sensory component of reflex arc.

Results in autonomous/LMN bladder

- There will be loss of bladder sensation and reflex contraction
- Normal urination is lost
- Person will have incontinence

Features

- Continuous dribbling of urine
- Considerable residual urine
- High risk of infection

If there is significant damage to sensory fibers, there will be large atonic overdistended bladder with overflow incontinence.

Other features

- Feature of cauda equina lesion
- Presence of saddle anesthesia

 Note

In posterior column lesions, peripheral neuropathy, there will be painless over. Distension of urinary bladder.

Atonic bladder: Large distended/dilated urinary bladder—either due to loss of nerve supply or due to chronic obstruction.

SYRINGOMYELIA

Syringomyelia—fluid-filled cavity in the spinal cord.

Hydromyelia—dilatation of central canal of the spinal cord.

Characteristic Features

Long cavities surrounded by gliosis in the brainstem. Cavities extend from central part of the spinal cord up to medulla.

Common sites of cavity

- Lower cervical cord. Upper thoracic region
- Medulla, pons up to internal capsule can be affected. Rarely lumbar and sacral cord can be affected.
- May be due to developmental anomalies or traumatic transverse lesion of the cord.

Spinal cord abnormalities in a patient of Syringomyelia

- Enlarged in the transverse plane
- ↑ in the AP diameter of spinal canal
- Protein contents of CSF is ↑
- Cavity affects less resistant gray matter than white matter
- Cavity can erode anterior horn cells.

Medullary extension

- Posterolateral medulla near spinal nucleus of Vth nerve and nucleus ambiguus.
- Later can involve—corticospinal tract, sensory fibers.
- Hemorrhage into syringomyelia cavity can occur.

Aetiopathogenesis

Communicating Syringomyelia

Cavity communicates with the IV ventricle associated anomalies

- Chiari type I malformation
- Craniovertebral anomaly
- Basal arachnoiditis
- Dandy-Walker syndrome (closure of foramen of Luschka and Magendie)

  Above lesions prevent course of CSF from IV ventricle to subarachnoid space

  ↓

  Pressure wave down to central canal

  ↓

  Dilatation

- Dilatation of cavity—ependymal loss
- Divarication of fibers—upwards or downwards—along the central canal.

Noncommunicating Type

Syringomyelic cavity does not communicate with the IV ventricle

- Often due to spinal injury with or without paraplegia
- Spinal tumor
- Spinal arachnoiditis.

Syringobulbia

- Brainstem may be progressively involved
- Syngobulbia may be the presenting symptoms of the disease
- *Can have*
  - Trigeminal pain
  - Vertigo
  - Facial, palatal/or laryngeal palsy.

Morvan's syndrome

- Progressive loss of pain ulceration and loss of soft tissue.
- Resorption of phalanges, muscle atrophy of hand, feet with perforating ulcers.

Differential diagnosis of syringomyelic symptoms: Leprosy, hereditary sensory motor neuropathy.

CLINICAL FEATURES OF SYRINGOMYELIA

Mode of onset: Insidious, may follow episodes of coughing, sneezing, straining.

Sensory symptoms and signs
Unilateral

- At first involves decussating fibers of sensation from dorsal root.
- Pain, heat, cold sensations are interrupted.

Dissociated sensory loss

- Ulnar borders of hand
- Upper part of forearm
- Chest, back and arm or one side   } Half cafe
- Lower border across the chest
- If the lesion is in the center or extends to other side, symptoms become bilateral.

Suspended anesthesia

At the level of syrinx: Loss of pain and temperature with preservation of touch over

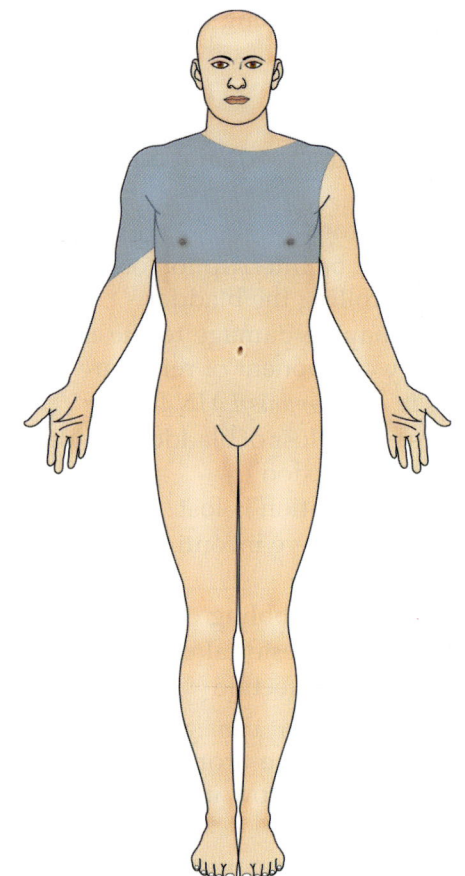

Fig. 4.16: Suspended Jaquet type of anesthesia in syringomyelia

corresponding part of the body with normal sensation above and below that body part.

As the lesion extends

- Involves radial side of upper limb, back and downwards over thorax.
- Postcolumn—last to get affected.
- Patient can have painless burns/ulcers and not feeling hot water
- Spontaneous pain: Burning, aching, shooting pain like lightening pain of tabes dorsalis.
- Horner's syndrome—due to involvement of descending sympathetic chain.

Motor symptoms and signs

- Wasting of small muscle of hands—unilateral or bilateral—along with involvement

of forearm, arm, shoulder and upper intercostals.

- Fasciculations—rare.
- Contractures may develop.
- Lower limb weakness with stiffness and difficulty in walking. There will be development of UMN signs in the lower limb.
- Later there will be loss of bladder and bowel control.
- *Associated features*
  - Kyphoscoliosis
  - Charcot's joints

BASILAR INVAGINATION

- Top of C2 vertebra invaginates into the base of the skull.
- Odontoid process is projected into the foramen magnum and can cause narrowing.
- It can cause pressure effect on upper spinal cord and lower brainstem.

Basilar invagination: Upward displacement of top of C2 with normal base of the skull and foramen magnum.

Basilar impression: Similar displacement as above due to softening of base of the skull.

Causes

- Congenital
- Acquired
  - Rheumatoid arthritis
  - Osteogenesis imperfecta
  - Klippel-Feil syndrome
- Associated abnormalities
  - Syringomyelia
  - Hydrocephalus.

Platybasia

Flattening of the base of the skull due to increase in the basal angle of the skull (wider angle between the skull base of the anterior fossa and the clivus). It is usually associated with basilar invagination and can cause compression over the lower brain.

Features

- Posterior headache
- Lower cranial nerve dysfunction
- Spastic quadriparesis
- Cerebellar signs
- Downbeat nystagmus

Associated other features

- Syringomyelia
- Obstructive hydrocephalus.

ARNOLD-CHIARI MALFORMATION

Due to Malformation of Skull

Consists of downward displacement of the cerebellar tonsils through the foramen magnum.

Type 1: Herniation of cerebellar tonsils 3 mm below foramen magnum

Can cause headache, neck pain, ataxia, syringomyelia of cervical cord, displacement of lower brainstem.

Type 2: Displacement of cerebellar cortex and brainstem including medulla

- Paralysis below the spinal defect
- Lumbar and sacral meningomyelocele

Type 3: Herniation of cerebellum into high cervical meningomyelocele

Type 4: Rare will have primary cerebellar agenesis

Features

- Headache posterior aspect
- Lower cranial nerve palsy
- Spastic quadriparesis
- Cerebellar features with downbeat nystagmus
- Scoliosis
- Lhermitte's sign
- Can have central cord syndrome

Dandy-Walker syndrome

- Congenital defect
- Fluid filled spaces around with the absence of vermis in between two cerebellar hemispheres
- There will be enlargement of 4th ventricle.

KLIPPEL-FEIL SYNDROME

A form of craniovertebral anomaly.

Characteristic triad

- Low posterior hair line
- Short neck
- Limited neck movement
- Etiology—unknown
- There is failure of cervical vertebral segmentation—during 3rd to 8th weeks of gestation.

Types

Type 1: Many of cervical vertebrae are fused into single block

Type 2: Fusion of cervical vertebrae with failure of segmentation of one or two cervical vertebrae.

Type 3: Segmentation defect of lower dorsal/lumbar vertebrae with type 1 or type 2 anomaly.

Clinical presentation

- Due to compression of nerve roots and spinal cord.
- Cervical cord involvement—may be high cervical cord—at early age.
- Even minor trauma can precipitate high cervical cord abnormality.
- Occurrence of cervical spondylosis exacerbates pre-existing abnormality.
- Presence of mirror movement.

Other coexisting defects: VSD, deafness, short stature.

Investigations

- X-ray cervical spine
- MRI: Cervical spine
- Occasionally syringomyelia can be associated.
- Symptoms and signs of craniovertebral anomaly is aggravated by
  - Trauma to the neck
  - Carrying load on the head
  - Cervical spondylosis.

APPROACH TO A PATIENT OF DIFFICULTY IN WALKING

Normal control of body position and equilibrium is maintained by

- Visual system
- Vestibular system
- Posterior column—proprioception.
- And above 3 structures (minimum of 2 are required) along with cerebellum which is acting as a coordinating center are required for maintenance of posture.

Normal formation of steps and locomotor function: Purpose or goal of walking/generation of steps is determined by cerebral cortex.

Brainstem center for locomotor function

- Midbrain
- Pontine tegmentum
- Subthalamic region.
- Structures like ventromedial part of spinal cord and reticular activating system also take part in locomotor function.

Normal balance is controlled by

- Vermis and central part of cerebellum
- Vestibular nucleus.

Causes of Difficulty in Walking and Gait Abnormality

Non-neurological causes

- Severe fatigue
- Arthritis
- Deformity of lower limbs and feet
- Abnormality of refraction/reduce vision of the eye, e.g. cataract.

Neurological causes

- Metabolic/toxic/drug induced, e.g. alcohol, phenytoin overdosage
- Labyrinthine/vestibular—peripheral and central cause
- Disease of spinal cord—myelopathies.
- Disorders of sensory system—sensory ataxia
- Disorders of cerebellum.
- Disorders of muscles—myopathies.

- Disorders of cerebral cortex/basal ganglia and connections
  - Multi-infarct state
  - Normal pressure hydrocephalus
  - Progressive supranuclear palsy
  - Late stages of idiopathic parkinsonism
  - Parkinsonism plus syndromes
  - Rarely psychogenic

Drop attack

Sudden fall (loss of postural tone) without loss of consciousness
- Site of lesion—3rd ventricular lesion
  - Colloid cyst of 3rd ventricle
  - Obstruction to the CSF flow.

Gait Abnormalities

Freezing of gait (initiation/ignition defect)
- Frontal lobe disease
- Parkinsonism
- Multisystem atrophy
- Progressive supranuclear palsy
- Corticobasal degeneration.
- Freezing of gait—sudden difficulty in moving forward in spite of intention to walk. Feet appear as though stuck to the ground.

Disorders of frontal lobe: Can cause gait apraxia.

Normal Pressure Hydrocephalus

Features
- Memory loss
- Urinary incontinence
- Difficulty in walking—gait abnormality.

Different types of loss of balance/fall depending on the structures involved
- Falling backwards—progressive supra-nuclear palsy
- Falling forwards—late parkinsonism.
- Falling more in the dark—sensory ataxia.
- Sway/fall to one side—same side disease of cerebellum
- Truncal ataxia—vermis lesion
- Vertigo with falling to one side—same side—labyrinthine disease.

Gait Abnormalities

Apraxia of gait
- Occurs in—frontal lobe disease.
- Person is unable to lift the leg as if legs are glued to the ground (magnetic gait).

Waddling
- Abnormal type of gait due to proximal weakness of hip girdle muscles.
- Weakness of gluteus medius causes exagge-rated swing of pelvis due to lack of splin-ting action of gluteus medius.

Antalgic gait
- Occurs in person with pain in the lower extremity.
- They avoid leaning weight on the affected side. Person is usually limping while walking.

Astasia-abasia
- Functional disorder
- Unable to stand upright (astasia) and unable to walk (abasia)
- Rarely can occur in thalamic CVA and NPH.

Causes of Foot Drop
(Inability to Dorsiflex the Foot)

Unilateral foot drop
- L_4–L_5 radiculopathy
- Sciatic neuropathy
- Lower limb sacral plexopathy
- Common peroneal nerve palsy.

Bilateral foot drop
- All causes of peripheral neuropathy
- Charcot-Marie-Tooth disease.
- Distal myopathy
- MND
- Friedreich's ataxia.

CEREBELLUM

Part of Cerebellum

Cerebellar hemisphere: Takes part in appendi-cular skeleton coordination.

Vermis
- Small median portion

- Predominantly involved for gait and axial skeletal function

Flocculonodular lobe—mainly connected with vestibular connections.

Functions of Cerebellum

Major functions
- Determines coordination of movement
- Controls rate, range and force of movement
- Facilitatory control over the tone.

Connections of Cerebellum

Inferior cerebellar peduncle (Restiform body)—connected with spinal cord and medulla.

Middle cerebellar peduncle (brachium pontis)
- Connected with cerebellovestibular fibers
- Pontocerebellar fibers
- Corticopontocerebellar pathways

Superior cerebellar peduncle (brachium conjunctivum): Connected to rubral and dentatothalamic pathways.

Archicerebellum
- Oldest part of cerebellum
- Connected with vestibular functions
- Floccules, nodulus and part of vermis

Paleocerebellum
- Corresponds to anterior lobe
- Connected with spinocerebellar tracts and called spinocerebellum
- Maintains equilibrium and muscle tone.

Neocerebellum (posterior lobe)
- Recently developed part of cerebellum
- Consists of cerebellar hemisphere
- Connected with afferent fibers from cerebral cortex (parietal lobe)
- Concerned with skilled movement
- Connected to corticopontocerebellar pathways
- Sends output to thalamus and motor cortex and red nucleus.

Clinical aspects of cerebellar dysfunction
Titubation
- Anteroposterior, to and fro nodding movement of head. Trunk can be involved.

- Occurs in lesion of vermis.
- *Lesion of vermis*: Vermis lesion can occur in chronic alcoholism and medulloblastoma.
- Lesion of vermis causes gait and truncal ataxia

Dyssynergia: Cerebellum—coordinates smooth movements of muscles by organizing and regulating the muscle actions.

In cerebellar dysfunction
- Person's skilled and speed of movement becomes abnormal.
- Movement become erratic, jerky and disorganized.

Test for dyssynergia
- Repeated rapid movements like repeated quick tapping of the hand becomes defective.
- Dysmetria (finger–nose and finger–finger incoordination with intension tremor)
- In cerebellar dysfunction—there will be abnormality in judging and gauzing the distance of movement. Coordination between agonists and antagonists become abnormal.

Hypotonia: Normally there will be tonic output from cerebellar nuclei, fascilitating the motor cortex. This loss of fascilitation leads onto hypotonia.

Pendular knee jerk
- Elicit the knee jerk—normal number of oscillations is usually around 3 full to and fro swings. In cerebellar dysfunction it will be more than 3 swings.
- Pendular knee jerk occurs due to combination of hypotonia and defective check reflex response.

Pronator drift in cerebellar dysfunction
- It is a manifestation of hypotonia
- In cerebellar dysfunction—there will be drifting of outstretched arm outwards in the same plane (patient closing the eyes).

Other manifestations of cerebellar hypotonia
- Tapping the outstretched arm/wrist while testing for pronator drift.
- There will be oscillations up and down due to hypotonia.

Demonstration of pronator drift in the lower limb (see also chapter on motor system)
- Patient is in prone position. Bend the knee so as to keep the leg vertically upwards. There will be oscillations of leg and lateral deviation of the leg—deviation of the leg to the side of lesion.
- Rebound phenomenon is manifestation of impaired check reflex.

Tests for Coordination

Finger nose test
- Keep the upper limb in a state of full abduction.
- Note steadiness, and accuracy of movement of upper limb when it is brought towards the nose.

In cerebellar disease
- The limb will be brought in wavering movement.
- For lower limb incoordination: Knee heel test.

Features of Cerebellar Dysfunction

Hemispheric lesion
Features
- Hypotonia
- Dyssynergia
- Dysdiadochokinesis
- Drift of limb and past pointing will be towards the affected side.
- Fast phase of nystagmus towards the side of lesion.

Vermis lesion: Gait and truncal ataxia.

Causes of diffuse cerebellar lesions
- Spinocerebellar ataxia
- Drugs—alcohol, phenytoin toxins
- Paraneoplastic syndrome

Unilateral cerebellar disease
- Cerebellar tumors
- Abscess
- Infarct/hemorrhage.

APPROACH TO A PATIENT OF ATAXIA

Ataxia Suggests Imbalance
Key Points
- Cerebellar ataxia is not associated with dizziness/vertigo. They only present with imbalance.
- Ataxia associated with dizziness/vertigo is usually a feature of vestibular disease.
- Ataxia which aggravates on darkness/ when eyes are closed is a manifestation of sensory ataxia.
- Patient with proximal muscle weakness of lower limb can also have imbalance in walking and on examination they will have muscle power decrease.

Approach to a Patient of Cerebellar Ataxia

Acute onset: Unilateral cerebellar ataxia
Causes
- Lateral medullary syndrome
- Cerebellar infarct hemorrhage
- Cerebellar abscess
- Demyelinating disease
- Trauma—subdural hematoma

Other associated findings with acute unilateral cerebellar lesions
- Headache
- Signs and symptoms of raised intracranial tension
- Lower cranial nerve palsy
- Altered sensorium due to brainstem compression.

Subacute/chronic unilateral cerebellar ataxia
Causes
- Multiple sclerosis
- Craniovertebral anomalies
- CP angle mass lesion
- Cerebellar mass lesions Gliomas/secondaries.

Bilateral cerebellar ataxia

Acute onset

- Acute alcohol intoxication
- Viral encephalitis
- Postinfectious: ADEM, e.g. varicella infection
- Phenytoin overdosage.

Subacute onset

- Alcoholism
- Chemotherapeutic drugs
- Paraneoplastic syndrome—carcinoma lung, breast and ovary.

Chronic cerebellar ataxia

- Hereditary/degenerative disorder: Spinocerebellar degeneration
- Paraneoplastic syndrome
- Hypothyroidism
- CNS syphilis
- Alcoholic cerebellar degeneration
- Phenytoin toxicity

Hereditary Ataxias
(Spinocerebellar Ataxia)

Genetic Disorder

Usual features

- Gait abnormality
- Incoordination of movements of hands and eyes with speech abnormality.

Structural abnormalities

- Cerebellum and its connections
- Peripheral sensory abnormalities
- Spinal cord lesions

Diagnosis

- Characteristic clinical features
- Positive family history

Rule out following disorders in a patient of hereditary ataxia:

- Alcoholism
- Vascular disease
- Vitamin deficiency (B12)
- Demyelinating disorder
- Neoplastic lesion of cerebellum
- Paraneoplastic syndrome

Types of Hereditary Ataxias

Autosomal dominant

For example

- Cerebello olivary atrophy
- Inherited OPCA
- Marie's ataxia

Autosomal recessive

For example

- Ataxia teliengiectasia
- Friedreich ataxia
- Refsum's disease

Episodic ataxia, ataxia with spasticity. X-linked ataxia and ataxia associated with mitochondrial disorders are other forms of hereditary ataxias.

Refsum's disease

Features

- Ataxia
- Neuropathy
- Retinopathy
- Deafness
- Icthyosis

Ataxia telangiectasia

Features

- Ataxia
- Telangiectasia
- Immune deficiency

FRIEDREICH'S ATAXIA

Hereditary degenerative disorder

- Autosomal recessive disease
- Commonest hereditary ataxia.

Structures involved

- Cerebellum and cerebellar nuclei
- Corticospinal tract
- Spinocerebellar tract
- Posterior column
- Peripheral nerve
- Cranial nerve nuclei 9th, 10th, 11th and 12th

Clinical features

- Age of onset: 2nd and 3rd decade of life
- Strong family history.

Presenting symptoms
- Insidious onset and progressive
- Difficulty in walking and swaying and slurred speech.

Cerebellar features
- Limb, truncal and gait ataxia
- Scanning speech
- Nystagmus
- Titubation

Pyramidal signs
- Knee jerk (may be brisk) and ankle jerk absent
- Plantar extensor
- Distal muscle weakness

Sensory features
- Posterior column sensory loss with loss of vibration and proprioception.
- Axonal neuropathy may be present.
- Sphincters—usually intact.

Associated features
- Skeletal—scoliosis, pes cavus
- Cardiac—cardiac conduction defect
- Cardiomyopathy with murmurs
- Rare—diabetes mellitus type 2, mental retardation
- Usual cause of death—cardiac abnormality.

MOTOR NEURONE DISEASE

Characterised by degeneration of upper motor neurons/anterior horn cells and cranial nerve nuclei.

Structures spared
- Higher mental function
- Sensory system
- Bladder and bowel function
- Cerebellum
- Ocular movement

Different clinical types
- Amyotrophic lateral sclerosis
- Progressive bulbar palsy
- Progressive muscular atrophy
- Primary lateral sclerosis
- Pseudobulbar palsy

Other forms
- Familial spastic paraplegia
- Spinal muscular atrophy.

Features

Amyotrophic lateral sclerosis
- Involvement of upper motor neurons (lateral sclerosis)
- Involvement of anterior horn cells (amyotrophy—muscle atrophy secondary to neuronal dysfunction).

Signs
- Motor weakness of limbs
- Muscle cramps
- Fasciculations with wasting of muscles
- Signs of LMN involvement of upper limb
- Signs of UMN involvement of lower limb.
- Hypertonia, exaggerated deep reflexes and extensor plantar—bilateral
- Cranial nerve dysfunction
- Pseudobulbar features

Rule out following disorders while diagnosing amyotrophic lateral sclerosis
1. Compression of cervical cord
2. Thyrotoxicosis with bulbar weakness
3. Multifocal motor neuropathy with conduction block
4. Poliomyelitis.

Rare presentation Amyotrophic lateral sclerosis with parkinsonism with dementia.

Progressive muscular atrophy: Characterised by features of only LMN involvement.

Primary lateral sclerosis (only UMN signs): Can have corticobulbar and corticospinal tract involvement with changes.

Absence of fasciculation and absence of pyramidal cells in the precentral gyrus.

Progressive bulbar palsy—brainstem cranial nerve nuclei are involved.

Pseudobulbar palsy (already described above).

Madras motor neuron disease
- Younger age of presentation (10–20 years)
- Found in patients of Indian origin
- Weakness and wasting of distal limb muscles.

- Pyramidal involvement.
- Sensory neural hearing loss.
- Cranial nerve 7th, 10th dysfunction.
- Other features—bilateral optic atrophy.
- Bulbar muscle weakness.

Monomelic MND
- Younger age presentation.
- Weakness and wasting of upper limb.
- Progression may not occur.
- Fasciculations—rare
- Shoulder girdle muscles may be spared.

Differential diagnosis of monomelic MND
1. Initial presentation of ALS
2. Spinal muscular atrophy
3. Cervical cord disease
4. Brachial neuritis
5. Multifocal motor neuropathy with conduction block.

Guam disease
- Present in Guam island
- Possibly due to consumption of neurotoxic substance
- Features of amyotrophic lateral sclerosis, parkinsonism and dementia occurring together or in isolation.

DD of LMN MND: Multiple motor neuropathy with conduction block, spinal muscular atrophy.

DD of UMN MND: Multi-infarct state.

Spinal Muscular Atrophy
- Lower motor neuron disease.
- Starts at early stage.

Type I
- Werdnig-Hoffmann disease
- Infantile type
- May be present before birth and in infancy
- LMN weakness causing death—1st year of life.

Type 2
- Chronic childhood type
- Begins in childhood and progressive

Type 3
- Kugelberg-Welander type
- Juvenile spinal muscular atrophy
  Spinal muscular atrophy patients have proximal weakness and fasciculations.

Minipolymyoclonus
- Involuntary tremor like movements of small joints. Found in patients with spinal. Muscular atrophy and degenerative anterior horn cell disease—possibly due to frequent fasciculations.

Differences between spinal muscular atrophy *vs* progressive muscular atrophy (*see* below).

Familial (Hereditary) Spastic Paraplegia
- Progressive weakness and stiffness of lower limb—predominantly distal weakness (UMN type).
- Later in the course—urinary incontinence
- Rarely posterior column disease/mental retardation/cerebellar ataxia.
- Optic atrophy
- Respiratory involvement rare.

Table 4.4: Differences between spinal muscular atrophy and progressive muscular atrophy		
	Spinal muscular atrophy	*Progressive muscular atrophy*
• Family history	Present	Absent
• Age of onset	Younger age (1st and 2nd decade)	Usually 5th decade
• Type of involvement	Only LMN	LMN ± UMN
• Bulbar muscles	Not involved	Usually involved
• Progression	Slowly progressive	Rapidly progressive
• Prognosis	Relatively better	Worse

AUTONOMIC NERVOUS SYSTEM

Parasympathetic Nervous System

Parts

1. General visceral efferent fibers of cranial nerves 3, 7, 9, 10 and 11
2. Sacral segments S2, S3, S4
   - Supply the urinary bladder, descending colon
   - Genitalia, rectum and anus.

Cranial nerve nuclei

- Edinger-Westphal nucleus
- Superior and inferior salivatory nuclei
- Dorsal motor nucleus of vagus and nucleus ambiguus

Peripheral parasympathetic ganglia

- Ciliary ganglion
- Otic ganglion
- Submandibular and sphenopalatine ganglion

Sympathetic Nervous System

Central connections: Sympathetic nervous system fibers connect with cerebral cortex, amygdala, hypothalamus, basal forebrain, ventral striatum, brainstem and spinal cord.

Sympathetic system

- Preganglionic fibers
- T1–L3 segments of spinal cord
- Fibers terminate in the sympathetic ganglion chain, pre-vertebral plexus, etc.
- Post-ganglion fibers supply the viscera.

Sympathetic chain

- 22–24 ganglia from cervical region to coccyx
- Superior cervical ganglion lie at C2–C3 level behind internal carotid artery.
- Supply and terminate as internal carotid and cavernous plexus.
- Superior, middle and inferior cervical ganglia supply—structures within the head, thorax and upper extremities.

Bed side tests for autonomic nervous system

1. *For postural hypotension*: Recording of blood pressure after standing for 2 minutes.

If systolic blood pressure decreases by 20 mm of Hg or diastolic blood pressure decreases by more than 10 mm of Hg.
2. *Sustained handgrip*: Maintain the sustained handgrip (30% of handgrip for 3 to 4 minutes).
3. *Immersion of hand in ice cold water*: Immerse the hand in ice cold water for 1 to 3 minutes.
   - Normally diastolic blood pressure goes up by 10–15 mm of Hg by the above maneuvers
   - If it does not increase by 10 mm of Hg—suggestive of autonomic dysfunction.

   Other tests
   - Abnormal pupillary reflexes
   - Abolition of sinus arrhythmia
   - No heart rate variation with respiration.

PERIPHERAL NEUROPATHY

Common Causes of Peripheral Neuropathy

Deficiency Disorders

- Folic acid and B12 deficiency
- Pyridoxine deficiency

Infection related

- Leprosy
- HIV infection
- Lyme's disease

Drug-induced and toxins

- INH/phenytoin
- Lead/arsenic
- Alcohol

Metabolic disorders

- Diabetes mellitus
- Amyloidosis
- Porphyria.

Endocrine disorder

- Diabetes mellitus
- Hypothyroidism } Entrapment neuropathy
- Acromegaly

Vasculitis: Primary/secondary vasculitis

Neoplastic: Paraproteinemia, lymphoma

Hereditary: Hereditary neuropathy.

Different types of nerve fiber involvement

Types of nerve fibers
- Myelinated
  - Large
  - Small

Large myelinated: Motor fibers

Large myelinated—sensory fibers: Conduct touch, vibration and joint sense.

Small myelinated and unmyelinated fibers: Conduct pain and temperature.

Autonomic fibers: Small diameter fibers.

Conditions which mimic peripheral neuropathy
- LMN type of MND
- Myopathy
- Neuromuscular junction disorder.

GENERAL ASPECTS OF PERIPHERAL NEUROPATHY

In Large Fiber Neuropathy

- More deep reflex loss
- Motor involvement
- Loss of proprioception
- Pain and temperature—not involved
  - e.g. uremia
  - B12 deficiency
  - Diabetes mellitus.

Small Fiber Neuropathy

- Affects predominantly pain and temperature
- Produces burning pain
- No motor loss
- Deep tendon reflexes preserved
  - e.g. amyloidosis
  - Diabetes mellitus
  - Hereditary sensory neuropathy
- In axonopathy—length dependent reflex loss.
- In demyelinating neuropathy—slight sensory loss with global reflex loss.

Important Clinical Aspects Regarding Peripheral Neuropathy

- CIDP, porphyria cause recurrent neuropathy.

- Peripheral neuropathy with significant autonomic neuropathy occurs due to diabetes mellitus, porphyria and amyloidosis.
- Small fiber neuropathy causes predominantly pain and temperature loss (e.g. diabetes mellitus, amyloidosis).
- Large fiber neuropathy causes loss of proprioception—B12 deficiency.
- Mononeuropathy multiplex (asymmetrical involvement) can occur due to diabetes mellitus, vasculitis and Hansen's disease.
- Peripheral neuropathy and upper motor neuron signs can occur together in AIDS, subacute combined degeneration of spinal cord, chronic liver disease and Friedreich's ataxia and paraneoplastic syndrome.

History in a Patient of Peripheral Neuropathy

Patient may Present with Following Symptoms

- Motor fiber involvement: Motor weakness.
- Sensory fiber involvement—sensory symptoms.
- Autonomic fiber involvement—autonomic symptoms.

Ask onset and duration of symptoms
- *Acute onset*: Up to 4 weeks
- *Subacute onset*: 4–8 weeks
- *Chronic onset*: 8 weeks to months to years.

Motor symptoms
Muscle weakness
- Distal/proximal or both
- Associated wasting
- Symmetrical/asymmetrical.

Sensory symptoms
- Swaying in the dark
- H/o tingling and numbness
- Loss or decreased sensation
- Burning type of pain
- Painless ulcer
- Usually distal
- Symmetrical/asymmetrical

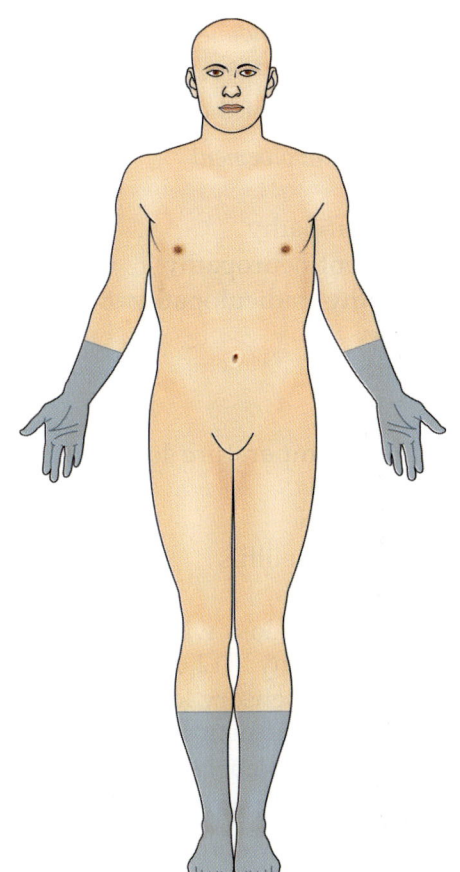

Fig. 4.17: Distribution of sensory loss in peripheral sensory loss (glove and stocking type of sensory loss)

Autonomic symptoms
- Dizziness on standing
- Impotence
- Sexual dysfunction
- Bladder dysfunction.

Other history
- History of hepatitis, renal disease
- History of exposure to drugs and toxins.
- History of fever with weight loss
- History of nutritional intake, type of diet, malabsorption/ileal disease.
- History of joint pain and rash.
- History of diabetes mellitus.
- History of any drug precipitating the attack.
- History of exacerbates and remission.
- Painless ulcers, deformities.

Past history
- Similar episodes before
- Past exposure to drugs and toxins
- Previous gastric surgery.

Personal history
- Weight loss
- Loss of appetite
- Intake of alcohol
- Smoking
- Exposure to commercial sex workers.

Family history
- Similar illness in the family members
  - Nutritional history: Type of diet-strict vegans and
  - Malabsorption—folic acid or B12 deficiency
  - History of connective tissue disorder: Vasculitis with neuropathy
  - History of diabetes mellitus: Diabetic neuropathy.
  - History of drugs which is causing sudden onset of motor weakness and autonomic disturbance: Porphyria
- History of exacerbation and remissions:
  - CIDP
  - Porphyria.
- History of painless ulcer over the pressure areas—sensory neuropathy with loss of pain and temperature, e.g. leprosy.
- Painful neuropathy, e.g. diabetes mellitus
- Painless neuropathy, e.g leprosy.

Past history
- Previous episodes: CIDP/porphyria
- Exposure to drugs and toxins—drug-induced neuropathy.
- Previous gastric surgery—B12 deficiency.

Personal history
- Weight loss/loss of appetite—systemic illness.
- Alcohol—alcohol-induced/deficiency neuropathy
- Smoking—can cause bronchogenic carcinoma—paraneoplastic neuropathy

- History of exposure to commercial sex workers: HIV-induced neuropathy.

Family history
- History of peripheral neuropathy: Possible B12 deficiency/nutritional neuropathy
- Hereditary neuropathy.

Approach to a Patient of Peripheral Neuropathy

Onset and duration
Acute
- <2 weeks duration
  - Porphyria
  - Vasculitis
  - Diabetic amyotrophy
- AIDP: Strictly not peripheral neuropathy

Subacute
- 2–6 weeks
  - All of the above causes
  - Drug-induced

Chronic
- >6 weeks
  - Due to deficiency
  - Metabolic
  - Endocrinal
  - Systemic disease like connective tissue disease/malignancy
  - Hereditary causes of neuropathies.

Predominantly proximal involvement
- AIDP
- Porphyria—shoulder involvement
- Diabetic amyotrophy

Only/predominantly motor
- AIDP
- Diphtheria
- Porphyria
- Paraneoplastic
- Lead
- Guillain-Barré syndrome

Predominantly sensory
- B12 deficiency
- Alcohol, diabetes mellitus, drug like INH, vincristine.

Predominantly autonomic: Diabetes mellitus, porphyria, amyloidosis.

Symmetrical: Most of the polyneuropathies.

Asymmetrical involvement
Consider
- Mononeuropathy
- Entrapment neuropathy
- Plexopathy/radiculopathy
- Leprosy
- Vasculitis

Sensory loss
- Pain and temperature loss—small fiber involvement
  - e.g. leprosy
  - Diabetes mellitus
  - Amyloidosis
- Proprioceptive loss with swaying—large fiber neuropathy: B12 deficiency
- Predominant sensory loss without weakness: Small fiber neuropathy:
- Drugs, toxins, diabetes mellitus
- Burning type of pain—small fiber neuropathy.

Other significant history
Fever with weight loss
- Systemic illness
- HIV related
- Systemic vasculitis
- Paraneoplastic

Exposure to drugs and toxins
- Various drugs causing neuropathy
- Exposure to lead, mercury/arsenic, tri-ortho-cresyl phosphate and thallium.

H/o liver and renal disease: Chronic liver disease and CKD-associated neuropathy.

General Physical Examination in Peripheral Neuropathies
- Built and nourishment
- Pallor, icterus, cyanosis, clubbing, edema and lymphadenopathy

Vital signs
- Pulse

- Blood pressure
- Respiratory rate
- Temperature

Pallor—anemia
Possible B12 deficiency
- Systemic disease
- Internal malignancy
- Drugs like lead, arsenic
- Paraproteinemia

Icterus
Megaloblastic anemia with ineffective erythropoiesis
- Chronic liver disease
- Systemic disease involving liver
- Cyanosis—part of systemic disease
- Clubbing—part of systemic disease, e.g.
  - Bronchogenic carcinoma
  - Chronic liver disease
  - Malabsorption syndrome
  - POEMS syndrome

Specific General Examination Findings in Peripheral Neuropathy Disorders

Face
- Hair changes—discoloration/graying—B12 deficiency
- Hair discoloration and hair loss: Thallium toxicity
- Lateral 1/3 of eyebrow loss: Leprosy, hypothyroidism
- Malar rash: SLE
- Bilateral parotid swelling: Sjögren's syndrome/diabetes mellitus/HIV infection
- Oral cavity
  - Candidiasis: HIV infection
  - Blue line over the gum: Lead toxicity
  - Pigmentation: B12 deficiency
  - Severe pallor: Anemia
  - Ulcers: Connective tissue disease.

Skin—diffuse pigmentation
- Drugs—anti-malignant
- B12 deficiency
- POEMS syndrome

- Rain drop pigmentation—areas of pigmentation and decreased—pigmentation—arsenic toxicity
- Hypopigmented maculo-anesthetic patch—leprosy
- Subcutaneous nodules: Neurofibroma/deposits of malignancy.
- Vitiligo-associated autoimmune disorders.

Hand and extremities
- Pigmentation of knuckles: B12 deficiency
- Mees' lines: Transverse ridges at the base of nail
  - Arsenic toxicity
  - Thallium toxicity
- Look for changes of connective tissue disorders and vasculitis
- *Also look for*
  Pes cavus
  Kyphoscoliosis } Hereditary neuropathy
- *Features of*
  - Chronic liver disease
  - Chronic kidney disease
  - Bone tenderness—myeloma
  - Sarcoidosis.

Vital signs
- *Pulse*: Rate variation can occur with autonomic neuropathy.
- *Blood pressure*: Variation occurs with autonomic neuropathy.
- Postural hypotension occurs with autonomic neuropathy.

Systemic Examination in Peripheral Neuropathy

Higher Mental Function Involvement
Dementia/memory loss: Can occur due to:
- B12 deficiency
- HIV infection
- Porphyria
- Degenerative disorders

Cranial nerves involvement occurs in following types of peripheral neuropathies
Multiple cranial nerves: Polyneuritis cranialis
Causes
- Vasculitis

- Diabetes mellitus
- Sarcoidosis

2nd cranial nerve: Look for:
- Papilledema: GB syndrome
- Optic atrophy: B12 deficiency/Hereditary neuropathy
- Retinitis pigmentosa: Refsum's disease

3rd, 4th, 6th nerve involvement
- Diabetic ophthalmoplegia
- GB syndrome

7th cranial nerve involvement
- Leprosy
- Diabetes mellitus
- Sarcoidosis
- Lymphoma
- GB syndrome

Motor System Examination

Attitude of Limbs
- Observe for wrists drop/foot drop
  - Unilateral/bilateral
- Unilateral foot/wrist drop can occur in mononeuropathies
- Bilateral wrist/foot drop occurs in polyneuropathies.

Nutrition: Look for wasting of limb or parts of limb.

Upper limb
- Small muscle wasting and claw hand: Ulnar and median nerve involvement.
- Wasting can occur in part of limb depending on the nerve involved.
- For example, mononeuritis.
  - In polyneuropathy/peripheral neuropathy: There can be distal wasting of limb.
  - In L5, S1 lesion: Mononeuritis of lateral popliteal nerve—foot drop and wasting of lower part of the lower limb.

Typical wasting in peroneal muscular atrophy (CMTD): Wasting of distal part of the fore arm and thigh—inverted champagne bottle appearance (peroneal muscular atrophy).

Proximal part of thigh—wasting—diabetic amyotrophy.

Wasting of deltoid—can occur in brachial neuritis (neuralgic amyotrophy).

 Note

- *Wasting of one limb—can occur in mononeuritis multiplex: Rule out.*
- *Monomelic MND in such circumstances.*

Tone: There will be hypotonia—with peripheral neuropathy.

Power
- Test for individual group of muscle or particular muscle group supplied by that corresponding nerve.
- Test the power of individual small muscle of hand.
- Look for: Wrist drop—extensor weakness of wrist
- Foot drop—extensor weakness of foot
- Look for clawing of hand due to wasting of small muscles of hand.

Coordination: Test in the upper limb and lower limb depending on the muscle power.

Involuntary movement
- Not common in peripheral neuropathies.
- Fasciculations are a feature of neuronopathies not neuropathy.

Sensory system examination
- Test of all modalities of sensation depending on the dermatomal pattern.
- If all modalities are lost—in a glove stocking manner—typical of polyneuropathy.
- If all modalities are lost in particular dermatomal distribution—radiculopathy or mononeuropathy.

Type of sensation involved
- Early temperature and painloss, e.g. leprosy.
- Early vibration sensory loss: Diabetic neuropathy.
- Early proprioceptive loss: Large fiber neuropathy.

- Patchy—asymmetrical distribution of sensory loss—mononeuritis multiplex.

Reflexes

- Superficial reflexes are lost if the corresponding dermatome or nerve involved.
- Deep reflexes are lost if the damage occur to the corresponding nerve.
- Deep reflexes are preserved till late in leprosy because of the late involvement of large fibers.
- Plantar becomes extensor in patient with B12 deficiency with subacute combined degeneration of spinal cord.

Autonomic signs

Look for autonomic signs

- Postural hypotension
- Fixed heart rate.
- Abnormal papillary response.

Signs of cerebellar dysfunction

Peripheral neuropathy with cerebellar involvement.

Causes

- Alcoholism
- Phenytoin administration
- Hypothyroidism
- Paraneoplastic syndrome
- Friedreich's ataxia
- Severe B12 deficiency
- Refsum's disease

Involvement of bladder and bowel dysfunction: Look for bladder retention/incontinence—can be involved in peripheral/autonomic neuropathy.

Look for peripheral nerve thickening: Supraorbital, posterior auricular, ulnar, lateral popliteal.

Causes of nerve thickening

- Leprosy
- Neurofibromatosis
- Diabetes mellitus
- Amyloidosis
- Hereditary sensory motor neuropathy
- Refsum's disease.

Gait

- Patients with peripheral neuropathy will have Romberg's sign positive (due to involvement of proprioception.)
- Patients with peripheral neuropathy will be having stamping gait (may be high stepping due to associated foot drop).

Other system examination: For evidence of cardiovascular/respiratory and gastrointestinal tract disease.

PLEXOPATHY

Brachial Plexopathy

Brachial plexus formed by ventral rami of lower 4 cervical nerves and T1 (C5, C6, C7, C8 and T1).

Different Causes of Brachial Plexus Involvement

- Immunologically mediated
- Acute brachial plexitis (neuralgic amyotrophy)
- Neoplastic involvement of brachial plexus
  - Pancoast tumor
  - Secondary from bronchogenic carcinoma
  - Lymphomatous infiltration
  - Primary tumor of the nerve.

Neuralgic amyotrophy

- Painful condition: Occurs after injury/illness or inoculation of serum into the deltoid.
- Usual segments affected: C5, C6, C7—may be unilateral.

Genetic/autoimmune factors play a role.

Features

- Marked wasting of shoulder girdle
- Muscles—supraspinatus, infraspinatus, deltoid and trapezius affected.
- Wasting occurs after 2–3 weeks, progresses for months and slowly recovers over the years.
- Sensory loss can occur in the distribution of circumflex nerve.
- Inflammation of the nerve root occurs causing weakness and wasting of muscles.

Lumbar/lumbosacral plexopathy

- 1 to 4 lumbar spinal nerves form lumbar plexus along with contribution from T12.
- Sacral 1 to 4 form sacral plexus along with lumbar nerves L4 and L5.

Causes of lumbosacral plexopathy

- Malignant disorders
  - Carcinoma cervix
  - Carcinoma endometrium
  - Ovarian carcinoma
  - Testicular and colonic prostate malignancy
- Diabetes mellitus
- Psoas abscess
- Retroperitoneal hemorrhage
- Fracture pelvis

Chronic Inflammatory Demyelinating Polyneuropathy (CIDP)

- Considered to be chronic form of AIDP.
- Can present with symmetric weakness of upper limb and lower limb >8 weeks.
- Both proximal and distal weakness.
- Chronic course with exacerbations and remission.
- Causes purely motor, occasionally minimal sensory symptoms.
- Deep tendon reflexes are absent, can have autonomic involvement.
- Associations—external ophthalmoplegia.
- Investigations—CSF protein. NCV shows-demyelinating form. CIDP—responds to corticosteroids.
- *DD of CIDP*: Multifocal motor neuropathy with conduction block.

Multifocal Motor Neuropathy with Conduction Block

Features

- Asymmetrical weakness with atrophy
- Can start as single, nerve involvement as wrist drop/foot drop.
- Can have multifocal weakness.
- No UMN signs. No bulbar involvement.
- No sensory involvement.

- Mimics progressive muscular atrophy type of MND.

Investigations

- There is neuronal conduction block
- CSF protein is increased
- Antiganglioside GM1 antibody positive.

Treatment: IV immunoglobulin.

 Note

Bilateral symmetrical sensory loss with UMN involvement: B12 deficiency.

Table 4.5: Differences between axonal and demyelinating neuropathy	
Axonal	*Demyelinating*
• Insidious	Acute/insidious
• Glove and stocking sensory loss	Minimal sensory loss
• Deep reflexes—elicitable	Absent
• Recovery very slow	Quick
• Residual deficiency common	Less common
e.g.: Diabetes mellitus	e.g.: CIDP
HIV infection	AIDP
Alcoholism	HMSN
B12 deficiency	

Features of Certain Clinically Important Neuropathies

Diabetes Mellitus

Different types of diabetic neuropathy

- Distal sensory/sensory motor neuropathy
- Proxymal neuropathy: Diabetic amyotrophy
- Truncal neuropathy
- Cranial neuropathy
- Autonomic neuropathy
- Mononeuropathy

Diabetic distal sensory and sensory motor neuropathy

- Glove and stocking distribution of symptoms.
- Most common type of diabetic neuropathy.
- Both sensory and motor affected.
- Can result in trophic ulcers, Charcot's joints.

Diabetic amyotrophy

- Acute onset of pain in the low back, hip and thigh—unilateral.
- Weakness and wasting of quadriceps.
- Usually associated with significant weight loss.
- Usually recovers with minimal weakness may persist.
- Cervical and thoracic nerve roots can also be involved.

Truncal neuropathy

Presents as severe pain over the trunk in the distribution of intercostal nerves can resemble tabetic crises.

Diabetic autonomic neuropathy: Common in uncontrolled diabetes.

Manifestations

- Postural hypotension
- Circumoral gustatory sweating
- Abnormality of pupil
- GIT: Nocturnal diarrhea, gastroparesis
- Dryness of mouth and eye
- Cardiac arrhythmias.
- Erectile impotence

Diabetic cranial neuropathy

- LMN type of facial palsy
- Unilateral/bilateral
- Ophthalmoplegia: 3rd, 4th and 6th nerve palsy.
- Pupil is spared as superficial pupillo-constrictor fibers are spared.
- Any other cranial nerve can also be involved.

Mononeuropathy of diabetes

- Any peripheral nerve—like ulnar or median can be involved.
- Can cause mononeuropathy multiplex.

 Note

In some patients of diabetic neuropathy after initiation of insulin aggravation of symptoms of neuropathy can occur.

Neuropathy due to Vitamin B12 Deficiency

- Presents as distal sensory neuropathy with long fiber involvement.
- Loss of vibration and proprioception
- Preservation of pain and temperature.
- Associated with spinal cord involvement
- Exaggerated knee jerk with loss of ankle jerk and plantar extensor.
  (subacute combined degeneration of spinal cord).
- *Associated features*: Anemia, knuckle pigmentation, optic atrophy, higher mental function abnormalities.

Leprosy

Types of Neuropathy

- Mononeuropathy: Ulnar or median— causes claw hand
- Mononeuropathy multiplex.
- 7th nerve palsy
- Symmetrical sensory, motor neuropathy.
- Associated features: Maculo-anaesthetic patch
- Nerve thickening
- Trophic ulcers
- There will be early loss of pain and temperature sensation due to small fiber involvement with preservation of deep reflexes due to relative sparing of large fibers till late.

Pure Neuritic Form of Leprosy

Predominantly seen in India and Asian region.
Features

- Skin lesions are usually absent
- There will be enlargement of large nerves and their branches
- Present as either mononeuritis or mononeuritis multiplex associated with sensory loss in the distribution of the nerves.
- Skin smear is negative for AFB and lepromin test is positive
- Nerve biopsy demonstrates tuberculoid/borderline leprosy

Porphyria
- Acute onset of weakness of proximal and distal muscles
- Initial involvement of proximal muscles with shoulder and arm
- Can also involve bulbar musculature
- No sensory disturbance.
- Significant autonomic disturbance

Associated features
- Acute abdominal pain.
- Higher mental function abnormalities.

Amyloid neuropathy
- Generalised axonal neuropathy. Can be multifocal. Can have sensory motor neuropathy.
- Severe autonomic involvement.

Diphtheritic neuropathy
- After 2–3 weeks of development of diphtheritic symptoms
- Palate and pharyngeal paralysis. Can present like acute Guillain-Barré syndrome.
- Accommodation reflex is lost

Associated feature: Myocarditis.

Paraneoplastic neuropathy
- Gradually progressive sensory symptoms
- Loss of large fiber sensation causing sensory ataxia.
- Common association—small cell carcinoma lung.

Associated features: Higher mental abnormalities.

Antibody in CSF / serum: Anti-HU antibodies.

Hereditary neuropathy
- Insidious onset and slowly progressive
- Positive family history
- Thickening of nerves
- Skeletal deformities—pes cavus and scoliosis
- Features of peripheral neuropathy.

CMTD (Charcot-Marie-Tooth disease)
- Most common type of hereditary neuropathy.

- Occurs at 2nd and 3rd decades of life.
- Significant motor weakness—distally with foot drop and loss of deep tendon reflexes.
- Can have objective sensory loss.
- Typical wasting—of distal groups of muscles inverted champagne bottle appearance.

CMT type 2: Predominantly axonal neuropathy.

CMT type 3: Dejerine-Sottas: Hereditary demyelinating sensory motor neuropathy.

Refsum's disease: Distal sensory motor neuropathy.

Features: Retinitis pigmentosa, cerebellar ataxia, cardiac conduction defect, sensory neural hearing loss.

Neuropathy Associated with Para Proteinemia

- Axonal neuropathy—distal sensory or sensory motor neuropathy.
- Secondary amyloidosis can have small fiber neuropathy.
- Rarely demyelinating polyneuropathy can occur.
- May be part of POEMS syndrome: Polyneuropathy, organomegaly, endocrinopathy, monoclonal protein increase and skin changes.

Neuropathy associated with HIV infection

HIV infection can cause neuropathy due to
- HIV infection itself
- Associated with CMV infection
- Due to B12 deficiency
- Due to anti-retroviral drugs, e.g. Stavudine

Different types of HIV neuropathies
1. *Polyneuropathy*
   - Distal bilaterally symmetrical
   - Glove and stocking distribution
2. Cytomegalovirus related polyradiculopathy
3. *During seroconversion*
   - AIDP can occur
   - CIDP can occur at any time during the course of illness.

- In patients with AIDP secondary to HIV infection: CSF shows lymphocytosis compared to Guillain-Barré syndrome.
4. Radiculopathy can occur due to CMV infection.
5. Mononeuropathy/Mononeuropathy multiplex can occur either due to vascular involvement or CMV related.
6. Autonomic neuropathy.

Lead neuropathy
- History of chronic exposure to lead.
- Pure motor neuropathy—with wrist or foot drop
- Sensory system: Normal
- *Associated features*
  - Blue line over the gum (Burton's line).
  - Peripheral smear: Basophilic stippling of RBCs
  - Abdominal colic
  - Encephalopathy.

Arsenic neuropathy
- History of chronic exposure to arsenic.
- Acute onset: AIDP-like presentation or chronic sensory motor neuropathy.

Associated features: Mees' lines: Transverse lines over the base of fingers or toes.

Rain drop pigmentation: Areas of depigmentation and hyperpigmentation of skin due to loss of superficial epidermal layers.

Charcot's Joints (Neuropathic Joint)
Progressive destructive arthritis associated with loss of pain sensation, proprioception. Joints are subjected to repeated trauma—progressive cartilage and bone damage.

Usual joints involved: Tarsal and tarsometatarsal joints, wrist, ankle and elbow joints.

Common causes: Diabetes mellitus, leprosy, syringomyelia, Charcot-Marie-Tooth disease, tabes dorsalis.

Mechanisms: Abnormal autonomic nervous system: Dysregulated blood flow to the joint and resorption of bone. Loss of pain and proprioception with repeated microtrauma. It is associated with ligamental tear and bone fracture.

Clinical manifestations
- Joint becomes progressively enlarged—due to bony overgrowth and synovial effusion. Loose bodies can become palpable.
- Subluxation, joint instability, crepitus and joint becomes totally disorganised. Pain is usually absent. Can develop infection, ulceration and osteomyelitis.

Peripheral Nerves
Median Nerve (Root C5, C6, C7, C8, T1)
Hand muscles supplied by median nerve
Thenar eminence
A: Abductor pollicis brevis (most superficial)
O: Opponens pollicis
F: Flexor pollicis
Median nerve supplies thenar eminence muscles and 1st and 2nd lumbricals.

Ulnar Nerve (Root Value C8, T1)
Supply
- Flexor carpi ulnaris
- Medial half of flexor digitorum superficialis and profundus
- Palmaris brevis
- 3rd and 4th lumbricals
- Palmar and dorsal interossei
- Two parts of adductor pollicis

Hypothenar eminence
A: Abductor digiti minimi
O: Opponens digiti minimi
F: Flexor digiti minimi

Small Muscles of the Hand
Following muscles are supplied by the ulnar nerve
1. *Hypothenar eminence*
   A: Abductor digiti minimi
   O: Opponens digiti minimi.
   F: Flexor digiti minimi
2. *Lumbricals*: 3rd and 4th lumbricals

3. *Interossei*: All interossei (palmar and dorsal interossei)

4. *Adductor pollicis*: Mainly two parts.

Action of lumbricals: Flexion at metacorpophalangeal joints (writing muscles).

Testing lumbricals: Patient is asked to flex the fingers which are kept in extended position with extension at the metacarpophalangeal joint.

Action of interossei

Palmar interossei: Action: Adduction of fingers.

Testing palmar interossei: Card test: Unable to hold the card between the fingers (if paralysed).

Dorsal interossei: Action—abduction of fingers (may also extend middle phalanx).

Test: Unable to abduct the fingers against resistance (if paralysed).

Adductor pollicis

• Action—adduction of thumb

• Testing adductor pollicis (along with 1st palmar interosseous)

• If paralysed: Unable to hold the paper piece between the thumb and palm. Or book test (Froment's sign).

Froment's sign: Person is asked to grasp the book between the thumb and palm.

Normal: Thumb remains straight due to the action of adductor pollicis, 1st palmar interossei and flexor pollicis longus.

In ulnar nerve lesion: There will be flexion of the thumb due to intact flexor pollicis longus and paralysis of adductor pollicis and 1st palmar interossei.

 Note

Rarely abductor pollicis brevis is supplied by branch of ulnar nerve.

Tests for ulnar nerve

• For palmar interossei: Card test

• For dorsal interossei: Abduction of fingers

• For adductor pollicis and first palmar interossei: Book test (Froment's sign).

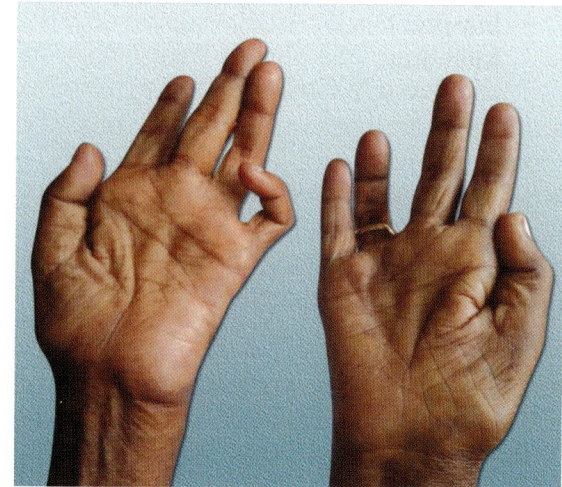

Fig. 4.18: Bilateral wasting of small muscles of the hand

Muscles Supplied by the Median Nerve (C5, C6, C7, C8, T1) in the Hand

1. *Thenar eminence*:

   A: Abductor pollicis brevis (most superficial)

   O: Opponence pollicis

   F: Flexor pollicis brevis

2. 1st and 2nd lumbricals

Tests for abductor pollicis brevis (pen test): Patient is asked to raise the thumb vertically above the original position so as to touch the pen against resistance (pen test).

 Note

Abductor pollicis brevis is the first muscle involved in carpal tunnel syndrome as it is most superficial.

Tests for Median Nerve

For lumbricals—flexion of fingers at MCP joint: Testing the lumbricals: *see* above.

Flexor digitorum profundus (lateral part)

• Action—flexion of distal interphalangeal joints.

• *Testing*

  – Support the middle phalanx

  – Ask the patient to flex the terminal phalanx against resistance.

- Supply: Lateral part—median nerve
- Median part—ulnar nerve.

Pointing Index

Occurs due to lesion of the median nerve.

Testing: Patient is asked to clasp the two hands.

In median nerve lesion
- Index finger on the affected side fails to flex.
- Due to lesion of the median nerve—lateral part of the flexor digitorum profundus fails to act, whereas medial half of the muscle is intact with its action with normal action of the ulnar nerve.

Flexor pollicis longus: Person is not able to flex the terminal phalanx of the thumb against resistance. (Examiner should hold the proximal phalanx firmly to avoid the action of short flexors).

Opponens pollicis: Patient is asked to touch the little finger with the thumb.

Flexor pollicis brevis: Flexion of metacarpophalangeal joint of thumb.

Testing: Keep interphalangeal joint of the thumb extended. Ask the patient to flex the metacarpophalangeal joint of the thumb which is extended.

Flexor digitorum superficialis
- Supplied by the median nerve
- Examiner places his finger on the middle phalanx and apply resistance while the patient is asked to flex the middle phalanx.
- Action—flexion of proximal IP joint of 4 fingers.

Ape thumb (*Simian thumb*)
- Thumb is in line with the other metacarpals, due to paralysis of opponens pollicis.
- Person cannot move the thumb from other fingers—due to injury to the median nerve.

Policeman receiving tips (*Obstetrical/Erb's paralysis*): Arm hanging by the side of the body and internally rotated, forearm extended at elbow and fully pronated. Paralysis and atrophy of deltoid, biceps and brachialis. Arm cannot be raised from the side lesion at C5–C6.

Carpal Tunnel Syndrome
- Entrapment neuropathy of median nerve.
- Median nerve is compressed when it passes through the carpal tunnel.

Causes
- Hypothyroidism
- Rheumatoid arthritis
- Diabetes mellitus
- Other contributing factors:
  - Obesity
  - Pregnancy
  - Genetic factors.

Clinical Features

Symptoms
- Present as pain and numbness of hand, aggravated during sleep—pain can aggravate up to shoulder.
- During sleep—wrists are held flexed and curved.
- Sleeping on one side may also contribute.
- *Motor involvement*: Abductor pollicis brevis is most commonly involved: Most superficial muscle. Wasting can be made out.

 Note

Rarely abductor pollicis brevis can be supplied by ulnar nerve.

- Other muscle involvement is compensated by long forearm muscles.
- Sensory loss over the thenar eminence is less common as sensory branch of the median nerve passes over the carpal tunnel.

Phalen's test
- Patient is asked to keep his wrist in flexion with back of two hands together in front of the patient for one minute. Observe for development of paresthesia/pain in the distribution of the median nerve.

- Indicates median nerve compression in carpal tunnel syndrome.

Claw hand: Due to lesion of ulnar nerve or combined lesion of ulnar and median nerve causing paralysis of lumbricals and interossei.

Characteristics:

- Hyperextension of metacarpophalangeal (MCP) joint and flexion of proximal and distal interphalangeal (IP) joints.
- Extension of MCP joint is due to unopposed action of extensor digitorum—extends proximal phalanx only.
- Flexion of PIP and DIP joints due to paralysis of interossei (main extensors of these joints) with over action of long flexors.

Ulnar Paradox: If the lesion of the ulnar nerve occurs proximally at the elbow—deformities are less due to involvement of long flexors.

Pseudoclaw hand

- Occurs due to paralysis of extensors of metacarpophalangeal, joints due to paralysis of posterior interosseous nerve.

- It can mimic ulnar palsy with involvement of little fingers and then other fingers.

 Note

Occasionally posterior interosseous nerve continuation called Froment-Rauber nerve can innervate 1st, 2nd and 3rd dorsal interossei and lesion of that nerve causes paralysis of interossei (rare anatomical variation) and can cause claw-like hand.

Cutaneous Innervation of Hand

Median nerve

- Palmar surface of thumb, index and middle finger and half of ring finger, nail bed of these fingers.
- Lateral part of palm—palmar cutaneous branch of median nerve, which leaves the nerve proximal to wrist crease. Has got a separate facial groove and sparred in carpal tunnel syndrome.
- Posterior aspect of fingertips of thumb, index, middle finger and half of ring finger is supplied by median nerve.

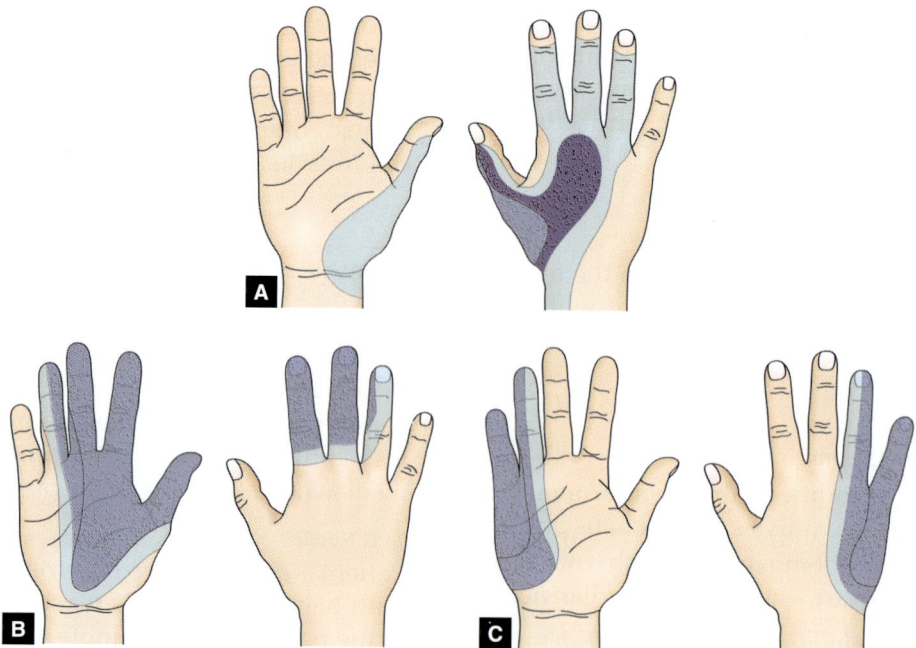

Fig. 4.19A to C: Distribution of sensation by cutaneous nerves in the hand: (A) Radial nerve; (B) Median nerve; (C) Ulnar nerve

Ulnar nerve: Supplies medial one hand half of palm with little finger and medial part of ring finger, and corresponding posterior aspect of palm.

Radial nerve: Posterior aspect of palm with thumb, index, middle and half of ring finger, except fingertips and small area at thenar eminence.

Tardive Ulnar Palsy

- Occurs in long standing cubitus valgus/ supracondylar fracture of humerus.
- Due to stretching and traction of nerve during movement.
- Occurs over 20–30 years (tardive—slow).
- Results in ulnar nerve damage with atrophy of 1st dorsal interosseus.

Tinel's sign: Percussion over a peripheral nerve produces paresthesia over the distribution of peripheral nerve indicates localized nerve pathology/nerve irritation.

Unilateral (phrenic nerve) palsy
- May be asymptomatic
- Can have exertional dyspnea.

Bilateral diaphragm palsy
Features
- Exertional dyspnea and orthopnea
- Difficulty in coughing, sneezing and sniffing
- Paradoxical movement of abdomen occurs during respiration.

Paradoxical movement of abdomen: Abdomen moves inwards during inspiration.

APPROACH TO PATIENT OF MUSCLE DISEASE AND MUSCLE END PLATE

Muscle disease may occur due to
- Abnormalities of structure of the muscle
- Abnormal metabolism of the muscle
- Abnormality of channels: Channelopathies

Muscle involvement may also occur due to
- Abnormalities of neuromuscular junction
- Peripheral nerves
- Motor neuron/anterior horn cells.

Classification of muscle disorders
Hereditary
- Muscular dystrophies
- Congenital myopathies
- Channelopathies
- Mitochondrial myopathies
- Metabolic myopathies

Acquired causes
- Endocrine myopathies
- Drug-induced myopathies
- Inflammatory myopathies
- Immune-related myopathies
- Systemic infections and illness
- Toxic myopathies

Approach to a Patient of Muscle Disease

Symptoms of muscle disease
- Muscle weakness
- Muscle fatigability
- Muscle pain
- Muscle atrophy/hypertrophy
- Muscle cramps
- Muscle contracture
- Myotonia
- Myoglobinuria

History of presenting illness
Muscle weakness: Enquire following details:
- Onset and duration
- Part affected
- Distributing muscle weakness
- Episodic/constant
- Related to exercise
- Precipitating factors
- H/o drug intake.

History of sensory, cranial nerves and cerebellar involvement (*see* under examination). History of systemic illness including cardiovascular, respiratory symptoms.

Past history
- Similar episodes
- Systemic illness

- Drug history
- History of taking treatment details.

Personal history
- Appetite and weight loss
- Smoking
- Alcoholism
- H/o exposure to drugs/toxins
- Sexual transmission

Family history
- History of muscle disorders in the family
- H/o using wheelchairs—patient's family members
- H/o using sticks/support for walking
- H/o skeletal deformities

Other important history
Systemic illness
- Fever
- Joint pain
- Rash
- Respiratory symptoms
- Cardiovascular
- Higher mental function abnormalities
- Thyroid, parathyroid and adrenal symptoms.

Muscle weakness
Acute onset, e.g.
- Inflammatory disorders
- Chronic—degenerative disorder
- Episodic myasthenia
- Nonprogressive—congenital myopathies
- Single episode—drug induced
- Exacerbations/remissions—polymyositis.

Importance of age of onset of muscle weakness
- At birth—congenital myopathies
- At around the age of 3 years: Duchenne dystrophy
- Adolescent and later: Facio scapulohumeral/limb girdle type of muscular dystrophy

Childhood onset
- Dermatomyositis
- Duchenne/Becker type.
- Facioscapulohumeral/limb girdle type

Adult onset
- Polymyositis
- Distal myopathies
- Drugs/toxins.

Muscle weakness
Ask for distribution of muscle weakness:
Different groups of muscle involved in muscle weakness
- Facial
- Ocular
- Bulbar
- Cervical
- Trunk muscles
- Shoulder girdle
- Forearm
- Pelvic girdle
- Legs and foot
- Respiratory

Muscle weakness may involve
- Upper limb: Distal
             Proximal
- Lower limb: Distal
             Proximal

Muscle weakness due to cranial nerve involvement
- Slurred speech
- Difficulty in swallowing
- Double vision

Precipitating factors for muscle weakness:
- Exercise
- Drugs
- Excessive ingestion of carbohydrates
- Cold exposure
- Fever

Exercise: Worsening of myasthenia.
Drugs: Aminoglycosides—worsening of NM junction disorders.
Excessive ingestion of carbohydrate: Hypokalemic periodic paralysis.
Cold exposure: Worsening of myotonia.
Fever—worsening of muscle weakness—in carnitine palmityl transferase deficiency.
DD of myopathies depending on the distribution of muscle weakness.
Limb girdle weakness: Most myopathies (hereditary and acquired) except distal myopathies.
Involvement of muscles of proximal arm + muscle of distal leg (scapuloperoneal).
Facioscapulohumeral/scapuloperoneal type of dystrophies.

Weakness of muscles of distal arm with proximal leg muscles:

Inclusion of body myositis and myotonic dystrophy.

Ptosis + ophthalmoplegia + pharyngeal involvement: Oculopharyngeal type.

Ptosis + Facial weakness + No pharyngeal involvement—mitochondrial myopathy.

Facial weakness and no ophthalmoplegia: Myotonia/Facioscapulohumeral dystrophy

Bulbar muscle weakness

- Myasthenia gravis
- Thyrotoxicosis
- Oculopharyngeal muscular dystrophy

Predominantly distal: Muscle weakness: Inclusion body myositis/myotonia/distal-myopathy.

Pain + Muscle weakness+ Myoglobinuria: Drugs

- Toxins
- Glycogen storage disorder

Neck extensor weakness

- Dropped head syndrome
- e.g. polymyositis
  Painful muscle weakness with involvement of neck muscles, proximal muscle weakness, no ocular muscle weakness: polymyositis.

Fatigability

- Usual presenting feature of myasthenia
- Patient becomes progressively fatigued after exercise
- Associated with episodic muscle weakness

Episodic muscle weakness: Not related to exercise: Consider periodic paralysis.

Myopathy associated with pain

- Usually suggests inflammatory disorders
- Occasionally with metabolic myopathies

Examples of myopathy associated with pain

- Inflammatory myositis
- Drugs/toxins
- Hypothyroid myopathy
- Infective disorder—like viral infection
- Myotonic disorder

- Mitochondrial myopathy
- Polymyositis

Muscle cramps

- Usually affects calf muscles.
- It is due to rapid firing of motor units.

 Note

Muscle cramp is not a usual manifestation of muscle disease except in Duchenne muscular dystrophy.

Disorders associated with muscle cramps

- MND
- Peripheral neuropathy
- Sodium and calcium abnormalities
- Physiological—pregnancy.

Muscle contracture

- Resembles muscle cramps but it is prolonged
- It is increased by exercise
- It can cause stiffness of joints
- It is due to shortening of muscle fibers with thickening and not due to fibrous contracture.
- Emery-Dreifuss and Bethlem type of muscular dystrophy presents with early muscular contractures.

Muscle stiffness

- Muscle stiffness in the trunk and limbs can result in muscle spasm along with
- Abnormal posturing of the body parts. It can occur in stiff man syndrome/paraneoplastic syndrome.

Myotonia

- Difficulty in relaxation after forceful muscle contraction.
- After shaking the hand there will be difficulty in relaxation.
- Difficulty in opening of the eyelid after forcibly closing the eyes.
- Due to repetitive repolarisation of muscle membrane
- Improved with repeated exercise
- Myotonia ↑ after exposure to cold
- Paramyotonia—worse after exercise

- Exposure to cold worsens both myotonia and paramyotonia

Myoglobinuria: Occurs due to muscle destruction

- Urine—coke/red colored
- Can develop acute kidney injury

Causes

- Drugs toxins (statins, alcohol), etc.
- Neuroleptic malignant syndrome
- Heat stroke
- Metabolic myopathy
- Viral myositis
- Inflammatory myopathies

General Physical Examination in Muscle Disease

Severe pallor: Rule out systemic disease

Clubbing: Systemic disease

Cyanosis: May be due to respiratory failure due to muscle weakness

Jaundice: Part of systemic disease

Edema: Associated with systemic disease/ due to CCF secondary to cardiomyopathy

Specific Features on General Examination in a Muscle Disease

- Alopecia: SLE
- Lateral eyebrow loss—hypothyroidism
- Frontal balding—myotonic dystrophy
- Cataract—myotonic dystrophy
- Atrophy of facial muscles—facial scapulo-humeral dystrophy
- Heliotroph rash—dermatomyositis
- Butterfly rash: SLE
- Mauskopf face: Systemic sclerosis
- Exophthalmos: Thyrotoxicosis
- Ptosis: Myasthenia
- Oculopharyngeal dystrophy
- Mitochondrial myopathy
- Neck-goiter-thyroid disease
- Neck muscle weakness:
  - Myasthenia
  - Polymyositis
  - Myotonic dystrophy

- Shawl's sign: Dermatomyositis
- Lymph nodes—systemic disease
- Skin—bruising—excess corticosteroids
- Pigmentation—Addison's disease
- Erythema nodosum in sarcoidosis
- Hand deformities—connective tissue disorders
- Lower limb deformities Bowing of limbs } due to muscle disease or osteomalacia

Vital signs

- *Pulse*: Abnormalities can occur due to cardiac arrhythmias with muscle disease.
- Blood pressure abnormality can occur due to endocrine disorders.
- *Respiration*: Rate and depth of respiration becomes abnormal due to respiratory muscle involvement/diaphragm weakness.

CNS Examination in Muscle Disorder

Mental state examination

- Consciousness—usually normal.
- Orientation to time, place and person—normal.
- Intelligence and memory: May be affected in Duchenne muscular dystrophy.
- Speech can have dysarthria due to facial muscle involvement.
- Prolonged speaking—voice can decrease in myasthenia.

Cranial nerve examination

- Cranial nerve and nucleus are not involved
- Muscles supplied by cranial nerve can be affected.
- *Check for*
  - Orbicular oris
  - Tongue muscles
  - Palate muscles
  - Ocular muscles for
    - Ptosis
    - Ophthalmoplegia

Muscular dystrophies involving muscles supplied by cranial nerves

- Facial muscles—facioscapulohumeral dystrophy
- Ptosis and ophthalmoplegia:
  - Myasthenia gravis
  - Oculopharyngeal dystrophy
  - Myotonic dystrophy
  - Mitochondrial myopathy.
- Bulbar muscle involvement
- Bulbar myasthenia
- Neck extensors: Myasthenia gravis
- Muscle of neck—polymyositis
- Neck flexors—myotonic dystrophy

 Note

Ptosis and ophthalmoplegia are not a feature of facio-scapulohumeral type of muscular dystrophy and polimyositis.

Motor System Examination

Muscle bulk

- Atrophy—chronic muscle disease
- Normal—early muscle disease
- Myasthenia gravis till late normal bulk

Bulk is increased

- True hypertrophy:
  - Physical reconditioning
  - Myotonia congenita
  - Anabolic steroids
- Pseudohypertrophy (calf muscles, shoulder muscles):
  - Duchenne/Becker/limb girdle dystrophy
- Focal muscle enlargement can also occur due to
  - Inflammation
  - Neoplasm
  - Tendon rupture
  - Cysticercosis

 Note

Muscle appears enlarged in amyloidosis, sarcoidosis, hypothyrodism.

Muscle tenderness occurs in

- Rhabdomyolysis
- Inflammatory myopathies

Tone

- Usually decreased in all myopathies.
- Impaired relaxation in myotonic disorders
- For example, action—myotonia after hands-haking—difficulty in relaxing
- Percussion myotonia: Percussion over the following structures
- Over the tongue—there will be dimpling over the tongue
- Over the thenar eminence—produces dimpling.

Muscle power: Check for grades of muscle power.

Check specifically for following groups of muscles

- Facial, ocular, bulbar, neck muscles
- Forearm and hand muscles
- Muscles around the trunk, muscles of shoulder and muscles around the hip.
- Quadriceps, muscles of leg and foot.

Tests for myasthenia

For ocular muscle fatigability

- Ask the patient to look constantly upwards—observe for slow development of ptosis.
- Frequent blinking test also can be done. Patient may also c/o diplopia with the use of eyes.

Bulbar muscle weakness

- Head and neck extension movement—repeated till fatigability.
- Single breath count test can also be done.

Fatigability of limb muscle

Upper limb—abduction test: Raise the arm up to 90 degrees and check shoulder adduction and abduction. Move one arm up and down with shoulder adduction and abduction and compare with the other for the limb fatigue.

Ice pack test in myasthenia

- Application of ice pack for 2–5 minutes to the eye with ptosis (prevent the ice burns to the eye). Observe for improvement of ptosis. Decrease of temperature inhibits acetylcholinesterase activity.

- Coordination: Get affected due to power loss.

Involuntary movements

- Not a feature of muscle disease.
- Fine tremors—occurs in thyrotoxicosis.

Reflexes

- Superficial reflexes usually normal.
- Can get affected if corresponding muscle is involved.
- Deep reflexes
  - Usually normal till late in muscle disorders.
  - Absent—late muscle disease
  - Delayed relaxation—hypothyroidism
  - Can become exaggerated in thyrotoxicosis.

Sensory system—usually normal in primary muscle disease. If involved consider; alcoholism, para neoplastic, HIV infection, etc.

Cerebellar system usually normal. If involved:

- Toxin induced: Alcoholism
- Paraneoplastic syndrome
- HIV infection
- Hypothyroidism
  Bowel and bladder usually normal in primary muscle disorder.

If involved consider: Peripheral nerves/spinal cord involvement.

Skull and spine can have scoliosis and exaggerated lumbar lordosis in Duchenne muscular dystrophy.

Gait: Waddling gait in proximal (hip muscle) weakness.

Other Systemic Examination

Cardiovascular system: Involved in

- For CCF: Duchenne/Becker's dystrophy.
- Polymyositis
- Myotonic dystrophy

- Cardiac arrhythmias: Duchenne dystrophy
- Cardiomyopathy: Duchenne dystrophy
- Kearns-Sayre syndrome—conduction block.

Respiratory system: For

- Respiratory failure
  Occurs early—myotonic dystrophy. Late stages of all myopathies.

Abdominal examination

Hepatosplenomegaly

- Amyloidosis
- Sarcoidosis
- Systemic illness

Musculoskeletal contractures

- All myopathies of long-standing duration
- Early contracture: Bethlem myopathy and Emery-Dreifuss muscular dystrophy.

Systemic disease

Rule out

- Sarcoidosis
- Amyloidosis
- Endocrine disorder
- Collagen disease
- Mitochondrial disease.

Diagnosis of muscle disease depending on the muscle atrophy

Periscapular muscle wasting with winging of scapula:

- Facioscapulohumeral dystrophy
- Limb girdle type of dystrophy

Wasting of quadriceps with wasting of forearm muscles:

- Inclusion body myositis
- Atrophy of distal muscles—distal myopathies.

Differential diagnosis of muscle weakness apart from muscle disease:

• Fever, body ache with respiratory symptoms	Viral fever polymyositis
• Obesity, hypertension with easy bruisability	Excess corticosteroids Cushing's syndrome

Muscle weakness with other CNS symptoms	CVA/other CNS disease
↑Muscle weakness with exercise	Myasthenia
Positive family history with muscle weakness	Hereditary myopathy
Pain abdomen, renal calculi and polyuria	Hypercalcemia
Pain in the neck/low back pain/root pain	Spondylosis/disc disease
H/o intake of certain drugs/statins alcohol	Drugs/toxins induced muscle weakness
Weight gain, fatigue, muscle weakness	Hypothyroidism/cortisol excess

Causes of Proximal Muscle Weakness

Inflammatory
- Polymyositis
- Dermatomyositis.

Endocrine
- Hypothyroidism
- Hyperparathyroidism
- Osteomalacia
- Cushing's syndrome
- Addison's disease.

Metabolic: Hypokalemia

Drugs
- Statins
- Fibrates
- Zidovudine

Toxin: Alcohol

Infection
- Retroviral infection
- Cytomegalovirus
- Epstein-Barr virus.

Differential diagnosis of acute onset muscle weakness
- Vascular disease: CVA
- Infective disorder: Poliomyelitis
- Metabolic: Periodic paralysis
- Demyelinating: Transverse myelitis/multiple sclerosis

- Primary muscle disease: Polymyositis/rhabdomyolysis.
- Neurological: AIDP
- May be parasitic: Toxoplasmosis/trypanosomiasis

Differential diagnosis of muscle weakness due to basic muscular disorder

Endocrine and metabolic disorders
- Thyrotoxicosis
- Hypothyroidism
- Cushing's syndrome
- Hypercalcemia
- Hypokalemia

Drug-induced myopathy and toxins: Statins
- Corticosteroids
- Alcohol
- Zidovudine
- Penicillamine.

Neuromuscular disease: Myasthenia gravis/Eaton-Lambert's syndrome.

Inflammatory myopathy
- Polymyositis
- Dermatomyositis
- Inclusion body myositis

Degenerative disorder: Muscular dystrophies. Metabolic disorders of muscle.

Certain systemic diseases associated with muscle weakness

Infections
- HIV infection
- Epstein-Barr virus
- Poliomyelitis

Electrolyte abnormalities
- Hypercalcemia
- Hypocalcemia
- Hypokalemia
- Hyponatremia

Endocrine disorders
- Acromegaly
- Vitamin D deficiency
- Hyper/hypothyroidism

- Cushing's syndrome
- Hypoparathyroidism

Drug and toxins
- Alcohol
- Steroids
- Statins

Rheumatological
- Polymyalgia rheumatica
- Systemic sclerosis.

Specific clinical abnormalities in certain muscle disorders

Duchenne muscular dystrophy
Look for
- Thoracic scoliosis
- Lumbar lordosis
- Ileotibial band
- Gower's sign
- Pseudohypertrophy—calf muscles
- Learning difficulty and memory defect
- Dilated cardiomyopathy
- Becker's dystrophy—congnitive dysfunction less common.

Facioscapulohumeral dystrophy
- Absence of pectoralis
- Popeye effect of limb
- No involvement of ocular muscles and no ptosis
- Positive Beevor's sign
- Muscle biopsy—shows inflammatory pattern
- Sensory neural hearing loss.

Popeye effect: Wasting of biceps and triceps with less involvement of deltoid and forearm muscles. This results in popeye appearance.

Myotonic dystrophy
- Frontal balding
- Cataract
- Hatchet face
- Distal muscle weakness
- Myotonia
- Ovarian and testicular dysfunction
- Wasting of flexors of neck: Swan neck appearance of neck.

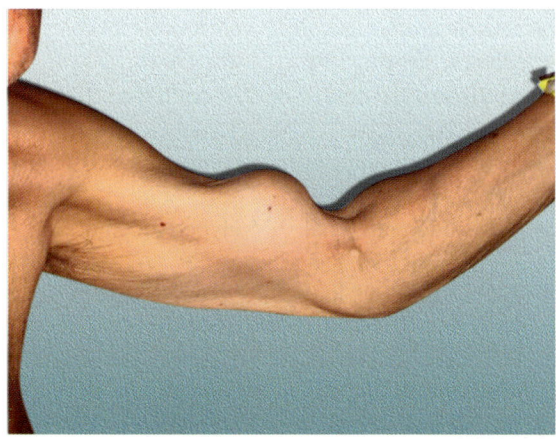

Fig. 4.20: Popeye effect

Hatchet face
- Wasting and hollowing of temporal and jaw muscles
- Drooping of lower lips
- Sagging of lower part of face.

Difference between neuropathy/myopathic weakness

Neuropathic weakness	Myopathic weakness
Distal weakness	Usually proximal weakness
Unilateral/bilateral	Usually bilateral
Fasciculations may be present	Fasciculations absent
Tendon reflexes are lost early	Tendon reflexes are preserved till late
Early muscle atrophy	Later muscle atrophy

Thyroid myopathy
Hyperthyroidism
Features
- Proximal muscle weakness
- Respiratory, bulbar and oesophageal muscle involvement.
- Exaggerated deep reflexes
- Fasciculations

Other associations
- Myasthenia gravis
- Graves' ophthalmopathy
- Acquired periodic paralysis.

Lab parameters
- No CK raise
- Normal EMG

Hypothyroidism
- Proximal muscle weakness
- Muscle cramps and stiffness can occur
- Delayed relaxation of ankle jerk. (Hung up reflex: Woltman's sign)
- Muscle enlargement is present (Hoffman's syndrome)
- CK is significantly raised.

Myasthenia Gravis

Type of disease: Autoimmune disorder

Structure involved: Neuromuscular junction

Characteristic antibody
- Autoantibody to acetylcholine receptors at neuromuscular junction.
- Autoantibody to muscle specific kinases (anti-MSK Ab)

Associated conditions
- Thymoma/thymic hyperplasia
- Autoimmune disorders
  - Hashimoto's thyroiditis
  - SLE
  - Rheumatoid arthritis

Pathogenesis: Autoantibodies to acetylcholine receptors with loss of acetylcholine receptors. There is impairment of neuromuscular transmission.

Clinical features
- Sex involved—female predominant
- Common symptoms—muscle fatigue and weakness
- Type of muscle weakness—episodic and fluctuating, more as the muscle is progressively used.

Muscles involved
- Extraocular muscles
- Causes ptosis/diplopia
- Unilateral/bilateral

Other features
- Difficulty in chewing

- Slurred speech
- Dysphagia
- Proximal weakness
- Respiratory difficulty

Above symptoms appear as the muscle is progressively used.

Characteristic clinical points: In myasthenia gravis, deep tendon reflexes are preserved in spite of muscle weakness except in a patient of Eaton-Lambert syndrome—muscle weakness is associated with loss of deep tendon reflexes (due to associated neuropathy).

Bed side tests for myasthenia: See under muscle disorder.

Ocular myasthenia: Only ocular muscle weakness without involvement of other muscles even after 3 continuous years.

Bulbar myasthenia:
- Involves muscles supplied from brainstem (medulla)
- Associated with anti-MSK antibody.

Differential diagnosis of weakness of cranial nerves and paralysis of limbs:
- Eaton-Lambert syndrome
- Hyperthyroidism
- Botulism

Acute onset ocular muscle weakness with limb weakness:
- Neurotoxic snakebite
- Miller-Fisher variant of Guillain-Barré syndrome.

Conditions which present with progressive ocular muscle weakness:
- Oculopharyngeal muscular dystrophy
- Intracranial mass lesion at superior orbital fissure.
- Progressive external ophthalmoplegia.

Drugs which can cause myasthenia like features: Penicillamine.

Drugs which exacerbate myasthenic weakness:
- Aminoglycoside
- Penicillamine.

Eaton-Lambert syndrome
- Associated with small cell carcinoma of lung
- Present as:
  - Proximal lower limb muscle weakness
  - Ocular muscle weakness with diplopia and ptosis.

Differentiating feature of Eaton-Lambert syndrome which are not present in myasthenia gravis
- Male sex/smokes/advanced age
- Absence of deep tendon reflexes
- Presence of autonomic features:
  - Impotence
  - Dry mouth
- Incremental response to nerve stimulation and exercise.

Differential diagnosis of myasthenia gravis
- Eaton-Lambert syndrome.
- Intracranial mass lesion—at superior orbital fissure/midbrain
- Graves' disease
- Muscular dystrophy—Oculopharyngeal
- Mitochondrial myopathy: Progressive external ophthalmoplegia
- Kearns-Sayre syndrome
- Botulism
- Drug-induced myopathy.

Mitchondrial Myopathies

Kearns-Sayre syndrome
- Younger age less than 20 years
- Retinitis pigmentosa
- Progressive external ophthalmoplegia
- May have complete heart block
- Higher CSF protein
- Cerebellar ataxia

Chronic progressive ophthalmoplegia
- A form of mitochondrial ophthalmoplegia
- Progressive weakness of extraocular muscles.

MELAS syndrome
- Mitochondrial encephalopathy
- Lactic acidosis
- Stroke-like episodes

Hypokalemic periodic paralysis
- Younger age—usually less than 25 years of age
- Males more affected than females

Features:
- Episodic muscle weakness
- Precipitated by high carbohydrate and sodium containing meals
- Present as proximal limb weakness
- Muscles usually not involved—ocular, brainstem supplied and respiratory muscles.

Differential diagnosis: Thyrotoxic periodic paralysis (if more than 30 years of age).

Lab abnormalities
During the attack
- Low serum potassium level
- Nerve conduction—reduced amplitude of motor conduction
- EMG: No electrical activity in involved muscles.

OCCLUSION OF CORTICAL VENOUS SINUSES

Occlusion of Venous Sinus Produces Venous Infarct

General Features of Cortical Venous Infarct
- Altered sensorium
- Headache
- Convulsions
- Neurological deficit

Specific features related to individual sinus occlusion
Superior saggital sinus thrombosis
- Papilledema
- UMN paraplegia
- Bladder involvement
- Cortical sensory loss

Occlusion of cavernous sinus
- Proptosis
- Ophthalmoplegia with involvement of 3rd, 4th and 6th cranial nerves.

- Involvement of ophthalmic division of 5th nerve.

Occlusion of transverse sinus
- Papilledema
- Hemiplegia
- Cranial nerve palsy: 9th, 10th and 11th nerve.

Common causes of thrombosis of cortical venous sinuses:
- Postpartum state
- Pregnancy
- Hypercoagulable state
- Vasculitis
- Trauma to the head
- Pyogenic meningitis

Investigations

- Blood counts
- ESR
- Blood culture/sensitivity
- Work up for hypercoagulable state
- CR/MRI: Angiogram with venous phase for cerebral edema and venous occlusion.

Different CT signs of cortical venous sinus thrombosis:
- *Empty delta sign: See* chapter on Radiology.
- Hyperdense straight sinus: *See* chapter on Radiology.

MULTIPLE SCLEROSIS

Disease Description

Demyelinating Disorder
- Multiple sites of CNS involvement
- Usually associated with optic neuritis
- Exacerbations and remissions

Risk factors
- Women > Men
- Deficiency of vitamin D
- Smoking
- Exposure to Epstein-Barr virus.

Other possible associations
- High salt intake
- Associated with HLA DRB1 gene.

Pathogenesis and pathology
- Inflammatory infiltration surrounding the white matter
- Destruction of myelin
- Gliosis and scarring
- Loss of neurons.
- Consequences—can result in axonal destruction
- Block in the neuronal conduction
- Block in the neuronal conduction can be aggravated by increased temperature and exercise.

Clinical features
- W > F
- Recurrent attacks
- Multiple sites of involvement.

Usual features
- Fatigue
- Motor involvement
- UMN type of motor paralysis.
- Sensory involvement
- Paresthesia
- Anesthesia
- Level of sensory loss below a certain level
- Lhermitte's symptoms (due to plaque at cervical cord level)
- Cranial nerves:
  - Trigeminal neuralgia with signs of nerve involvement
  - Optic neuritis/retrobulbar neuritis (usually unilateral)
  - Internuclear ophthalmoplegia.
- Cerebellar ataxia
- Neurogenic bladder

Other features
- Occasional involvement of higher mental functions in the form of memory loss, loss of cognition and depression.
- Sudden exacerbations and remissions (a few weeks to months)

Uhthoff's Phenomenon

- Transient increase in the neurological dysfunction with increase in the body temperature.

- For example, febrile illness—causes decrease in the neuronal conduction.
- Occasionally feature of LMN-like loss of reflex—due to disturbance in the conduction at the cord level.

Features which are not common in multiple sclerosis

- Fever
- Loss of consciousness
- Convulsions
- Central speech defect
- Involvement of peripheral nervous system
- Involvement of extrapyramidal system
- Dementia.

Differential diagnosis

- HIV infection
- Vasculitic syndrome
- APLA syndrome
- B12 deficiency
- CNS syphilis
- Lymphoma of central nervous system.

Course of the illness

- RRMS
  - Relapsing remitting multiple sclerosis.
  - Recurrent exacerbations and remissions
- SPMS
  - Secondary progressive multiple sclerosis.
  - Initial exacerbations and remissions
  - Later progressive deterioration.
- PPMS
  - Primary progressive multiple sclerosis.
  - No recurrent exacerbations and remission.
  - Slow progression of the disease from the beginning.
- PRMS
  - Progressive relapsing multiple sclerosis.
  - There is progression from the beginning with acute exacerbations.

Investigations

- CSF
  - Mononuclear pleocytosis

  - Increase in the intrathecal IgG in the CSF. Raise in the intrathecal IgM carries adverse prognosis.
  - Presence of oligoclonal band
- Evoked potentials: Abnormal visual evoked potential is more diagnostic compared to somatosensory potential.
- MRI: Hyperintense lesions—periventricular perpendicular to the lateral ventricles (Dawson's fingers).

Distribution of lesions

- Cerebellum
- Spinal cord
- Corpus callosum
- Periventricular white matter

Diagnosis of multiple sclerosis

- Multiple site of involvement of CNS
- Multiple attacks with a gap of >1 month
- Optic neuritis/retrobulbar neuritis (usually unilateral)
- Abnormal visual evoked potentials
- Typical MRI lesions.

CAUSES OF UPPER LIMB MONOPARESIS

1. *Intracranial*: CVA involving MCA branch occlusion involving precentral gyrus. Intracranial tumor involving upper limb area in the cortex
   Demyelination—in the cortex
   In cortical lesions there may be associated UMN facial weakness.
2. *Extracranial spinal cord*
   - Cervical cord involvement
   - Causes
     - Trauma
     - Disc prolapse
     - Tumors
   - Anterior horn cell disorder
     - Poliomyelitis
     - Monomelic MND
   - Brachial plexus/root lesions
     - trauma
     - brachial plexus neuritis
     - Pancoast's tumor (C8, T1)

- Peripheral nerve lesion and mononeuritis multiplex
3. *Rare—functional disorder*

 Note

Occasionally injury to the radial/median nerve can cause upper limb weakness. Endocrine disorders like diabetes mellitus and hypothyroidism (compression of nerve can cause single limb weakness).

Causes of acute onset of single limb weakness (either upper or lower limb)

- CVA
- Trauma
- Todd's paralysis
- Poliomyelitis
- Demyelination.

Causes of UMN/spastic single limb weakness

Upper limb—UMN
1. Cortical lesion
2. Brainstem lesion
3. Compressive lesion of cervical cord
4. Demyelinating lesion of the brain/spinal cord.

Lower limb—UMN
1. Cortical lesion
2. Brainstem lesion.
3. Compression of thoracic/lumbar cord
4. Demyelinating lesion of brain/spinal cord.

Causes of lower limb monoparesis

Intracranial
- CVA involving ACA territory
- Demyelination/tumor involving cortical lower limb area
- Extracranial; monomelic MND, poliomyelitis
- Trauma/tumor/disc lesion involving lumbar cord
- Lumbar plexopathy/mononeuritis. Multiplex involving lower limb nerves.

Approach to Hemiplegia

History

Complains of weakness of one half of the body.

Enquire following history in a patient of hemiplegia

Onset and duration and progression
- Acute (24–48 hours)
- Subacute (days to weeks)
- Chronic (months to years)

Part affected
- Upper limb and lower limb on one side
- Distal or proximal
- Stiffness of limbs, incoordination of limbs on the affected side
- Involuntary movements.

History of cranial nerves involvement
- Facial deviation to one side.
- Closing the eye possible/not possible on one side
  (Rarely—tongue and palate can be transiently involved in acute CVA)
- Patient may complain of field of vision decrease if hemianopia is present.

History of sensory involvement on the affected side: Enquire whether there is decrease or complete loss of sensation on the affected side including same side of face: e.g. hemi-anesthesia.

Symptoms of incoordination: Occasionally symptoms of incoordination may be present due to cerebellar involvement on the side of hemiplegia, e.g. ataxic hemiparesis.

Involvement of bowel/bladder in the form of incontinence/retention of urine.

History of headache, vomiting, altered sensorium, convulsions including speech disturbance

To diagnose the etiology of hemiplegia
- History of fever, rash, joint pain, subcutaneous swellings (lymph nodes).
- History of trauma to the head
- History of cardiac symptoms
- History of respiratory symptoms
- History of hypertension, diabetes mellitus and IHD
- History of taking medication.

Past history: History of TIA. Similar episodes, hypertension, diabetes mellitus and IHD.

Personal history: Loss of appetite and weight, smoking, alcohol intake, history of exposure to commercial sex workers.

Family history: Of cerebrovascular accident, CNS disorder

Consanguinity between parents.

Treatment history

- Antihypertensives, diabetes mellitus, IHD medications
- History of taking aspirin
- History of taking antiepileptic medications
- History of taking anticoagulants
- Taking: Benzathine penicillin.

Approach to a Patient of Hemiplegia

Onset, duration and progress of weakness

Acute 24–48 hours: CVA, vasculitis, trauma

Subacute (days to weeks): Infective, trauma, subdural hematoma, demyelination.

Chronic (months to years):

- CNS—space occupying lesion
- CNS neoplasms
- Vascular like AV malformation
- Chronic SDH
- Degenerative

Part affected

- Involvement of both upper limb and lower limb affected equally and severely: Internal capsular lesion.
- Upper limb is more affected than the lower limb: Middle cerebral artery occlusion.
- Lower limb is more affected than the upper limb: Anterior cerebral artery occlusion.
- Only upper limb is affected with face—faciobrachial monoplegia—MCA branch occlusion or Heubner's artery—recurrent branch of ACA occlusion.
- Patient complains of symptoms of incoordination of limbs suggestive of cerebellar symptoms on the affected side of hemiplegia—consider ataxic hemiparesis.
- Patient can complain of involuntary movement on the hemiplegic side

May be due to

- Focal convulsion—cortical lesion
- Fasciculation—e.g. MND
- Tremor of Parkinsonism—e.g. hemiplegic parkinsonism.

Enquire the history of cranial nerve involvement

1. Deviation of angle of mouth to the unaffected side.
2. Eye closure on the affected side

If the facial palsy is of UMN type (upper part is spared—eye closure possible)

- Facial palsy and hemiplegia on the same side, e.g. internal capsule and corona radiata and cortical lesion on the opposite side.
- If the facial palsy (LMN) is on the opposite side of hemiplegia—crossed hemiplegia consider: Brainstem—pontine lesion.
- In brainstem lesion—there will be LMN palsy of 3rd, 4th, 6th and 7th cranial nerve on one side (on the side of lesion) with hemiplegia on the opposite side.

📖 *Note*

- *Occasionally UMN facial palsy in acute conditions can be severe and can involve upper part of face behaving like LMN facial palsy.*
- *If hemiplegia and facial palsy is on the same side— even if upper part of face is involved. Consider it as UMN type and the lesion is usually in the opposite internal capsule.*
- *In acute CVA—transiently there can be involvement of palate and tongue on the same side of hemiplegia.*
- *Patient may also complain of decrease of vision in one half of visual field in each eye if there is hemianopia.*

Sensory involvement

- Enquire whether there is decrease or absence of sensation on the affected side.
- For example, hemianesthesia.

Cerebellar symptoms: History of incoordination on the affected side: For ataxic hemiparesis.

History of bowel/bladder involvement in a hemi-plegia
Possibilities
- ACA occlusion
- Due to altered sensorium
- Massive cerebral edema
- Brainstem involvement.

 Note

Patient might have been catheterized due to inability to walk—may not be because of actual bladder involvement.

History of headache, vomiting, altered sensorium, convulsions including speech disturbances
Headache and vomiting
- Due to raised intracranial tension—due to cerebral edema.
- For example, intracerebral hemorrhage, subarachnoid hemorrhage.

Convulsions
- Cortical lesion
- For example, encephalitis/intracerebral hemorrhage
- Cortical mass lesion
- Cortical infarct

Altered sensorium: See later.
Speech disturbances
- Aphasia/dysphasia: Due to left MCA occlusion with right hemiplegia.
- Slurring of speech: Can be due to facial palsy/central speech defect.

History of trauma to the head: Can cause acute/subacute/chronic subdural hematoma causing hemiplegia.

History of fever
- Usually suggests infective pathology
- Fever with rash—may be exanthematous viral fever causing meningoencephalitis fever, rash with joint pain—infective/inflammatory disorder, e.g. viral exanthema and primary/secondary vasculitis.
- *Fever—may also be due to*
  - Pyogenic meningitis
  - Cerebral abscess

- TB meningitis
- Syphilis
- Retrovirus related illness
- Infective endocarditis
- Internal malignancy

History of cardiac symptoms
- Consider atrial fibrillation with embolization with CVA
- AF may be due to: RHD/congenital heart disease, IHD with LV clot
- CVA can also occur due to
  - Dilated cardiomyopathy
  - Infective endocarditis.

Respiratory symptoms with hemiplegia
Consider
- Tuberculosis
- Bronchogenic carcinoma
- Pneumonia/lung abscess.

Respiratory symptoms can occur after hemi-plegia due to aspiration pneumonia.

History of diabetes mellitus/hypertension and IHD
- Suggestive of risk factors for CVA/multi infarct state.
- History taking medications—*see* under treatment history.

Past History

History of TIA
Types of TIA
- Embolic
- Lacunar
- Low flow (atherosclerotic vessel)

Depends on the vascular territory involved: Carotid/vertebra basilar.

Embolic TIA: Cardioemboli/artery to artery embolisation.

Cardioembolic
- AF with left atrial clot
- IHD with LV intramural clot
  Dilated cardiomyopathy with LV clot
- Infective endocarditis

- Left atrial myxoma
- Paradoxical embolization.

Features of cardioembolic TIA

Different sites of occlusion each time

- Not stereotyped defect each time
- Larger clot with major vessel occlusion
- Symptoms and signs of cardiac disease.

Likely embolisation of cardiac cause occurs as a result of intermittent atrial fibrillation with clots getting dislodged during normal LA contraction.

Possible sites of occlusion of cerebral vessels in cardioembolic CVAL

- Most common MCA territory (may be left sided)
- Next common site: PCA territory.
- Cardioembolic stroke: Less likely to occur with ACA territory

Artery to artery embolism

- Occurs from common carotid or internal carotid artery.
- Causes stereotyped TIA
- Evidence of atherosclerotic vascular disease and carotid narrowing.
- Associated with hypertension, diabetes mellitus and smoking.
- Recurrent episodes of hemiplegia occurring and recovering—suggests recurrent CVA and occasionally demyelinating disorder.
- History of diabetes mellitus/hypertension/IHD-risk factor for CVA.
- Rarely MELAS syndrome can present with recurrent stroke-like episodes.

Personal History

Loss of appetite and weight—suggests systemic disease.

- For example, tuberculosis
- Retroviral illness
- Internal malignancy

Smoking—risk factor CVA

Alcohol intake: Hemiplegia can occur due to head injury and SDH.

Exposure to commercial sex workers

- Risk for syphilis—causing endarteritis and hemiplegia
- Risk for HIV infection and its complications causing hemiplegia (CNS TB, cryptococcal infection, toxoplasmosis, PML, primary CNS lymphoma).

Family history: CVA can occur in family members and may be due to common risk factors of CVA/CARASIL/CADASIL syndromes.

Treatment history

Ask for history for intake of

- Antihypertensive, anti-diabetic and IHD medications.
- Aspirin, clopidogrel—for previous TIA/IHD.
- Anti-coagulants—for atrial fibrillation, prosthetic valve (risk for intracerebral hemorrhage).
- Taking injection benzathine penicillin—suggestive of RHD with atrial fibrillation.
- Previous history of intake of steroids with improvement—possible demyelinating disorder.

Examination of a Patient of Hemiplegia

General Physical Examination

Pallor

- Due to anemia—can be due to systemic disease.
- May aggravate CNS hypoxia in a patient of CVA.

Icterus: Suggests systemic disease with CNS involvement.

Causes

Systemic disease with CNS involvement with icterus

- Disseminated TB/fungal infection or retroviral infection.
- Parenchymal liver disease with hepatic encephalopathy
- Wilson's disease.
- Vasculitis syndromes
- Disseminated malignancy/lymphoma

Clubbing: Systemic disease which causes clubbing involving nervous system.

Cyanotic heart disease
Cerebral abscess in Fallot's tetralogy.
Infective endocarditis with embolization.

Systemic respiratory disease like
- Bronchiectasis causing cerebral abscess
- Lung abscess causing cerebral abscess
- Bronchogenic carcinoma causing secondaries in the brain.

Hepatic disorders: Cirrhosis/hepatoma can involve CNS.

Cyanosis
- Cardiac and respiratory disorders causing central cyanosis with CNS involvement.
- For example, type 2 respiratory failure causing CO_2 narcosis
- Chronic lung disease with polycythemia causing CVA.

Lymphadenopathy: Conditions causing generalized lymphadenopathy involving nervous system.

Pedal edema
- Part of systemic disease
- Edema of lower limb on the hemiplegic side—due to vasomotor paralysis or occurrence of DVT.

Vital Signs

Pulse rate: Bradycardia can be due to cerebral edema.

Rhythm: Irregularly irregular s/o AF with embolization.

Volume: Alteration may be due to associated cardiac condition.

Thickening of vessel wall: Suggests atherosclerosis.

Other evidence of atherosclerosis
- Presence of locomotor brachialis
- Thickening of superficial temporal artery.
- Carotid pulsation—may be feeble on one side with bruit (opposite to hemiplegic side).
- Palpate: Dorsalis pedis—for thickening and decrease pulsation.

Palpate all peripheral pulses—absence of peripheral pulse may be suggestive of cardiac embolization.

Also look for xanthomas/xanthelasmas as indirect evidence for hyperlipidemia and atherosclerosis.

Blood pressure: Record the blood pressure not on the paralysed side—recording of BP on the paralysed side may give a false recording due to autonomic disturbance with vasomotor paralysis (decrease of blood pressure).
May also become a wrong recording due to alteration in the tone/limb girth.

Higher blood pressure—indicative of accelerated hypertension/reactionary hypertension (no evidence of target organ damage).

Respiratory rate and rhythm: Rate and rhythm can be abnormal due to cerebral edema: Brainstem involvement or/and brainstem CVA.

Temperature: Increased;
- Febrile illness causing CVA
- Hyperpyrexia—pontine hemorrhage
  Hypothermia: Myxedema coma

Other Important General Examination Findings
- Oral candidiasis: HIV infection
- Look for skin manifestation of HIV
- Healed scar/chancre of syphilis
- External markers of TB (phlycten)
- Manifestation of connective tissue disorder—rash, skin ulcers, etc.
- Markers of endocarditis
- Petechiae/purpura—can be due to bleeding/clotting disorder
- Subcutaneous nodule: Neurocysticercosis.
- Polyarthritis—connective tissue disease.

Systemic Examination: CNS

Mental state examination
Altered sensorium—in a hemiplegic may be due to
- Massive infarct involving one cerebral hemisphere

- Bilateral hemispherical lesion
- Brainstem involvement
- SIADH causing hyponatremia
- Cerebral edema
- Due to seizure episodes.

Occurrence of speech disturbance

Aphasia—due to involvement of speech center—left side lesion with right hemiplegia.

Dysarthria—due to UMN/LMN facial palsy with hemiplegia.

Occasionally dysarthria may also be due to central speech defect.

In left-sided hemiplegia with right cortical lesion—look for hemineglect on the left side.

Subacute/chronic hemiplegia—can have memory loss

Possible multi-infarct/diffuse vascular disease/ICSOL

Emotional incontinence—can occur due to multi-infarct.

Handedness: In right handed individual: Left cortical involvement causing aphasia.

Cranial Nerve Examination

Look for gaze preference

- If eyes are deviated towards the side of hemiplegia—irritative lesion on the opposite side—cortex.
- If the eyes are deviated away from the hemiplegic side—paralytic lesion of the opposite cortex.

 Note

Opposite of above eye position occurs in brainstem lesions (see under gaze palsy).

Look for UMN facial palsy on the side of hemiplegia.

3rd, 4th, 6th, 7th and 12th LMN cranial nerve palsies on the opposite side of hemiplegia suggest crossed hemiplegia with lesion in the brainstem on the side of cranial nerve palsy.

Other cranial nerves in a hemiplegic patient

- Transiently palate and tongue can be affected on the hemiplegic side.

- Sternomastoid can be paralysed on the side of lesion.
- 6th nerve palsy may be a false localizing sign.

2nd cranial nerve including fundus examination

- Look for homonymous hemianopia—in internal capsular lesion.
- Pupillary asymmetry can occur due to uncal herniation
- Ophthalmic fundus—papilledema—due to cerebral edema/mass lesion
- Subhyaloid hemorrhage (made out by horizontal level of blood—in patient sitting position—in subarachnoid hemorrhage while looking at fundus).
- Choroid tubercles—in disseminated TB.
- Hollenhorst plaque—cholesterol emboli-atherosclerotic CVA
- Roth spot—infective endocarditis.
- Bleeding spots—bleeding/clotting disorder.
- Papillitis—demyelinating disorder.
- Optic atrophy—degenerative disorder.
- Changes of hypertension, diabetes mellitus and arteriosclerosis.
- Toxoplasma/CMV retinitis: In HIV patients.

Motor System Examination

Attitude of the limb: Upper limb is adducted, semi-flexed and semi-pronated (due to flexor hypertonia) and lower limb is extended and externally rotated (extensor hypertonia in the lower limb).

Nutrition

- Not affected in acute hemiplegia
- Subacute/chronic hemiplegia can have wasting due to disuse atrophy/LMN lesion.

Tone

- In neuronal shock—there will be hypotonia
- In all other UMN type of lesions—spasticity will be present
- In LMN type, e.g. MND there will be hypotonia.

Power

- Grade the power in all group of muscles.

- Distal weakness in more than proximal weakness—pyramidal tract lesion.
- Trunk muscles are not involved in a hemiplegic due to bilateral representation.

Coordination
- Coordination is affected due to powerloss (less than grade 3 power)/tone alteration
- If the power is more than grade 3 and if incoordination is present on the affected side—indicates cerebellar involvement, e.g. ataxic hemiparesis.

Involuntary movements
- Tremors—can be present in hemiplegic parkinsonism.
- Fasciculations—suggestive of MND.

Sensory system: Look for evidence of hemianesthesia.

Reflexes
Superficial
- Corneal and conjunctival reflex—will not be affected (bilateral representation)
- Abdominal reflexes—lost on the affected side.
- Cremasteric reflex—lost on the affected side.
- Plantar-extensor—affected side (after the period of neuronal shock).

Deep reflexes
- Initially all deep reflexes are lost on the affected side—due to neuronal shock.
- After recovery from neuronal shock all deep reflexes become exaggerated.
- There can be associated clonus on the affected side due to hyperreflexia and hypertonia.

Elicit Hoffman's, finger flexion and Wartenberg's sign on the affected side.

 Note

Superficial reflexes are polysynaptic and they are under facilitatory control of the pyramidal tract and they are lost in UMN lesions. Deep reflexes are under the inhibitory control of the pyramidal tract and they become exaggerated in UMN lesions.

Primitive reflexes: Usually absent in unilateral lesion. Present in multi-infarct state.

Cerebellar signs: Usually not present.
If present on the hemiplegic side: Consider ataxic hemiparesis.

Bladder/bladder involvement: If involved—*see* above under history analysis.

Signs of meningitis: If present—suggestive of TB/syphilis/HIV/viral infection.
- Palpate the carotid for pulsation and compare with the opposite side and auscultate for bruit over the carotid (on the side of the lesion).
- If carotid is totally occluded on one side auscultate opposite orbit for the bruit.

 Note

Ideally internal carotid on the side of the lesion should be palpated against the tonsillar bed (requires wearing of gloves and local anaesthetic).

Other Systems Examination
CVS
- For evidence of RHD
- Hypertensive heart disease
- IHD
- AF
- Endocarditis
- Cardiomyopathy (degenerative disorder)
- Arrhythmias/conduction block
- Congenital heart disease.

Respiratory system: For evidence of TB, pneumonia, mass lesion, etc.

Abdominal examination: For hepatosplenomegaly for systemic cause.

Gait if the patient is able to walk: Look for circumduction gait.

Look for following additional features in a prolonged bedridden patients
- Presence of bed sore
- Nasogastric tube (due to altered sensorium/brainstem lesion) with its complications

- Deep vein thrombosis
- Pressure palsy: Radial nerve/lateral popliteal nerve on the affected side.
- Aspiration pneumonia: In a patient of altered sensorium

Final neurological diagnosis should include the following features
- Clinical
- Anatomical site of lesion
- Pathology
- Aetiology
- Present functional status of the patient.

Key Points

- If hemiplegia, hemianesthesia and hemianopia occur together. It is called dense hemiplegia. And lesion is in the internal capsule.
- Can caused by the occlusion of MCA or anterior choroidal artery.
- There can be hemiplegia without cranial nerve palsy.

Causes of hemiplegia without cranial nerve palsy:
- Cortical involvement
- Minimal UMN facial palsy resolved
- Involvement of medullary pyramid
- Spinal cord involvement.

Differential Diagnosis of Hemiplegia

Features suggestive of CVA
- Sudden/acute onset.
- Headache/vomiting, convulsions
- Pertaining to vascular territory
- Cannot be explained with any other aetiology.
- Associated hypertension, IHD and diabetes mellitus and cardiac disease.

Sudden/Acute Onset

Embolism

Features of embolic CVA
- Sudden onset and occurs during physical activity.

- Associated with cardiac disease/IHD/AF
- Sudden onset with maximum deficit at the onset with recovery.

Features of hemorrhagic CVA
- Usually occurs during physical activity
- Sudden onset headache, convulsions, vomiting and altered sensorium
- History of hypertension and head trauma (subdural hematoma)
- Excruciating headache: Subarachnoid hemorrhage with vasospasm.

Features of thrombotic CVA
- Gradually progressive neurological deficit (stroke in evolution)
- Less common headache, vomiting
- History of HT and diabetes mellitus and TIAS
- Can occur during sleep

Differential Diagnosis of Hemiplegia

Hemiplegia: Sudden Onset

Causes

CVA

If fever with convulsions
- Viral meningoencephalitis
- TB endarteritis
- Fungal infection of CNS
- Occasionally syphilitic
- HIV with opportunistic infection
- Pyogenic meningitis
- Head injury
- Hemorrhage into the intracranial tumor

 Note

Endarteritis obliterans can cause sudden onset hemiplegia (TB/syphilis).

Hemiplegia: Days to Weeks

Presence of headache/fever/weight loss
- TB of CNS
- HIV infection involving CNS
- Fungal infection of CNS
- Cerebral abscess

Headache convulsions with subcutaneous nodules: Intracranial space occupying lesions, e.g. cysticercosis.
- Previous history of head injury: Subdural hematoma.
- History of visual involvement, multiple parts of CNS is involved—demyelinating disorder.

Chronic Onset: Prolonged History

Headache, vomiting with hemiplegia with or without convulsions
- Intracranial space occupying lesions, e.g. neurocysticercosis
- Primary or secondary neoplasms of CNS.
- History of previous head trauma—chronic SDH.
- History of intermittent headache, neurological symptoms—possible AV malformations.
- History of hypertension, diabetes mellitus, IHD, smoking bilateral pyramidal signs— possible multiple infarct.
- Prolonged history of without recovery with only motor involvement—degenerative disorder, e.g. MND.

Causes of Hemiparesis

Acute onset (24–48 hours)
Vascular: Cerebrovascular accident involving
- Cortex
- Corona radiata
- Internal capsule
- Brainstem

Vasculitis: Tuberculosis
- Syphilis
- Retroviral illness/with opportunistic infection
- Primary vasculitis

Hemiparesis (days to weeks)
- Infective: Tuberculosis—tuberculoma
- CNS—fungal infection
- Cerebral abscess
- Neurocysticercosis
- Trauma—subdural hematoma

- Demyelination—multiple sclerosis
- Primary/secondary CNS tumors

Chronic (weeks to months to years)
- Trauma—chronic subdural hematoma
- Vascular—A-V malformation
- Neoplastic—primary neoplasms of brain
- Degenerative—MND

Points to Remember
- Occasionally unilateral lesion of cervical cord can cause hemiparesis without cranial nerve involvement.
- Involvement of medullary pyramid can cause hemiparesis without cranial nerve involvement.
- After an attack of poliomyelitis—it can result in LMN lesion mimicking MND (after 30–40 years).
- After an electric shock injury—can result in LMN disease.
- If the lesion is bilateral at cervicomedullary junction—can involve both upper limbs.

Different Terminologies while Describing Hemiplegia

Crossed Hemiplegia: In brainstem lesions: Features of LMN cranial nerve palsy on the side of lesion with opposite side hemiplegia.

Dense hemiplegia
- Occurs in internal capsular lesions
- Features—combination of hemiplegia, hemianesthesia and hemianopia.

 Note

Occasionally hemiplegia with very less power (grade 0 to 2) is also called dense hemiplegia.

Cruciate hemiplegia: Occurs in lesions of cervicomedullary junction.

Features: One side upper limb weakness with opposite lower limb weakness.

 Note

Cervicomedullary junction lesion can present with only bilateral upper limb involvement.

Double Hemiplegia
- Not commonly used term
- In patients with cerebral palsy with bilateral involvement, one side more involved than the other.

Conditions which mimic stroke (stroke mimics)
- Hemiplegic migraine
- Todd's paralysis
- Hypoglycemia (can present with hemiplegia)
- Hyperglycemia (can present with hemiplegia)
- Multiple sclerosis
- Intracranial mass lesions:
  (can cause sudden bleed and vasospasm)
- Subdural hematoma
- Hysterical conditions

Differential diagnosis of TIAs
- Syncope
- Seizure
- Hypoglycemia
- Migraine
- Labyrinthine dysfunction
- Transient global amnesia
- Anxiety and depressive disorder

Hemiplegia alternans: (alternating hemiplegia of childhood)
- Occurs in children
- Developmental disorder of the nervous system.
- Mutation in the ATP1A2 gene
- Neuronal and cardiac tissue is involved.
- Recurrent attacks of hemiplegia on one side and the other side.

Ipsilateral hemiplegia
- Lesion above brainstem
- For example, classical internal capsular CVA.
- *Features*: UMN facial palsy with hemiplegia—on the opposite side of the lesion.

Carotid hemiplegia: Due to occlusion of the internal carotid artery results in opposite side hemiplegia with ipsilateral blindness due to occlusion of ophthalmic artery.

PARAPLEGIA

Causes of Paraplegia

Depending on the onset

Acute (24–48 hours)
Intracranial causes
- Unpaired anterior cerebral artery occlusion
- Superior sagittal vein thrombosis
- Rarely acute hydrocephalus

Extracranial causes
- Acute transverse myelitis
- Guillain-Barré syndrome
- Spinal epidural abscess
- Anterior spinal artery occlusion
- Trauma to the spine
- Intervertebral disc herniation
- Demyelinating disorder
  - ADEM
  - Multiple sclerosis
  - Neuromyelitis optica

Subacute (weeks to months)
Slowly progressive compressive lesion of spine/spinal cord
Tuberculosis
- Tumors
- Trauma
- Syringomyelia
Chronic
- Peripheral neuropathy
- CIDP
- Spinal muscular atrophy
- MND
- Myopathy/muscular dystrophy
- Hereditary spastic paraplegia
- Toxin/infection—HILV induced
- Lathyrism
- Fluorosis

Causes of Paraplegia Depending on the Etiology

Infective causes
Viral myelitis
- Herpes simplex virus

- Cytomegalovirus
- Epstein-Barr virus

Bacterial
- Spinal epidural abscess
- TB/brucellosis

Parasitic: Toxoplasmosis

Inflammatory
- Multiple sclerosis
- ADEM ⎫
- Acute transverse myelitis ⎬ para-infectious
- GB syndrome ⎭

Vascular
- Occlusion of the anterior spinal artery
- Vasculitis
- Trauma: Hematomyelia
- AV malformation.

Mechanical
- Intervertebral disc prolapse
- Vertebral fracture
- Neoplasms
- TB/brucellosis of spine

Toxin induced
- Lathyrism
- Alcohol

Other causes
- Periodic paralysis
- Intracranial causes
- Psychogenic
- Fluorosis

Compressive Lesions of Spinal Cord

Common causes
- Infective: TB spine
- Traumatic injury to the vertebra, cord and hematomyelia
- Degenerative: Spondylosis of spine
- Neoplastic secondaries in the spine.

Other causes
Infective
- Spinal epidural abscess
- Brucellosis
- Syphilis

Disorders of vertebra: Craniovertebral anomaly

Intramedullary—syringomyelia

Neoplastic lesions
- Myeloma
- Lymphoma
- Leukemic infiltration
- Primary tumors of the vertebra/cord.

 Note

TB, syphilis can cause adhesive arachnoiditis.

Non-compressive Myelopathy

Causes
- Infectious—viral myelitis, HIV-related causes, HTLV induced.
- Post/parainfectious-postvaccinal myelitis
- Acute transverse myelitis
- ADEM
- *Demyelinating*
  - Multiple sclerosis
  - Neuromyelitis optica
- *Vascular*
  - Anterior spinal artery occlusion
  - AV malformation
  - Dissecting aneurysm of aorta
- *Vasculitis*: TB, syphilis, primary vasculitis.
- Deficiency/toxins—subacute combined degeneration of spinal cord.
- TOCP exposure
- Lathyrism

Degenerative disorders
- MND
- Spinal muscular atrophy
- Hereditary spastic paraplegia

Miscellaneous
- Chronic liver disease
- Paraneoplastic
- Fluorosis

Causes of paraplegia/quadriplegia depending on the part of the spine/spinal cord involved
Cervical
- Spondylosis

- Intervertebral disc prolapse
- Craniovertebral anomaly
- Tumors—primary/secondaries
- Syringomyelia

Thoracic
- TB spine
- Secondaries in the vertebra
- Primary—tumors of cord/vertebra

Lumbosacral
- Spondylosis/disc prolapse
- Epidural abscess
- Primary/secondaries in the vertebra.

Causes of Spastic Paraplegia

- Intracranial causes
- Compressive lesions of spinal cord
- Recovering transverse myelitis
- Recovering anterior spinal artery occlusion
- MND
- Erb's spastic paraplegia
- Tropical spastic paraplegia (HTLV-1 induced)
- Hereditary spastic paraplegia
- Lathyrism and endemic fluorosis

Causes of pure motor paraplegia with only spinal cord involvement
- Motor neuron disease
- Spinal muscular atrophy
- Hereditary spastic paraplegia
- Poliomyelitis
- Rare: Lathyrism
- Erb's/tropical spastic paraplegia

Causes of flaccid paraplegia
- Acute transverse myelitis: Acute phase
- Anterior spinal artery occlusion: State of spinal shock
- Spinal muscular atrophy
- Poliomyelitis
- GB syndrome
- Myopathy/muscular dystrophy
- Peripheral neuropathy.

Approach to Paraplegia

Patient will usually present with weakness of lower limbs.

Elicit following history
Motor weakness
Onset and duration
- Acute
- Subacute
- Chronic

Muscle weakness
- Symmetrical/asymmetrical
- Fluctuating/non-fluctuating
- Proximal/distal
- Painless/painful
- Presence of thinning or enlargement of limb
- Feeling of stiffness of limbs
- Presence of involuntary movement.
- Presence of muscle cramps
- Presence of muscle contracture

Enquire history of sensory disturbance
- Positive symptom—paraesthesia
- Negative symptoms—decrease/loss of sensation.
- Band like sensation around the trunk
- Horizontal level of sensory disturbance.
- Glove and stocking type of sensory disturbance.
- Unilateral loss of sensation
- Root pain, back pain, and funicular pain
- Dissociated sensory loss:
  - Only loss of pain and temperature
  - Only loss of touch
- Difficulty in walking in the dark.

Enquire history of cranial nerve disturbance
- Disturbance of 2nd cranial nerve
- Disturbance of 3rd, 4th and 6th cranial nerves.
- Disturbance of facial nerve.
- Disturbance of lower cranial nerves.
- History of involvement of bowel and bladder
- History of cerebellar disturbance.

Enquire also history of
- Fever at the onset of weakness
- Fever 2–3 weeks before the onset of weakness.
- History of headache, vomiting, convulsions and altered sensorium.
- History of taking medications/vaccinations
- History of cardiac and respiratory symptoms.
- History of hypertension, diabetes mellitus and IHD.

Past history
- Similar episodes before with exacerbations/remissions.
- History of trauma to the back exposure to drugs/toxins

Personal history
- Loss of weight
- Loss of appetite
- Nutritional deficiency
- Smoking, alcohol
- Exposure to commercial sex workers.

Family history
- History of similar illness in the family
- History of parenteral consanguinity.

Approach to a Patient of Paraplegia

Onset and Duration

Acute causes—*see* before
Subacute causes—*see* before
Chronic causes—*see* before

Motor Weakness

Bilaterally symmetrical

Causes
- Peripheral neuropathy
- GB syndrome
- Transverse myelitis
- Myopathies
- MND
- Hereditary disorders of spinal cord/muscle

Asymmetrical weakness (paraplegia)
- Cauda equina lesion
- Compressive myelopathy
- Poliomyelitis

Fluctuating weakness
- Myasthenia gravis
- Eaton-Lambert syndrome
- Periodic paralysis

Proximal > Distal
- GB syndrome
- Myopathies
- Muscular dystrophies
- Polymyositis
- Porphyria
- Diabetic amyotrophy

Distal > Proximal weakness
- Peripheral neuropathy
- Distal type of muscular dystrophy
- Myotonic dystrophy, inclusion body myositis
- MND

Painful muscle weakness
- Polymyositis
- Diabetic amyotrophy
- Osteomalacia

Presence of thinning of limbs
- Disuse atrophy with UMN lesion
- LMN lesion, e.g. cauda/root lesion/peripheral neuropathy
- Anterior horn cell disease
  - MND
  - Spinal muscular atrophy
  - Poliomyelitis

Presence of hypertrophy of limbs
For example, true hypertrophy—work hypertrophy
- Pseudohypertrophy
For example, Duchenne/Becker's muscular dystrophy
- *Occasionally*: In hypothyroidism calf muscle appear bigger: Hoffman's syndrome.
- In myotonia: True hypertrophy of muscle can occur.

Presence of stiffness of limbs

May be indicative of hypertonia

- Suggests pyramidal/extrapyramidal disorder
- Occasionally stiff man's syndrome.

Presence of involuntary movements of limbs-possibilities

- Presence of clonus—pyramidal tract disease.
- Presence of fasciculations:
  - MND
  - Spinal muscular atrophy
  - Poliomyelitis
- Extensor spasms: Pyramidal involvement
- Flexor spasms: Progressive disease of the spinal cord—involvement of pyramidal and extrapyramidal tract: Bad prognosis
- Mass reflex: Severe lesion of spinal cord with autonomic activity.

Presence of contracture: Emery-Dreifuss and Bethlem type of muscular dystrophy presents with early muscular contractures due to shortening of muscle fibers causing stiffening of joints.

Presence of muscle cramps

For example, peripheral neuropathy

- MND
- Electrolytes (hyponatremia)/hypocalcemia
- Rarely Duchenne type of dystrophy.

 Note

Muscle cramps are nor usual in muscle disease except in Duchenne muscular dystrophy.

Sensory disturbance

- Paresthesia and anesthesia
  - Due to peripheral neuropathy
  - Mononeuritis multiplex
  - Subacute combined degeneration
- Band-like sensation around the trunk/limb-posterior column pathology
- Horizontal level of sensory loss
- For example, compressive myelopathy
- Transverse myelitis

- Glove and stocking type of sensory disturbance, e.g. peripheral neuropathy
- Unilateral loss of sensation
- Root involvement
- Brown-Séquard syndrome
- Back pain, root pain, funicular pain—*see later*
- Dissociated anesthesia (pain and temperature loss with preservation of touch)
  - Intramedullary lesion
  - Peripheral neuropathy due to:
    - Hansen's disease
    - Amyloidosis
  - Anterior spinal artery occlusion.

Only loss of touch with pain and temperature intact:

Posterior column involvement:

- Tabes dorsalis
- Subacute combined degeneration
- Posterior spinal artery occlusion
- Large fiber neuropathy

Different types of pain associated with spinal cord disorders

Mechanical

- Aching and continuous localized on the spine, more on movement of spine
- Associated with local tenderness
- No radiation of pain

Pain of spondylosis: Pain on movement of spine.

Pain of infection, inflammation and malignant disorder of vertebra:

- Pain constant
- Severe
- More at night.

 Note

Vertebral pain of thoracic vertebra—consider non-degenerative disorder, e.g. TB spine, malignancy.

2. *Pain of muscle spasm*

- Localized over the muscle
- For example, paravertebral muscle spasm
- Tenderness over the muscle, pain is usually related to movement of muscle/spine.

3. *Funicular pain*
- Type of pain—burning
- Localization—may be diffusely felt in the trunk and extremities
- Fiber involvement—usually crossing fibers of spinothalamic
- Occasionally posterior column
- Lesion—intramedullary

4. *Root pain—as discussed above*

Enquire history suggestive of cranial nerve disturbance with paraplegia

7th nerve involvement—unilateral/bilateral
- GB syndrome
- MND

3rd, 4th and 6th involvement:
- Miller-Fisher variant of GB syndrome
- Diabetic neuropathy

2nd cranial nerve: Retrobulbar neuritis/papillitis
- Multiple sclerosis
- ADEM
- Neuromyelitis optica

Optic atrophy
- B12 deficiency
- Hereditary disorders with spinal cord involvement

Papilledema
- Meningioma—paracentral
- GB syndrome

Cerebellar Symptoms with Paraplegia
- Spinocerebellar degeneration
- Alcoholism
- High cervical cord lesion.

History of bladder and bowel involvement with paraplegia

Involvement of bladder and bowel

Involved
- Cord compressions
- Intramedullary lesion
- Peripheral neuropathy
- Transverse myelitis
- Paracentral lobule lesion

Bladder—not involved
- MND
- Spinal muscular atrophy
- GB syndrome
- Muscle disorders
- Disorders of neuromuscular junction.

History of fever—at the onset of weakness

Infective/parainfectious causes
- Viral myelitis
- Tuberculosis
- Brucellosis
- Spinal epidural abscess
- HIV infection

Systemic illness causing fever
- SLE
- Vasculitis
- Lymphoma, etc.

Fever 2–3 weeks before the onset of weakness
- ADEM
- Neuromyelitis optica
- Guillain-Barré syndrome

History of headache, vomiting, convulsions and altered sensorium
- Acute onset: CVA-ACA occlusion
- Cortical venous thrombosis
- Subacute/chronic—intracranial space occupying lesion
- For example, parasagittal meningioma

History of taking medications/vaccinations
- Taking anti-hypertensives, antidiuretics—suggestive of hypertension.
- Taking oral contraceptives: Risk factor for CVA/CVT.
- Taking anticoagulation: Risk factor for intracranial/spinal bleed
- Taking vaccination (nervous tissue vaccine)
  - Postvaccinal myelitis
- History suggestive of cardiac symptoms and hypertension:
  - Risk factor for CVA
  - Risk factor for ACA occlusion
  - Dissecting aneurysm of aorta

History of respiratory symptoms

Spinal cord involvement with respiratory disease

- Tuberculosis
- Bronchogenic carcinoma with secondary deposits
- Retroviral illness.

History of hypertension, diabetes mellitus and IHD-Risk factor for CVA

Past History

Similar episode with exacerbations and remissions

- Multiple sclerosis
- CIDP
- Myasthenia
- Periodic paralysis
- TIA of ACA territory

Previous history of trauma to the spine/spinal cord

- Vertebral pathology
- Post-traumatic syringomyelia

Exposure to drugs toxins

- Alcohol
- TOCP
- Lathyrism
- Fluorosis
- Drugs causing peripheral neuropathy

Personal History

- Weight loss ⎫
- Loss of appetite ⎬ systemic disease
- Nutritional history for B12 deficiency
- Smoking—risk factor for CVA, TB/malignancy
- Alcohol
  - Peripheral neuropathy
  - Myopathy
  - B12 deficiency
  - Hepatic involvement with myelopathy

Exposure to commercial sex workers

- For syphilis ⎫ involving spinal/cord
- HIV infection ⎭

Family History

- Similar illness in the family
  - Acute—viral illness
  - Chronic: Hereditary/degenerative disorder of spinal cord.

DIFFERENTIAL DIAGNOSIS OF PARAPLEGIA

Acute Paraplegia

Historical Approach

Intracranial pathology

- History of headache, vomiting, altered sensorium with lower limb involvement with hypertension and diabetes mellitus: Acute CVA—involving anterior cerebral artery.
- History of puerperium, volume depletion, fever, convulsions, paraplegia.
  - Suspect—cortical venous sinus thrombosis.

Acute Paraplegia

Extracranial Pathology

- Weakness of lower limbs, sensory loss of all modalities below a level with bladder involvement: Acute transverse myelitis.
- Sudden onset of weakness of lower limbs with no involvement of posterior column with history of hypertension, diabetes mellitus, cardiac disease: Anterior spinal artery occlusion.
- History of trauma to the back: Suspect vertebral/disc lesion.
- History of lifting heavyweight, back pain, root pain: Intervertebral disc prolapse.
- History of acute onset of pain in the back, fever with paraplegia: Spinal epidural abscess.
- History of infective episode 2–3 weeks before and then developed motor weakness of lower limbs with ascending paralysis without bladder/sensory involvement: Guillain-Barré syndrome (AIDP).
- History of fever, rash, altered sensorium, convulsions, bilateral 2nd nerve involvement symmetrical weakness, paraplegia: Acute demyelinating encephalomyelitis.

- History of multiple sites of lesions, retrobulbar neuritis, suspect multiple sclerosis.
- History of weakness of lower limbs, 2nd nerve involvement—bilateral—possible neuromyelitis optica.

Subacute and Chronic Paraplegia

- Slowly progressive weakness of lower limbs, back pain, root pain, bladder involvement and sensory involved—compressive pathology of the spinal cord: TB, tumor, trauma/disc prolapse.
- If presence of fever with above features: TB/brucellosis
- If severe weight loss: Suspect malignancy, HIV infection or tuberculosis
- Back pain, root pain: Degenerative spine disease.
- Slowly progressive weakness of lower limb, dissociated anesthesia may be with small muscle wasting of upper limb:
  - Intramedullary lesion
  - Syringomyelia.
- Glove and stocking type of sensory loss, bilateral symmetrical involvement, lower limb involvement more than upper limb: Peripheral neuropathy.
- History of memory loss, lower limb weakness along with peripheral neuropathy: Subacute combined degeneration of spinal cord.
- Slowly progressive weakness of lower limb, wasting, fasciculations, no sensory or bladder involvement
  - Motor neuron disease
  - Poliomyelitis
  - Spinal muscular atrophy
- Progressive weakness of lower limbs, positive family history, involvement of cerebellum, peripheral nerves, higher mental functions, cardiac involvement.
  - Spinocerebellar degeneration
- Progressive weakness of lower limb, stiffness of lower limbs, positive family history: Hereditary spastic paraplegia.

- Progressive weakness of lower limbs, proximal muscle weakness, no bladder/ or sensory involvement—suspect muscle disorder.
- Younger age, positive family history—muscular dystrophy.
- Proximal weakness, painful weakness, pharyngeal involvement: Polymyositis.

Neurocutaneous markers associated with paraplegia
- Short neck
- Low hairline
- Kyphoscoliosis
- Gibbus over the spine
- Tuft of hair/dimpling over the lower spine
- Pes cavus
  - Café-au-lait spot/neurofibromatosis
  - Bruit over the spine

Significance of neurocutaneous markers
- Short neck
- Low hair line } Craniovertebral anomaly
- Kyphoscoliosis: Spinocerebellar degeneration, synringomyelia.
- Gibbus over the spine: TB spine/post-traumatic
- Tuft of hair/dimpling over the spine: Spina bifida occulta with meningomyelocoele.
- *Pes cavus*
  - Spinocerebellar degenerations
  - Syringomyelia
- Neurofibromatosis/café-au-lait spot: Intradural compression by neurofibroma.
- Bruit over the spine: AV malformation.
- Specific general examination features associated with peripheral neuropathy (*see* under peripheral neuropathy)

Systemic Examination in a Patient of Paraplegia

Higher Mental Functions

Altered higher mental functions with paraplegia
- Intra-cranial causes
- CVA, cortical venous thrombosis, mass lesion in the paracentral region, ADEM

Other causes
- B12 deficiency
- HIV infection
- Trauma to the head and spine

Cranial nerve involvement with paraplegia
- 2nd cranial nerve
- 3rd, 4th and 6th cranial nerves ⎫
- 7th cranial nerves ⎬ *see* under history
- Lower cranial nerves ⎭

Motor system: Nutrition—look for wasting—LMN lesion.

Atrophy of distal part of limbs—inverted champagne bottle appearance—peroneal muscular atrophy.

Hypertrophy—pseudohypertrophy—muscular dystrophy.
Proximal thigh/quadriceps wasting—diabetic amyotropy.

Tone-spasticity
- UMN lesions—*see* under spastic paraplegia.

- Rigidity—less common—mainly in extra-pyramidal disorder
- Hypotonia—*see* flaccid paraplegia.

Power—grade the power—look for muscle power at different groups of muscles.

Important groups of muscles which decide the level of lesion in a paraplegic
- For example, upper abdominal weakness (T6–T9)
- Positive Beevor's sign—T10
- Lower abdominal weakness (T11–T12)
- Hip muscle weakness (L1, L2)
- Quadriceps weakness (L3)
- Foot drop: L5–S1
- Hamstring weakness (L5, S1 and S2)
- Plantar flexion weakness: S1 and S2

Coordination
- Incoordination—if present in the lower limb—judge whether it is proportional to the weakness.
- If disproportionate—possible associated cerebellar pathology.

Table 4.6: Different groups of muscles and their nerve supply which are involved in a patient of paraplegia

Muscle group	Muscle involved	Root involved
Hip		
Flexors	Iliopsoas, pectineus	L1 and L2
Abductors	Gluteus medius	L4, L5 and S1
	Gluteus minimus	
Adductors	3 Adductors: Longus	
	Magnus	
	Brevis	L2, L3 and L4
	Obturator	
	Gracilis	
Extensors	Gluteus maximus	L5 and S1
Knee:		
Flexors	Hamstrings	L5, S1 and S2
Extensors	Quadriceps	L2, L3 and L4
Foot:		
Dorsiflexion	Tibialis anterior	L4 and L5
Plantar flexion	Gastrocnemius and soleus	S1 and S2
Eversion	Peroneus longus and brevis	L5 and S1
Inversion	Tibialis posterior	L4 and L5
	Tibialis anterior	L4 and L5

- Involuntary movements—*see* under history taking.

Sensory examination
- Look for level of sensory loss
- At nipple level—lesion at T4 spinal cord segment
- At umbilical level—at T10 level
- At medial part of thigh—L1 level
- Over the patella—L3
- Dorsum of foot—L5
- Saddle area—S3, S4 and S5

Look for types of sensory loss
- Posterior column sensation—posterior cord pathology
- Spinothalamic sensation—intramedullary lesion
- Glove and stocking type: Peripheral neuropathy

Reflexes
- Superficial: Upper abdominal reflex—T6–T9
- Lower abdominal reflexes—T10 to T12
- Cremasteric—at L1 level.
- Plantar—S1 level
- Deep reflexes—knee jerk lost—L2, 3 level
- Ankle jerk lost—L5, S1 level.
- Bilateral extensor plantar: Bilateral pyramid tract involvement.
- Knee jerk and ankle jerk—exaggerated—bilateral pyramidal involvement.

Knee jerk: Brisk with ankle jerk lost and extensor plantar
Possibilities
- Subacute combined degeneration of spinal cord
- Friedreich's ataxia
- Taboparesis
- Paraneoplastic syndrome
- Conus medullaris + cauda equina lesion
- Ankle jerk loss—can also occur in peripheral neuropathy.

All reflexes are lost below a certain level
- LMN paraplegia
- Stage of spinal shock

Check—anal sphincter tone
- Loss of anal sphincter tone:
  - Lesion—S2, S3 and S4
  - Look for bulbocavernous reflex
  - If lost lesion: S2, S3 and S4
- Cerebellar signs
- Cerebellar involvement with paraplegia
- Possible spinocerebellar degeneration
- Alcohol induced
- Paraneoplastic
- Drug—phenytoin
- Phenytoin—causes peripheral neuropathy with cerebellar involvement.

Look for bowel and bladder involvement (look for bladder catheterization)

Examination—for spine
- Movement
- Tenderness
- Gibbus
- Paraspinal muscle spasm
- Bruit over the spine
- SLR for sciatic nerve compression
- Also look for: Decubitus ulcer
- Pressure palsy-L5–S1 → causes foot drop

Other system examination
- CVS
- RS } For evidence of systemic illness
- PA
- CVS: Hypertensive heart disease, IHD, valvular heart disease, atrial fibrillation
- RS: For evidence of TB, pneumonia and malignancy
- GIT examination: For systemic illness:
- Hepatosplenomegaly
- Lymphadenopathy
- Ascites

Approach to Quadriplegia

Quadriplegia is the term used to describe paralysis of all 4 limbs
Cause: Acute 24–48 hours
Intracranial
- Vertebral basilar CVA/TIA

- Bilateral CVA involving internal capsule—rare
- Brainstem lesion: Midbrain/pons

Extracranial causes
- Vascular: Vertebrobasilar insufficiency
- Anterior spinal artery occlusion
- Vasculitis
- AV malformation—bleed

Trauma
- Cervical cord/spine injury
- Cervical disc herniation

Demyelination
- Acute transverse myelitis
- ADEM
- Multiple sclerosis
- Neuromyelitis optica
- GB syndrome
- Metabolic: Hypo or hyperkalemic periodic paralysis
- Toxic: Neurotoxic bite

Subacute:
- Craniovertebral anomaly
- Syringomyelia
- Spondylotic myelopathy
- Tumors of the cervical spine or spinal cord
  - Primary
  - Secondary

Chronic
Chronic compression of the cervical cord
- CV anomaly
- Spondylosis
- Tumors

Deficiency: B12 ↓ subacute combined degeneration of spinal cord

Disorders of anterior horn cell
- MND
- Spinal muscular atrophy

Disorders of root/nerve
- Peripheral neuropathy
- CIDP

Disorders of muscle/myoneural junction
- Myopathies
- Muscular dystrophy

- Polymyositis
- Myasthenia gravis
- Eaton-Lambert syndrome

Toxins:
- Lathyrism
- Alcohol

Demyelinating: Multiple sclerosis.

Episodic Quadriparesis
- Periodic paralysis
- Myasthenia gravis
- Eaton-Lambert syndrome

Spastic Quadriparesis
- Bilateral supratentorial CVA (multi-infarct)
- Pontine lesion: Infarct/glioma
- Cervical cord compression
- Acute transverse myelitis at cervical level—after the stage of neuronal shock
- Anterior spinal artery occlusion after the stage of neuronal shock
- Multiple sclerosis
- Amyotrophic lateral sclerosis
- Lathyrism

Flaccid Quadriparesis
- Acute transverse myelitis
- Acute anterior spinal artery occlusion
- Progressive muscular atrophy
- Spinal muscular atrophy
- GB syndrome
- Peripheral neuropathy

Approach to a Patient of Quadriplegia
Patient presents with weakness of all 4 limbs.

History Elicitation
Motor symptoms
Similar to paraplegia with following additional features:
- Patient can present with small muscle wasting of upper limbs.
- Patient can have symptoms starting in one upper limb and then weakness of same side lower limb, opposite side lower limb

and opposite side upper limb in a U-shaped manner, called Elsberg phenomenon.
- Patient can have fluctuating weakness—causing quadriparesis.

History of Sensory Disturbance

Elicit in the similar way as of paraplegia with following extra features:
- Patient can present with neck pain and root pain radiating to upper limb.
- Person can complain of restricted neck movement.
- Person can have symptoms of vertebra basilar TIA:
  - Either due to craniovertebral anomaly
  - Cervical spondylosis.
- High cervical cord lesion can present with sensory loss over upper part of face.
- Patient can have Lhermitte's symptoms.
- Patient also can c/o occipital pain and sensory disturbance in high cervical cord lesion.
- Sacral sparing occurs in intramedullary lesion of cervical cord.

Cerebellar Involvement

- High cervical cord lesions, craniovertebral anomaly and vertebra basilar ischemia can cause quadriplegia with cerebellar involvement.
- Spinocerebellar degenerations can cause limb weakness with ataxia.

Bladder and Bowel Involvement

Quadriplegia: Intramedullary cervical cord lesion—early bladder involvement except syringomyelia—bladder late involved as it causes splitting of bladder fibers rather than dysfunction of them till late.

Following symptoms/history is not relevant to quadriplegia
- Cortical venous thrombosis—usually does not cause quadriplegia.
- Dissecting aneurysm of aorta—not cause of quadriplegia.

- Tuberculosis causing involvement of cervical cord—not common.

History of cranial nerve disturbance in a patient of quadriplegia
7th cranial nerve palsy
- Bilateral UMN 7th nerve palsy can occur due to: Multiple infarct causing bilateral UMN involvement of upper and lower limbs.
- Bilateral LMN 7th nerve palsy can occur in a patient with Guillain-Barré syndrome/ MND.
- Sensory loss over the upper part of the face: Due to involvement of descending tract of trigeminal nerve.
- Brainstem lesion/VBI: Can cause lower cranial nerve involvement.
- High cervical cord pathology: Can cause 9th, 10th, 11th and 12th cranial nerve involvement.
- Upper cervical cord lesion: Can cause Horner's syndrome.
- 2nd cranial nerve—same significance as under paraplegia except that papilledema— due to paracentral meningioma (causes paraplegia rather than quadriplegia).
- History of fever—same as for paraplegia
- History of headache, vomiting, convulsions— may not be relevant except bilateral pyramidal involvement.
- History of cardiac, respiratory symptoms, HT, DM and IHD—similar to paraplegia history of symptoms of brainstem involvement for vertebra basilar CVA.
- History of medications, vaccination: Same as paraplegia
- Past history: Same as paraplegia
- Enquire history of carotid or vertebrobasilar TIA in the past for multiple infarct/ brainstem CVA
- Rarely CV anomaly can present as vertebrobasilar TIA
- Family and personal history same as paraplegia.

General Physical Examination

- Same as paraplegia
- Vital signs: Same as paraplegia
- Neurocutaneous markers: Same as paraplegia

Higher Mental Functions

- Same as paraplegia
- Can have evidence of multi-infarct with pseudobulbar palsy type of features.

Cranial Nerve Involvement

- Same as paraplegia
- Sensory loss over the upper part of face-descending tract of Vth nerve involvement in higher cervical cord lesions.
- Bilateral Horner's in pontine lesions
- Bilateral UMN 7th in bilateral hemiplegia
- Lower cranial nerves: High cervical cord lesions.

Motor System

- Nutrition: Same as paraplegia.
- Wasting can occur in specific groups of muscle depending on the involvement of roots:
  - Deltoid wasting
  - Wasting of shoulder girdle
  - Wasting of small muscles of hand
  - Wasting of distal forearm: Peroneal muscular atrophy (inverted champagne bottle appearance)
  - Presence of clawhand
- Popeye effect: *See* under muscle disorder
- Sometimes pseudohypertrophy can be made out in infraspinatus, deltoid in patients of muscular dystrophies.
- Tone: Same as for paraplegia.
- Power: Grade the power
- Look for muscle power:
  - At shoulder
  - At elbow
  - At wrist
  - Small muscles of hand

- Lower limb groups of muscles
- Coordination: Same as paraplegia
- Involuntary movement: Same as paraplegia.

 Note

In syringomyelia observe for fasciculations of small muscles of hands MND and spinal muscular atrophy can have fasciculations of upper limb and trunk.

Sensory Examination

- Look for level of sensory loss starting from C_2
- High cervical cord lesions: Can have sensory loss of upper part of face.
- Syryngomyelia can have café/half café/suspended jacket type of sensory loss over the trunk.
- Sacral sparing of sensation occurs in intra-medullary cervical cord lesion.

Reflexes

- Abdominal, cremasteric reflexes are lost in UMN quadriplegia.
- Plantar bilaterally extensor in UMN quadriplegia.

Deep reflexes

- All deep reflexes are exaggerated above the level of C5 lesion.
- At C5 lesion: Biceps jerk is lost
  - Inverted supinator jerk is present
  - Triceps jerk becomes exaggerated
- At C6, C7 lesion: Triceps jerk is lost
- At C8 T1 lesion—small muscle wasting will be present
- Jaw jerk—brisk: If bilateral cortical lesion with lesion of internal capsule or above.
- Primitive reflexes become elicitable if bilateral corticospinal lesions with diffuse cortical involvement.

Cerebellar Involvement in a Quadriplegic

- Higher cervical cord lesion
- Spinocerebellar lesions
- *See* under paraplegia

Bowel and bladder lesions
- Early—intramedullary lesions
- Late—extrmedullary lesions
- Bladder—not involved—*see* under paraplegia.
- Examination of cervical spine:
  - For movements
  - Tenderness
- Other system examination—as for paraplegia.

Features of Different Levels of Cervical Cord Involvement

Lesion at foramen magnum
- Downbeat nystagmus
- Quadriplegia
- Occasionally cruciate hemiplegia
- Mirror movement.

High cervical cord/craniovertebral anomaly
- Low hair line
- Short neck
- Limitation of neck movements
- Quadriplegia
- Lower cranial nerve/cerebellar involvement

Other features of high cervical cord involvement
- Involvement of descending tract of Vth nerve.
- Horner's syndrome
- Can have diaphragm involvement

Cervical canal stenosis
- Sagittal diameter of the cervical canal inside the vertebra is less than 11 mm.
- Presents as cervical myelopathy.

 Note

Even if the lesion is higher up—in the cervical cord—C8 T1 can be involved because of venous stasis.

Whiplash injury
- Due to sudden movement of neck
- No actual trauma to the cord
- Damage to soft tissues
- Muscle and ligaments are stretched

- Sudden movement of head and neck—moves backwards and then forwards.
- Whiplash injury is usually transient with minimal pain. Rarely it can cause chronic pain or headache.

Key Points to Remember in Cervical Cord Lesion
- Downbeat nystagmus is a feature with C2 sensory loss: Lesion of foramen magnum
- Cruciate hemiplegia occurs in lesions of cervicomeduallary junction.
- Inverted supinator jerk with loss of biceps—C5, C6 lesion.
- C7 lesion is associated with loss of triceps jerk, intact biceps, exaggerated finger flexion reflex.
- Wasting of small muscles of hand occur in lesions of C8 T1 with or without Horner's syndrome.

 Note

Other features of cervical cord lesions: Discussed above.

Causes of Stroke in Young
Occurrence of CVA below the age of 45 years.
Occurrence of CVA at a younger age (pediatric age group):
- Cerebral venous thrombosis
- Congenital heart disease—due to embolization
- Polycythemia
- Infective endocarditis
- Younger adults: Cardiac embolization
  - AF due to RHD
  - Infective endocarditis
  - Left atrial myxoma.

Vasculitis
- Infective: Tuberculosis, syphilis, retroviral infection (endarteritis obliterans)
- Primary vasculitis: Primary vasculitis (including aortoarteritis)
- Connective tissue disorder, e.g. SLE

- Bleeding/clotting disorders:
  - Purpura—ITP
  - Disorders of coagulation—hemophilia.
- Procoagulant state—protein C and S deficiency
- Factor V Leiden deficiency
- APLA syndrome
- Other causes: Trauma
- Bleeding into intracranial tumors
- Intracranial space occupying lesions.
- Hematological disorder—sickle cell disease.

CSF EXAMINATION

Secretion and Circulation of CSF

- CSF is the ultra filtrate of the blood and it is the fluid present in the nervous system including brain and spinal cord.
- CSF is secreted from the choroid plexus of the ventricles.
- CSF also plays a role in the autoregulation of cerebral blood flow.
- It is present in the subarachnoid space surrounding the brain and spinal cord. It is present in the ventricles and central canal of the spinal cord.
- CSF is continuous with the perilymph of the bony labyrinth.

Circulation of CSF

- It is present in the two lateral ventricles.
- From lateral ventricles it reaches the 3rd ventricle.
- From the 3rd ventricles it reaches the 4th ventricle through aqueduct of Sylvius.
- From the 4th ventricles it reaches the subarachnoid space and also the central canal of spinal cord.

Normal CSF Pressure

- Opening pressure: 180 mm of CSF.
- Borderline CSF pressure increase: 180–200 mm CSF
- Abnormal CSF pressure increase: More than 200 mm CSF.

CSF Analysis

Color of CSF

- Normal CSF is crystal clear
- CSF cloudy—more number of cells
- Smoky CSF—presence of RBCs
- Blood in CSF-centrifuge the CSF—supernatant fluid becomes xanthochromic (yellowish).
- Xanthochromic CSF occurs due to—hemorrhage into the CSF
  - Presence of jaundice
  - High CSF protein occurs due to: Meningitis/encephalitis
- Very high CSF protein occurs due to:
  - Below spinal block (Froin's syndrome)
  - Guillain-Barré syndrome
  - Vicinity of neurofibroma
  - Tuberculosis or fungal infection
  - Meningeal carcinamatosis
- Clotting of CSF occurs due to:
  - Blood in the CSF
- High protein content of CSF—cobweb formation
- For example, tuberculosis.

Key Points about CSF Pleocytosis

- Very high CSF neutrophils (in thousands) can occur in bacterial, parasitic meningitis and cerebral hemorrhage.
- Lymphocyte predominant CSF (in hundreds) can occur in viral, tuberculosis or ADEM.
- Neutrophil predominant CSF (in hundreds) occur in chronic meningitis, metastasis.
- Early tuberculous meningitis can have neutrophil dominant CSF but less than 500 cells/cmm.

Neurofibromatosis

Type I: von Recklinghausen's disease.

Features
- Peripheral and spinal neurofibromas
- Optic gliomas
- Lisch nodules

- Café-au-lait macules
- Scoliosis and short stature
- Pheochromocytoma and other endocrine abnormalities

Type 2
- Bilateral acoustic neuromas
- Café-au-lait macules
- No endocrine abnormality

CENTRAL NERVOUS SYSTEM

Differential Diagnosis

- Sudden onset of neurological deficit, pertaining to a vascular territory with occasional recovery—consider CVA.
- Patient is a hypertensive, diabetes mellitus and IHD with past history of TIA with neurological deficit—consider
  - CVA (ischemic stroke)
  - Multi-infarct state
  - Lacunar stroke
- History of fever, convulsions, headache and neurological deficit—consider:
  - Meningitis
  - Meningoencephalitis
  - Cortical venous thrombosis
- History of severe headache, vomiting, convulsions, altered sensorium and a known hypertensive—consider hypertensive intracerebral hemorrhage.
- History of severe headache, neck pain, altered sensorium and after 48 hours developing neurological deficit (due to vasospasm)—consider subarachnoid hemorrhage.
- History of trauma to the head with altered sensorium and neurological deficit—consider traumatic intracranial hemorrhage like subdural/extradural hematoma.
- If there is history of fever, weight loss and neurological deficit:
  Consider vasculitis
  - Like infective: Tuberculosis/syphilis.
  - HIV related disorders
  - Noninfective primary/secondary vasculitis

- If there is history of neurological deficit with proceeding fever 2–3 weeks before: Postinfective/parainfectious demyelination, e.g. ADEM
- If history of weakness of limbs, no sensory loss, no bladder involvement with preceding diarrhea, consider AIDP.
- If there is history of exacerbations and remissions of neurological deficit:
- Consider demyelination, e.g. multiple sclerosis.
- If there is history of headache, projectile vomiting, convulsions with neurological deficit:
- Possible intracranial space occupying lesion
  - Infective like tuberculoma/cerebral abscess
  - Neoplastic lesions
- If there is LMN cranial nerve palsy on one side with limb involvement on the opposite side crossed hemiparesis—brainstem pathology.
- If there is history of weakness on one side associated with swaying with symptoms of incoordination on the affected side—consider ataxic hemiparesis.
- If there is history of dysphagia, dysarthria and cerebellar symptoms and lower cranial nerve symptoms: Posterior fossa/brainstem pathology.
- If there is history of swaying to one side or both sides—does not alter with closure of eyes—consider cerebellar dysfunction.

 Note

Vertigo is a symptoms of labyrinthine dysfunction and is not a symptom of cerebellar pathology.

Gradual onset of neurological deficit week to months
Consider
- Intracranial space occupying lesion
- Compressive pathology
- Sequelae of previous trauma

- If there is chronic progressive neurological deficit. No improvement, bilateral involvement, particular part of nervous system involvement with positive family history, consider: Degenerative disorder.
- If there is bilateral symptoms (sensory/motor) distal > proximal, lower limb more involved than upper limb: Consider peripheral neuropathy.
- If there is fluctuating neurological deficit with muscle fatigue and ptosis, consider disorder of neuromuscular junction disorder/periodic paralysis.
- If there is history of slowness of movement with tremors:
  - Possible parkinsonism: If unilateral onset—idiopathic parkinsonism.
  - Bilateral symptoms and signs. Possible arteriosclerotic parkinsonism.
- If there is history of frequent fall, difficulty in walking, consider following disorders
  - Progressive supranuclear palsy
  - Normal pressure hydrocephalus
  - Multi-infarct state
  - If there is associated with vertigo: Consider labyrinthine disorder.
  - If swaying one/both sides: Cerebellar dysfunction.

Hematology

APPROACH TO A PATIENT OF ANEMIC DISORDER

Symptoms and Signs Analysis of a Patient of Anemia

- History of decreased food intake, malabsorption, poor nutrition suggests nutritional deficiency.
- Evidence of blood loss, worm infestation, taking drugs like aspirin, NSAIDs, corticosteroids—leading to blood loss—suggestive of iron deficiency anemia along with koilonychia and platynychia.
- History of anemia, strict vegetarians, peripheral neuropathy, knuckle pigmentation, ileal disease—consider megaloblastic anemia—due to folic acid/B12 deficiency.
- History of anemia since childhood, jaundice since childhood, recurrent blood transfusions, jaundice, splenomegaly along with positive family history—consider congenital hemolytic anemia/hemoglobinopathies.
- History of anemia, bleeding tendency, recurrent infection, recurrent blood transfusions, no hepatosplenomegaly—consider primary aplastic anemia. Enquire history of radiation, chemical/drug exposure.
- History of anemia, bony pain, bleeding tendencies, evidence of infection, hepatosplenomegaly, lymphadenopathy—consider hematological malignancy—leukemia, lymphoma/paraproteinemia.

- History of anemia, splenomegaly, middle-aged adult, evidence of hemolysis—possible autoimmune hemolytic anemia.
- History of anemia, splenomegaly, hemolysis and tendency to clot along with pancytopenia—consider paroxysmal hemoglobinuria.
- Prolonged anemia, evidence of chronic systemic disease—consider anemia of chronic disease.
- Recurrent bleeding tendency since childhood, positive family history—consider bleeding or a clotting disorder.

Approach to a Patient of Hemolytic Anemia

Evidence of Congenital Hemolytic Anemia

Clinical

- Anemia
- Mild icterus
- Splenomegaly
- History of anemia, jaundice since childhood with hepatosplenomegaly, recurrent gallstones—consider hereditary spherocytosis.
- History of anemia since childhood, jaundice, recurrent infarction crisis, spleen not palpable—consider sickle cell disease.
- History of severe anemia since childhood, splenomegaly, survival not possible without transfusion/bone marrow transplantation—consider thalassemia major.

- Mild anemia, splenomegaly, transfusion not required, behaving like iron deficiency but not responding to iron—consider thalassemia minor.

Approach to a Patient of Suspected Hematological Malignancy

- Younger age/children—bony pain, infection, bleeding tendency, hepatosplenomegaly, bone tenderness, generalized lymphadenopathy—consider acute lymphoblastic leukemia.
- Adult onset to later ages, anemia, bony pain, bleeding (gum bleed) may also be present—can develop DIC and hepatosplenomegaly—possible—acute myeloid leukemia.
- 4th to 5th decade of life, pallor, massive splenomegaly—rule out CML.
- Elderly age, anemia, hepatosplenomegaly, lymphadenopathy of prolonged duration—consider CLL.
- Bimodal age of presentation, fever, weight loss, night sweats, rubbery lymph nodes (usually cervical) hepatosplenomegaly—consider Hodgkin's lymphoma.
- Middle age to elderly—hepatosplenomegaly, systemic involvement, B symptoms may not be present (common with HIV+ve status)—consider non-Hodgkin's lymphoma.
- Middle aged to elderly—bony pain, bone tenderness, pathological fractures—severe anemia—consider paraproteinemia.

 Note

Hepatosplenomegaly is usually not associated with multiple myeloma. Organomegaly is more a feature of Waldenstrom's macroglobulinemia.

Investigational Approach to an Anemic Disorder

Complete blood picture
- Hb%—to assess severity of anemia
- WBC count = very high—consider, leukemia/leukemoid reaction.

- Platelet count—very low may be suggestive of
  - Thrombocytopenic disorder
  - Part of pancytopenia
  - Part of DIC
  - Part of leukemia.
- Platelet count very high—suggestive of internal bleeding/may also suggest myeloproliferative disorder.
- If pancytopenia: Consider the following conditions:
  - B12/folic acid deficiency
  - Primary aplastic anemia
  - Aleukemic leukemia
  - PNH
  - Hypersplenism.

Peripheral smear
- Microcytic hypochromic: *See* later.
- Macrocytic: Hypersegmented neutrophils: Megaloblastic anemia
- Target cells: Thalassemia
- Spherocytes: Hereditary spherocytosis
- Sickle cells: Sickle cell anemia.
- Micro spherocytes—autoimmune hemolysis
- Abnormal cells: Hematological malignancy
- Pancytopenia: *See* above
- Anisopoikilocytosis—suggestive of possible hemolysis
- Tear drop cells: Possible myelofibrosis
- Leucoerythroblastic picture: Marrow irritation/myelofibrosis.

Evidence of hemolysis
- ↑Reticulocyte count—decreased haptoglobin and hemopexin
- Increased LDH
- If evidence of hemolysis is associated with:
  - Microcytic hypochromic anemia
  - Presence of target cells
  - Hb electrophoresis:
    - HbF pattern possible thalassemia major
    - HbA_2 pattern possible thalassemia minor.

- If presence of spherocytes with osmotic fragility is increased, consider hereditary spherocytosis.
- If peripheral smear shows the presence of sickle cells and Hb electrophoresis is HbS, consider sickle cell anemia.
- If presence of microspherocytes in the peripheral smear and Coombs test positive—autoimmune hemolysis.

Differential Diagnosis of Hematological Malignancy Disorders

- If peripheral smear—abnormal cells and
- Lymphoblast present—? ALL
- Myeloblasts present—? AML

No blasts in the peripheral smear

Very high WBC count, peripheral smear shows myelocytes and metamyelocytes. Low leukocyte alkaline phosphatase score cytogenetics reveals BCR, ABL positive—possible CML

- No blasts in the peripheral smear, very high WBC count with abnormal lymphocytes—possible CLL.
- Anemia, high ESR, blood counts may be normal, lymph node biopsy showing: Reed-Sternberg cell—Hodgkin's lymphoma (surface markers showing CD15, CD30).
- Anemia, very high ESR—abnormal lymphocyte infiltration into organs—NHL.
- Anemia, ↑ ESR, ↑ serum calcium, urine light chains present, serum protein electrophoresis showing M band—suggest myeloma.

Approach to a Patient of Anemia

Different Hematological Findings in Anemia

Microcytic anemia: Smaller RBCs (MCV <80 femtoliters (fl))

Causes

- Iron deficiency
- Sideroblastic anemia
- Thalassemia

- Lead poisoning
- Occasionally anemia of chronic disease.

Macrocytosis

- Larger RBCs (MCV > 100 fl)
- Size of the RBC is more than a small lymphocyte.

Causes

- Vitamin B12 and folic acid deficiency (MCV > 110 fl)
- Hypothyroidism
- Alcoholism
- Zidovudine therapy
- Chronic liver disease.

Normocytic Anemia

Causes

- Anemia of chronic disease
- Aplastic anemia
- Endocrine disorders
- Hemolytic anemia
- Drugs and toxin related
- Acute massive bleed

Disorders of RBCs

Normal RBC count

- Male: 4.5 to 5.5 million/cmm
- Female: 4–4.5 million/cmm

Normal Hb level

- Men: 16–18 gm/dl
- Women: Menstruating: 13–15 gm/dl
- Non-menstruating; 14–16 gm/dl.
- Normal RBC life span—around 120 days.

RBC indices

- Mean corpuscular volume (MCV) 90 ± 8 fl (90–100 fl)
- Mean corpuscular hemoglobin (MCH) 30 ± 3 pg
- Mean corpuscular hemoglobin concentration (MCHC) 38 ± 2 gm/dl
- Red cell distribution width 7.5 micrometer
- Reticulocyte count = 1–2%
- Anisocytosis—variation in the size of RBCs.
- Poikilocytosis—variation in the shape of RBCs.

Reticulocyte Count

- Normal reticulocyte count 1–2%
- Stain used—supravital dye
- Signifies: Recent RBCs that are released from the marrow
- If the reticulocyte count is less than 2–3 times the normal in an anemic patient—indicates insufficient response of the marrow.
- Corrected reticulocyte count:
  - Estimates marrow response to anemia
  - Corrected reticulocyte count: Patient's reticulocyte count × patient's Hb%/ normal Hb%.

Polychromasia

- Represents reticulocytes that are early released from the bone marrow.
- Color of the cell is due to staining of their remaining ribosomal RNA.
- These cells are larger than normal RBCs and with Giemsa stain, they stain—grayish blue.
- Significance of polychromasia:
  - Excessive stimulation of the marrow by erythropoietin
  - Bone marrow damage by malignant infiltration or marrow fibrosis.

Dimorphic picture: Combined appearance of micro and macrocytes, e.g. iron and folic acid/vit B12 ↓.

Schistocytes—RBCs are fragmented
- For example, microangiopathic hemolytic anemia/intravascular hemolysis
- Conditions associated: Sepsis syndrome.

Howell-Jolly bodies
- Found in patients with splenectomy/non-functional spleen.
- They are the nuclear remnants of RBCs which are not removed by the spleen.

Heinz body
- RBCs containing precipitating hemoglobin.
- For example, oxidative stress/unstable hemoglobin.

Target cells/Mexican hat cells
- Found in patients with
  - Thalassemia
  - Liver disease
- They are the dark centered RBCs with a rim of pallor surrounding the dark center with another outer rim of darker ring.

Tear drop cells
- Tear drop appearance of RBCs
- Found in patients with myelofibrosis

Acanthocytes (spur cells)
- RBCs containing projections which are irregularly placed.
- For example, abetalipoproteinemia.

Echinocytes (Burr cells): RBCs containing projections which are regularly placed, e.g. uremia.

Spherocytes: RBCs loose their central pallor and darkly stained found in hereditary spherocytosis, auto-immune hemolysis (micro spherocytosis).

Pappenheimer bodies: For example, RBCs containing iron granules. Found in hemolytic anemia, sickle cell anemia and sideroblastic anemia.

Sideroblasts: Nucleated erythroblasts with mitochondria with granules of iron surrounding the nucleus.

Basophilic Stippling (Punctate Basophilia)

Cytoplasm of the RBCs contain basophilic granules which can be demonstrated to be RNA, e.g. lead toxicity.

Leucoerythroblastic picture: Presence of nucleated RBCs and WBCs. Indicate marrow irritation, e.g. myelofibrosis.

Approach to a Patient of Anemia
Clinical Aspects of Anemia

General aspects of anemia: Symptoms and signs of anemia depending on the rapidity of its development:
- Blood loss up to 500 ml is well tolerated.
- Significant blood loss of about 1 liter—patient will develop palpitation and dizziness due to postural hypotension.

- Massive hemorrhage of more than 2 liters— person will develop hypovolemic shock.

Definition of anemia: Male: Hb% < 13 gm/dl, female: Hb% <12 gm/dl.

Iron Deficiency Anemia

Normal daily requirement of iron
- Adult male: 8 mg/day
- Menstruating female: 16 mg/day
- In pregnancy: Requirement increases by 4–6 mg/day.

Suspect iron deficiency anemia in the following circumstances
- History of blood loss including hookworm disease.
- Conditions associated with increased requirement of iron-like adolescence and pregnancy and excessive menstrual blood loss.
- Adult developing iron deficiency—always rule out blood loss from GIT.
- Conditions associated with chronic inflammatory conditions and malabsorption.
- Easy fatigability, pica, pallor, angular stomatitis, platynychia and koilonychias are the usual features of iron deficiency.
- Severe iron deficiency can result in Plummer-Vinson syndrome (with postcricoid web).

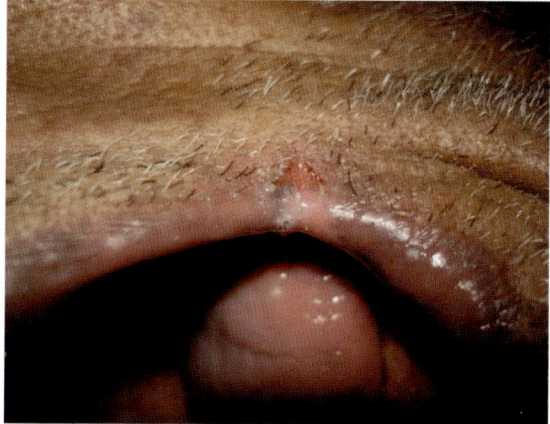

Fig. 5.2: Angular stomatitis

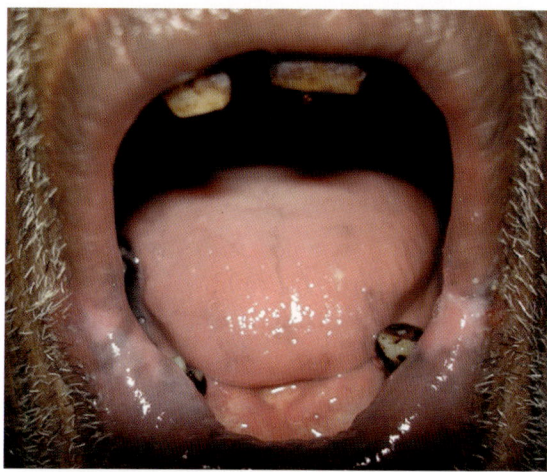

Fig. 5.3: Angular stomatitis and cheilitis

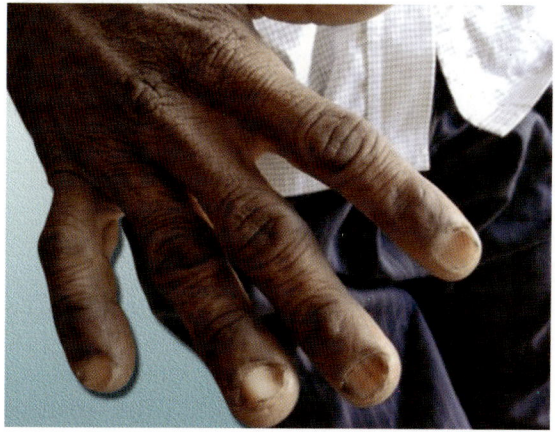

Fig. 5.1: Koilonychia in a patient of iron deficiency of anemia

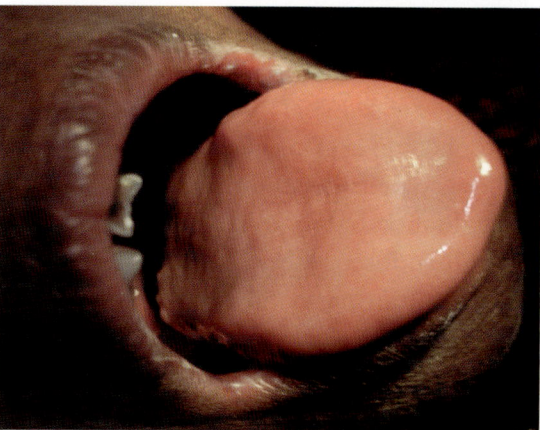

Fig. 5.4: Pale and bald tongue of iron deficiency anemia

Causes of iron deficiency
- Due to blood loss—from GIT, genitourinary and pulmonary disorders
  - Hookworm infestation
  - Physiological causes like menstruation and pregnancy.
  - Intravascular hemolysis.
- Due to increased demand
  - Adolescence
  - Pregnancy
- Due to ↓ intake and utilisation
  - Decreased nutritional intake
  - Malabsorption
  - Chronic inflammation.

Investigations of iron deficiency anemia
- Hb%—decreased
- Peripheral smear—microcytic hypochromic anemia.
- Platelet count increased—may suggest internal bleeding.

Establishment of iron deficiency
- Low serum iron (normal 50–150 μg/dl)
- Increased TIBC (total iron binding capacity: Normal 300–360 μg/dl)
- Decreased serum ferritin level (becomes less than 20 μg/dl).
- Bone marrow iron decreased or absent.

Transferrin saturation index
Saturation Index:
- Serum iron × 100 divided by TIBC
- If saturation <20%, indicates iron deficiency.

Evaluation of causes of iron deficiency
- Stool: Ova, cyst and occult blood
- Gynecological evaluation in females.
- Evaluation of blood loss
  - GI endoscopy
  - Genitourinary and pulmonary evaluation.
- Evaluation for malabsorption.

Other causes of microcytic hypochromic anemia
1. Thalassemia
   - Abnormal hemoglobin

- Serum iron is ↑, Ferritin ↑
- TIBC—normal
2. Sideroblastic anemia
   - Serum iron normal or ↑ and TIBC normal
   - Serum ferritin is ↑
3. Anemia of chronic disease
   - Normocytic normochromic anemia
   - Serum ferritin is ↑, TIBC ↓

Cause of microcytosis in iron deficiency: Iron plays a role in the maturation of RBCs and formation of hemoglobin. Hemoglobin occupies the major part of the RBCs and decides the RBC size. Whenever there is decreased iron, there is decreased hemoglobin. As a result there is decrease in the size of RBCs.

MEGALOBLASTIC ANEMIA

Megaloblastic anemia occurs due to the deficiency of either folic acid or vitamin B12.

Vitamin B12 (Cyanocobalamin)
- Normal serum B12 level: 180–200 pg/ml
- B12 is absorbed in the terminal ileum which requires intrinsic factor.
- B12 is mainly obtained from animal sources and bacterial synthesis.
- Liver is the main store for vitamin B12.
- Normal daily requirement of vitamin B12 is around 1.5 μg to 2.5 μg/day.
- B12 deficiency develops over years.

Megaloblastic Anemia

Suspect megaloblastic anemia in the following circumstances:
- Anemia and fatigability
- Strict vegetarians
- Recent knuckle pigmentation/whole body pigmentation.
- Anemia, peripheral neuropathy, spinal cord involvement and higher mental function abnormalities
- In patients with pancytopenia.

General Aspects of Megaloblastic Anemia

Usual causes

- Vitamin B12/folic acid deficiency.
- Other causes which affect the maintenance of vitamin B12 or folate.

Features

There will be defective DNA synthesis.

- Developing RBCs are significantly affected.
- Vitamin B12 deficiency causes neurological defect.
- Folate deficiency can cause peripheral neuropathy.

Structural abnormalities in megaloblastic anemia

- More prone to internal malignancy.
- Prone to develop cardiovascular disease like arterial/venous occlusion including IHD.
- All epithelial structures are affected—peripheral nerves and spinal cord is affected and can cause dementia and psychosis.
- Can result in infertility and neural tube defect in the fetus.
- Neurological involvement in vitamin B12 deficiency occurs due to abnormal myelination of nervous system.
- Pathogenesis of neurological involvement in vitamin B12 deficiency:
  - Decrease of S-adenosylmethionine and increase of methylmelanoic acid causing abnormal myelination.
  - Decrease of adenosylcobalamin (which is mitochondrial cofactor) with accumulation of methylmelanoic acid due to abnormal growth factor.

📝 *Note*

Large doses of folate can be helpful in the treatment of anemia of vit. B12 deficiency but not the neurological symptoms and may aggravate neurological abnormalities.

Cause of Macrocytosis

In B12 deficiency DNA synthesis is impaired but RNA synthesis is unimpaired. There will be accumulation of cytoplasmic components causing larger cells.

Causes of Vit B12 Deficiency

1. Due to defective absorption at terminal ileum
   - Malabsorption at terminal ileum (TB, Crohn's)
   - Intestinal resection, stagnant loop syndrome.
   - Fish tapeworm infestation
2. Decreased intake—strict vegetarians.
3. Malabsorption at the gastric level (due to intrinsic factor)
   - Atrophic gastritis
   - Intrinsic factor deficiency
   - Gastrostomy.

Folate deficiency

- Normal folate requirement: About 400 µg/day
- All cellular reactions require folate as coenzymes
- 5-methyltetrahydrofolate is the active physiological form and will be converted into tetrahydrofolate.
- Folic acid is mainly absorbed in the jejunum
- Green vegetables contain a large amount of folic acid.
- Deficiency of folate can occur in a few months.

Causes of folate deficiency

- Nutritional due to decreased dietary intake.
- Due to increased demand:
  - Adolescents with growth
  - Pregnancy
  - Lactation
  - Hemolysis
  - Hematological malignancies
  - Systemic disease: Liver disease
- Defective absorption—malabsorption disorder.
- Due to drugs and toxins: Alcohol, phenytoin, methotrexate.

Clinical features of megaloblastic anemia

- Due to anemia: Fatigability, pallor
- Due to ↑ melanin: Pigmentation of skin

- Due to epithelial involvement—glossitis, diarrhea.
- Due to ineffective erythropoiesis and hemolysis: Unconjugated bilirubin ↑ and jaundice.
- Due to pancytopenia
  - Infection (rare)
  - Bleeding tendency (rare)
- Due to neurological involvement
  - Dementia
  - Psychosis
  - Peripheral neuropathy.
- Spinal cord involvement (subacute combined degeneration of spinal cord).

Investigations

For vitamin B12 deficiency:
1. Serum B12 level is decreased (normal level—100 to 200 μg/L).
2. In early cobalamine deficiency serum homocysteine level and methylmalonoic acid is raised but these can also be raised in many other conditions—so not useful for diagnosis.

 Note

Neurological involvement can occur even without anemia in a patient of vitamin B12 deficiency.

For the causes of vit B12 deficiency

- For atrophic gastritis—upper GI endoscopy and biopsy.
- Pernicious anemia: ↑ serum gastrin level and anti-parietal cell and anti-intrinsic factor antibody detection.
- To rule out diseases of small intestine: Endoscopy and biopsy.

For folate deficiency

- Serum folate level is decreased
- Folate level of RBC is decreased.

For the causes of folate deficiency: Duodenal biopsy to rule out malabsorption syndrome and celiac disease.

Hematological abnormalities in megaloblastic anemia

- *Peripheral smear*
  - Macrocytic anemia (MCV >100 fl), MCV >110—more likely is associated with B12 deficiency.
  - Hypersegmented neutrophils (>5 lobes)
  - Pancytopenia may be present.
- *Bone marrow*
  - Megaloblasts present
  - Enlarged megakaryocytes.

ANEMIA OF CHRONIC DISEASE

Anemia of chronic disease occurs due to chronic infection/inflammation

- For example, chronic infection
- Rheumatoid arthritis
- Internal malignancy.

Pathogenesis

- Defective iron delivery and utilization by the bone marrow.
- Decrease in the production of erythropoietin and defective marrow response to erythropoietin.
- Due to the systemic illness—life span of the RBC becomes reduced.
- Inflammatory mediators produced by the liver (hepicidin) interferes with absorption and utilization of iron.

Characteristics

- *Type of anemia*: Normocytic normochromic/microcytic hypochromic.
- *Features*—usually mild and associated with features of systemic illness.
- Serum iron is normal or reduced with increase in the serum ferritin level.
- Significant decrease of Hb 2–3 gm/dl within 2–3 days—can occur in severe infection/inflammation.

HEMOLYTIC ANEMIA

General Aspects

- Hemolytic anemia may be acute/chronic and it may be hereditary/acquired.

- Some types of hemolytic anemia are common in certain geographical areas and certain ethnic groups.
- Suspect hemolytic anemia if there is combination of anemia, mild jaundice and splenomegaly.

Suspect hereditary cause for hemolysis or hemoglobinopathy in following circumstances
- Anemia and jaundice since childhood
- Presence of positive family history
- History of blood transfusion since childhood.
- Presence of gallstones.

Examples of acute hemolysis
- Autoimmune hemolysis
- Malaria
- Drug induced, e.g. primaquine induced in G6PD deficiency

Chronic hemolysis: Hereditary cause of hemolysis and hemoglobinopathies.

Different Types of Hemolysis

Extravascular hemolysis: In the spleen liver, bone marrow.

Intravascular hemolysis: In the circulation.

Laboratory Evidence of Hemolysis

- Hb%—decreased
- Reticulocytes count is increased
- Serum LDH level is increased
- Urine—urobilinogen is increased
- Serum—indirect bilirubin is increased
- Serum haptoglobin is decreased
- Bone marrow—erythropoiesis is increased.

Causes of Hemolytic Anemia and their Mechanism

- Antibody mediated—autoimmune hemolysis.
- Defect in the RBC membrane: Hereditary spherocytosis.
- Due to abnormal Hb: Thalassemia and other hemoglobinopathy.

- Due to defect in the RBC enzymes—G6PD deficiency.
- Due to acute infection—malaria and mycoplasma infection
- Due to drugs, e.g. primaquine.
- Mechanical abnormality in the circulation—prosthetic valve/calcified valve.
- Compliment mediated: PNH.
- Due to splenic destruction—hypersplenism.

Sickle Cell Anemia

Features and Clinical Diagnosis

- Anemia since childhood
- Recurrent attacks of vaso-occulsion resulting in painful crisis.
- Recurrent infarction of spleen causing autosplenectomy with loss of functions of spleen (occurs within 1st 5 years of life)
- Chronic leg ulcers.

Anemia is due to: Abnormal shape of RBCs which are destroyed by the spleen.

Chronic leg ulcer is due to:
- Due to occlusion of microcirculation in the distal part causing ischemia and infarction and then infection.
- Vaso-occlusion due to abnormal shape of the RBCs (sickled) not possible to negotiate the capillaries causing ischemia and infarction.
- Infarction can occur in the spleen, brain, bone, liver, kidney and lung.

Pathogenesis

Sickling of RBC occurs due to: Defect in the hemoglobin (At β globin chain at 6th position—glutamic acid is substituted by valine) resulting in HbS. During hypoxic states the above abnormality make the RBC membrane stiffen and sickled. Abnormal-shaped RBCs are destroyed in the spleen.

Different Circumstances Precipitating Increased Sickling and Crisis

- Hypoxia
- Infection and fever

- Excessive exercise
- Temperature change
- Acidosis
- Defect in the circulation—sluggish blood flow.

Different Types of Crisis in Sickle Cell Anemia

Painful crisis due to infarction of organs
- Causes severe pain
- Any organ system can be involved
- It can mimic:
  - Acute abdomen
  - Neurological manifestations
  - Hand and foot syndrome (infarction of digits—dactylitis)
  - Acute chest syndrome due to sickling within the lung
- Salmonella osteomyelitis can occur.

Hemolytic crisis—presents as severe hemolysis.

Aplastic crisis—caused by Parvovirus B infection.
- Parvovirus causes transient aplasia of the marrow. In persons with normal life span of the RBCs this causes a temporary decrease in the hemoglobin.
- In patients with hemolytic anemia because of the decrease in the life span of the RBCs, transient aplasia of the marrow caused by the parvovirus cannot compensate for the hemolysis resulting in severe aplastic crises

Splenic sequestration crisis—significant trapping of RBCs in the spleen
Manifest as severe anemia and requires emergency measures of transfusion/splenectomy.

Diagnosis of sickle cell anemia
- Evidence of hemolysis
- Peripheral smear—sickled cells
- Demonstration of sickling—inducing hypoxia—by keeping the coverslip over drop of blood on a slide, or by adding sodium metabisulphite.
- Hb electrophoresis demonstrates HbS.

Sickle cell trait
- Anemia—mild
- Usually asymptomatic
- Sickling crisis—rare

Sickle β thalassemia
- A double heterozygous state—can have anemia.
- Splenic infarction—less common.

 Note

Suspect sickle β thalassemia in a patient of sickle cell anemia if splenomegaly persists after 5 years of age.

HEREDITARY SPHEROCYTOSIS

Diagnosis

Suspect: Hereditary spherocytosis in the following circumstances
- Positive family history of hemolytic anemia (autosomal dominant disorder)
- Severe anemia/jaundice since childhood.
- Splenomegaly
- Gallstone at younger age.
- Defect—due to mutations in several genes of RBC membrane.
- There will be abnormalities in the cytoskeletal spectrin of RBC membrane making susceptible to hemolysis.
- Pregnancy and infection accelerate hemolysis.

Lab investigations
- Anemia with evidence of hemolysis
- Increase MCHC with normal blood counts
- Peripheral smear shows spherocytosis
- Increased osmotic fragility of RBCs.

Other causes of increased osmotic fragility
Autoimmune hemolytic anemia
Hypernatremia

Causes of decreased osmotic fragility
- Iron deficiency anemia
- Thalassemia
- Sickle cell anemia

Complications

- Growth retardation in children
- Hemolytic crisis
- Gallstones and cholecystitis.

G6PD deficiency

- Genetic defect of RBC enzyme
- Transmitted as X-linked disease
- RBCs are exposed to oxidative stress due to lack of NADPH and develop hemolysis.

Features

- May be asymptomatic throughout life
- May present as neonatal jaundice
- Develop hemolysis when exposed to infection and drugs.
- Can have hemoglobinuria when exposed to drugs.

Drugs which can precipitate hemolysis in G6PD deficiency

- Primaquine
- Dapsone
- Sulfamethoxazole/sulfasalazine
- Cotrimoxazole
- Methylene blue.

Lab features

- Evidence of hemolysis
- Presence of Heinz bodies in the peripheral smear
- Presence of blister—bite cells with RBCs appearing that parts are bitten
- G6PD level estimation which will be lower.

Autoimmune Hemolytic Anemia

Features

- Anemia can be severe
- Jaundice
- Splenomegaly
- Coombs' positive hemolysis (antibody mediated hemolysis)
- Hemolysis occurs due to the presence of antibody on the RBCs
- Autoimmune hemolytic anemia can be primary or secondary to
  - SLE
  - CLL

- Waldenström's macroglobulinemia
  - Lymphoma.
- Antibody mediated hemolysis may also be due to
  - Penicillin
  - Ceftriaxone
  - Piperacillin

Investigations

- Evidence of hemolysis
- Peripheral smear: Microspherocytes
- Positive Coombs' test.

Autoimmune hemolytic anemia responds to

- Corticosteroids
- Rituximab

Types of Autoimmune Hemolysis

Due to warm antibody

Causes

- Lymphoma
- Carcinoma colon/lung
- SLE/rheumatoid arthritis
- Drugs like penicillin intake

Due to cold antibody

Antibody of IgM type binds the RBC at 4 degree centigrade temperature.

Causes

- Mycoplasma pneumonia
- Low grade B cell lymphoma
- Paroxysmal cold hemoglobinuria.

THALASSEMIA

Normal Adult Hemoglobin

HbA: 2-alpha and 2-beta chains.

Fetal hemoglobin: HbF-2 alpha and 2-gamma chains.

Hemoglobin A2: 2-alpha and 2-delta chains.

Thalassemia are group of disorders—characterised by decreased biosynthesis of Hb chains.

Types of Thalassemia

Alpha thalassemia: Due to defective synthesis of alpha chains.

Beta thalassemia: Due to defective synthesis of beta chains
- Beta thalassemia major
- Beta thalassemia intermedia
- Beta thalassemia minor

Suspect β thalassemia major in following circumstances
1. Severe anemia in childhood
2. Typical thalassemic facies
3. Requires blood transfusion recurrently since childhood/bone marrow transplantation for survival
4. Associated with hepatosplenomegaly
5. Microcytic anemia not responding to iron therapy.

β thalassemia major

Defect: Defective synthesis of β chains with decreased production of beta chains.

Pathophysiology
- There is decreased β chain synthesis.
- There is unbalanced excess alpha chain synthesis which can precipitate and are toxic to RBCs and RBCs are removed by the spleen causing hemolysis.
- Severe anemia—causes erythroid hyperplasia due to erythropoietin release (marrow expansion) and hepatosplenomegaly.

Features of β thalassemia major
- Severe form of the disease causing severe anemia
- Chipmunk facies: Thalassemic facies (due to expansion of marrow cavity)
  - Frontal bossing
  - Malar prominence
  - Protuberant teeth
  - Growth retardation
  - Leg ulcers
  - Hepatosplenomegaly
  - Gallstones
  - CCF
  - Death in early life unless recurrently transfused.
  - Patients can develop transfusion related hemosiderosis and its complications.

β thalassemia—intermedia
- Mild to moderate anemia
- Transfusion may or may not be required

β thalassemia minor/trait
- Asymptomatic
- Mild anemia and splenomegaly—mimicking iron deficiency but not responding to iron therapy.

Lab investigations of thalassemia major
- Severe anemia
- Microcytic hypochromic type
- X-ray skull hair on end appearance due to marrow hyperplasia
- PS: Microcytic hypochromic anemia and presence of target cells
- Hb electrophoresis—presence of fetal hemoglobin.

Complications of β thalassemia major
- Growth retardation
- Severe anemia
- Aplasia of the marrow
- CCF
- Transfusion hemosiderosis.

β Thalassemia Minor

Suspect β thalassemia minor in the following circumstances
- Mild anemia—microcytic hypochromic—not responding to iron therapy
- Presence of anemia with splenomegaly since childhood
- Peripheral smear—target cells
- Raised HbA_2
- Positive family history.

Alpha Thalassemia

- There are 4 genes which contribute for 2-alpha chains.
- If one gene is deleted—patient is asymptomatic.
- If 2 genes are deleted (patient will have microcytic hypochromic anemia) resembling beta thalassemia minor.

- If 3 genes are deleted, it results in HbH disease—results in moderate hemolysis.
- HbH results in excess of beta chains which are nonfunctioning. Person requires folic acid, blood transfusion without iron supplementation.
- If all 4 genes are deleted—presents as Hb Bart's: Hydrops fetalis (baby is stillborn).
- Hb Bart's has got increased affinity to oxygen and oxygen delivery to the tissues becomes less. There will be asphyxia with CCF.

Paroxysmal Nocturnal Hemoglobinuria

Triad of features
- Anemia
- Pancytopenia
- Venous occlusion.

Other features
- Hemoglobinuria
- Abdominal pain due to venous occlusion or presents as hepatic vein occlusion or mesenteric vein occlusion.

Defect: Abnormal susceptibility of RBCs to complement resulting in hemolysis.

May progress to
- Acute myeloid leukemia
- Aplastic anemia.

Lab features
- Evidence of hemolysis
- Hemoglobinuria
- Bone marrow may be hypercellular and becomes hypocellular/aplastic
- CD 59 and CD 55 deficiency on RBCs.

Aplastic Anemia

Common features
- Pancytopenia
- No organomegaly
- Hypocellular bone marrow

Usual presenting features
- Due to anemia—easy fatigability
- Granulocytopenia—infection may be life-threatening.

- Due to thrombocytopenia—bleeding superficial/visceral bleed.

Usual complications
- Severe sepsis
- Intracranial bleed.

Signs
- Bleeding spots (oral cavity, mucosa, retina, skin)
- Evidence of infection
- Severe anemia
- No lymphadenopathy
- No hepatosplenomegaly

Lab investigations
- All 3 elements of blood are reduced (pancytopenia)
- Peripheral smear
  - Mild macrocytosis
  - Pancytopenia.
- Bone marrow
  - No abnormal cells
  - Increased fat content of the marrow
  - Hypocellular/acellular.

Severe Aplasia

Criteria
- Corrected reticulocyte count less than 1%
- Neutrophils <500 cells/cmm
- Platelets <20,000 cells/cmm

Causes of aplastic anemia
- Infection—previous viral hepatitis
- Exposure to drugs
  - Gold, NSAIDs
  - Chemotherapeutic agents.
- Exposure to chemicals, like benzene
- Paroxysmal nocturnal hemoglobinuria
- Exposure to radiation
- Constitutional disorders like Fanconi's anemia.

Other Causes of Pancytopenia
- With active (hypercellular) bone marrow
- Common causes:
  - Hypersplenism
  - Tuberculosis

- Megaloblastic anemia (B12/folate deficiency)
- SLE
- Severe infection.
- Rarer causes:
  - PNH
  - Lymphomas
  - Aleukemic/subleukemic leukemia

Pancytopenia with hypocellular marrow

- Aplastic anemia
- Occasionally myelodysplastic syndrome/leukemia/lymphoma.

MYELODYSPLASTIC SYNDROME

Disorder of Bone Marrow: Hemopoietic Stem Cell Disorder

Common Features

- Cell proliferation and differentiation becomes defective.
- Ultimately results in cytopenia
- Leukemic transformation (acute myeloid leukemia)

Risk factors: Exposure to benzine/radiation.

Cytogenetic abnormality

- Abnormalities of chromosome 5, 7, 20
- There may be loss of or partial loss of chromosome.
- Can also have an association with Trisomy 8.

Clinical Features

May be asymptomatic and can be detected on routine evaluation.

- Features of pancytopenia
- Splenomegaly.

Different Types of MDS

- Refractory anemia with unilineage dysplasia;
- Refractory anemia, neutropenia, thrombocytopenia
- Refractory anemia with ringed sideroblasts

- Refractory anemia with multilineage dysplasia
- Refractory anemia with excess blasts type I
- Refractory anemia with excess blasts type II
- MDS associated with isolated Del 5q
- Childhood MDS
- MDS unclassified

Secondary MDS can occur with

- Down's syndrome
- Chemotherapeutic agents

While diagnosing MDS—rule out

- Megaloblastic anemia: Folic acid/B12 ↓
- Drug toxicity
- Chemical toxicity
- Viral infection.

Lab investigation

- Pancytopenia
- Macrocytosis
- Occasional myeloblasts

Bone marrow

- Hypercellular
- Rarely hypocellular
- Dyserythropoiesis
- Presence of ringed sideroblasts/myeloblasts.

POLYCYTHEMIA VERA

Myeloproliferative Disorder

- Multipotent hemotopoietic progenitor cell undergoes proliferation—a clonal disorder.
- Increase in the production of RBCs, WBCs, and platelets.
- There is no increase in the serum erythropoietin level.
- Suspect polycythemia if Hb% is > 17 g/dl in males and if Hb% is > 15 g/dl in females.

Cytogenetic abnormality: Mutation in the JAK2 (Janause Kinase) leading on to kinase activation.

Clinical Features

- May be asymptomatic
- Polycythemia
  - Suffused conjunctiva

- Red ruddy complexion
- Tongue-purplish red
- Massive splenomegaly.

Can cause hyperviscocity symptoms

- Headache, vertigo, TIA, CVA, Budd-Chiari syndrome, hypertension, peptic ulcer, GI bleed.
- Acquagenic pruritis: Development of pruritis with hot water bath (due to increased density of mast cells and histamine release).
- Burning pain—extremities—erythromelalgia and digital gangrene.
- Suspect: Polycythemia vera, when RBCs, WBCs and platelets are increased with massive splenomegaly.

Lab Features

- Increase RBC mass
- Increase HB >20 gm/dl, ↑ Packed cell volume
- Normal arterial oxygen saturation.
- Lower serum erythropoietin level.
- Positive JAK 2 mutation.

Complications

- Hyperviscocity
- Vascular occlusion
- Splenic infarct.
- Bleeding into the GIT
- Later myelofibrosis
- Leukemic transformation

📝 *Note*

- *Polycythemia is the term used for any increase in Hb% >17 gm/dl in males and >15 gm/dl in females (Ht >45%).*
- *Erythrocytosis is the term used for increased in the RBC mass.*
- *Decrease in the plasma volume causes spurious or relative polycythemia.*

Causes of Secondary Polycythemia

- Cyanotic congenital heart disease including intracardiac shunt.
- Chronic respiratory diseases with hypoxia, e.g. chronic cor pulmonale.

- High altitude conditions
- Poisoning due to carbon monoxide
- Renal disease: Renal cysts
- Renal artery disease.
- Tumors: Hepatoma, renal cell carcinoma
- Cerebellar hemangioblastoma
- Uterine myoma
- Pheochromocytoma
- Drugs: Androgens
- Erythropoietin therapy

Essential Thrombocytosis

- Due to abnormality of multipotent hematopoietic progenitor cell
- Platelets are overproduced without a definite cause.

Features

- Detected to be having very high platelet count.
- May be on routine examination.
- There may be history of bleeding/thrombosis.
- Splenomegaly is milder compared to polycythemia vera.

Investigations

- Very high platelet count
- JAK 2 mutation positive
- Bone marrow—increased cellularity
- Megakaryocytic hyperplasia.

Complications

- Very high platelet count can cause bleeding due to acquired von Willebrand factor deficiency.
- Vascular occlusion.
- Evolve into progressive massive fibrosis.

MYELOPHTHISIC ANEMIA

Myelophthisic anemia usually occurs secondary to systemic disease: Causing secondary myelofibrosis/myelopthisis.

What is Myelophthisis

Bone marrow suppression secondary to marrow infiltration by inflammatory cells/neoplastic cells/granulomas.

Causes of Myelophthisis

- Infective disorders
  - *Mycobacterium tuberculosis*
  - Disseminated fungal infection
  - Infection due to HIV
- Radiation exposure
- Neoplastic disorders
  - Invasion of the marrow by the tumor cells:
  - For example, carcinoma of breast
  - Bronchogenic carcinoma
  - Myelofibrosis can also occur due to CML, myeloma, etc.

Features of myelophthisic anemia

- Severe anemia with pancytopenia
- Hepatosplenomegaly
- Marrow fibrosis
- Hemopoiesis occurs in extra medullary sites.

Laboratory investigations

Peripheral smear

- Leucoerythroblastic picture (nucleated RBCs, tear drop cells)
- Normocytic normochromic anemia
- Giant platelets—occur
- Bone marrow examination will demonstrate dry tap.

MYELOFIBROSIS

Clinical Diagnostic Features

- Hepatomegaly
- Massive splenomegaly
- Marrow fibrosis
- Extra medullary hemopoiesis

(Myelofibrosis is a diagnosis of exclusion after ruling out other disorders causing massive splenomegaly).

Aetiology

- Presence of JAK 2 mutation
- Abnormality of chromosomes 8, 9
- Growth factors like endothelial growth factors/transforming growth factors cause fibrosis.

Clinical Features

- Anemia, fatigue—weight loss
- Hepatospleomegaly (massive splenomegaly)
- Extra medullary: Hematopoiesis—can cause spinal cord compression, ascites, pulmonary hypertension.

Lab features

- Anemia—normocytic normochromic
- Peripheral smear—leucoerythroblastic picture
  - Tear drop cell
  - Leukocytosis and thrombocytosis
- Bone marrow
  - Dry tap due to increased reticulin
  - Can have hypercellular marrow
  - Increased size of megakaryocytes
- Other features
  - LAP score is increased
  - LDH↑

Complications

- Severe anemia
- Progressive marrow failure
- Complications due to extramedullary hematopoiesis
- Leukemic transformation.

DISORDERS OF WBCs

Neutropenia

- Decrease in the neutrophils
- Susceptible to infection
- Neutropenia can occur secondary to
  - Decreased production:
    - Deficiency: Vitamin B12 ↓
    - Alcohol induced

- Infective disorder:
  - Tuberculosis
  - HIV infection
- Drug induced:
  - Carbimazole
  - Zudovidine
  - Chloramphenicol
  - Cotrimoxazole
  - Carbamezapine
- Hematological—aplastic anemia
- Autoimmune: SLE, Felty's syndrome
- When neutrophil count—absolute is less than 1000 cells/cmm, there is increased susceptibility to infection.
- When absolute neutrophil count is less than 500 cells/cmm—endogenous organisms cause infection.
- When the count is less than 200 cells/cmm, there is absence of inflammatory response. And person can develop septic shock.

Eosinophilia

Increased number of eosinophils.

Causes

- Helminthiasis
- Hypereosinophilic syndrome
- Collagen disease
- Bronchial asthma
- Pulmonary eosinophilia
- Hodgkin's lymphoma

Types

Eosinophilia: Eosinophil count > 400 to 1,500 cells/cmm

Hypereosinophilia

Eosinophil count > 1500 cells/cmm (persisting for more than 6 months).

Causes

- Clonal abnormality (stem cell disorder)
- Chronic eosinophilic leukemia
- Myeloproliferative disorder
- Idiopathic hypereosinophilic syndrome

Tropical pulmonary eosinophilia

- Eosinophil count > 3000 cells/cmm
- Found in endemic area of filariasis
- It is an immune reaction to filarial antigen from *Wuchereria bancrofti / Brugia malayi*
- Increased level of IgG and IgE level
- Chest X-ray shows miliary mottling
- Responds to diethylcarbamazine and corticosteroids.
  Eosinopenia—can be due to corticosteroids.

Neutrophilia

Increased number of neutrophils.

Causes

- Bacterial infection
- Inflammation, burns, MI, collagen disease
- Myeloproliferative disorders
- Drugs—corticosteroids

Leukemoid Reaction

Features:

- Leukocytosis
- WBC count is usually less than 50,000 cells/cmm
- Mature forms like myelocytes and metamyelocytes are found in the peripheral smear.
- No abnormal cells in the marrow
- No organ infiltration
- Leucocyte ALP score normal
- Hb% and platelets are normal
- Leukocytosis subsides on treating the secondary cause
- Usually secondary to infection like pneumonia (neutrophilic) and tuberculosis (lymphocytic).

Monocytes

Monocytes differentiate into macrophages:

Causes of Monocytosis

- Tuberculosis
- Malaria

- Kala azar
- Internal malignancy

Monocytopenia
- Corticosteroids
- Aplastic anemia

Lymphocytosis
Causes
- Tuberculosis
- Brucellosis
- Infectious mononucleosis
- Lymphoma/leukemia

Lymphocytopenia
Causes
- HIV infection
- Protein energy malnutrition
- Severe combined immune deficiency

LEUKEMIAS
Suspect leukemia under following circumstances
- Severe anemia
- Bleeding tendency
- Bone tenderness
- Hepatosplenomegaly/generalized lymphadenopathy
- Evidence of infection.

Acute Leukemias
Acute Lymphoblastic Leukemia (ALL)
Clinically suspect ALL
- If younger age group
- Severe anemia, bleeding tendency and infection of acute onset.
- Bony tenderness.
- Hepatosplenomegaly and lymphadenopathy.
- *Occasionally*
  - Infiltration of the skin
  - Testicular enlargement
  - Nervous system involvement
- *Investigations*
  - Severe anemia

  - Thrombocytopenia
  - Very high WBC count (rarely normal or lower count)
  - Circulating lymphoblasts.
- *Bone marrow*: Malignant lymphoblasts >20%
- *Other abnormalities*
  - Increased uric acid
  - CSF—lymphoblasts
  - Chest X-ray-mediastinal mass
- *Aetiology*
  - Exposure to ionising radiation
  - Exposure to chemicals
  - Down's syndrome.

CHRONIC LYMPHOCYTIC LEUKEMIA
Suspect CLL
- If age group 55–60 years
- Generalised lymphadenopathy
- Hepatosplenomegaly
- Anemia and fatigue
- Above symptoms and signs will be for a longer duration (may be asymptomatic for a long time).

Lab features
- Anemia—mild to severe
- Very high WBC count (50,000–100,000 cell/cmm)
- Coombs' positive hemolytic anemia
- Peripheral smear-smudge or basket cell.
- B cells express CD5, CD19, CD23 and CD38 antigens

Bone marrow: Lymphocytosis, cells are distorted/smudge cells.

ACUTE MYELOID LEUKAEMIA
Diagnose acute myeloid leukemia under the following circumstances
- Older age group
- Acute onset fatigue
- Bleeding tendency and infection
- Fever
- Hepatosplenomegaly

- Lymphadenopathy
- Sternal tenderness

Other features
- Can present as tumor mass sites like skin, lymph node, testis, etc.
- Monocytic AML—gum hypertrophy
- Promyelocytic AML—DIC and bleeding
- Aetiological factors
  - Exposure to radiation and chemicals (Benzine/petroleum products) and
  - Alkalyting agents
  - Persons with Down's syndrome.

Lab investigations
- Severe anemia
- Very high WBC count
- Myeloblasts > 20% of marrow cellularity
- Myeloblasts contain Auer rods.
- Abnormal function and decreased number of platelets.
- Cytogenetic abnormality.

Table 5.1: Difference between lymphoblasts and myeloblasts		
	Lymphoblast	*Myeloblast*
Nucleoli	Less distinct	Distinct 2–4 nucleoli
Nuclear chromatin	Condensed	Finer/delicate
Cytoplasmic granules	More	Few fine/absence of granules
Myeloperoxidase stain	Negative	Positive
Auer rods	Absent	Present
Surface CD receptors	Present	Absent

CHRONIC MYELOID LEUKEMIA (CML)

Chronic myeloid leukemia is a disorder of clonal hemopoetic stem cell.

Age group involved: 50–60 years of age (not common in children).

Aetiology: Exposure to large doses of ionizing radiation may be a risk factor.

Genetic aspects
- Philadelphia chromosome—positive in 90% of patients of CML.

- Philadelphia chromosome: Reciprocal translocation of material between chromosome 22 and chromosome 9.
- Abelson oncogene: Present in the fragments of chromosome 9.
- A chimeric gene is formed when fragments of chromosome 9 joins remains of BCR (chromosome 22)
- Tyrosine kinase activity: Above mentioned chimeric gene codes for a protein with tyrosine kinase activity that protein is 210 kDa protein. Tyrosine kinase activity is important in the pathogenesis of CML.

Clinical Features
- May be detected to have splenomegaly on routine examination.
- May present as left hypochondrial discomfort, left hypochondrial mass and early satiety.

Characteristic Sign
- Massive splenomegaly
- Hepatomegaly
- Occasionally can have:
  - Infection
  - Vascular occlusion
  - Bleeding
  - Splenic infarction.

Different Phases of CML

Chronic phase: Bone marrow < 10% of blasts. Most cases are diagnosed at this stage.

Accelerated phase: Bone marrow > 10% up to 19% blasts. Symptomatic, basophilia may be present.

Blast crisis (Acute leukemic transformation—usually myeloid): Sudden worsening of symptoms with severe anemia, bleeding tendency, lymphadenopathy, hepatosplenomegaly.

Resistant CML: May not respond to treatment.

Lab Investigations
- Very high WBC count (> 50,000 cells/cmm).
- Peripheral smear:
  - Mature neutrophils

- Myelocytes
- Metamyelocytes
- Very few blasts (<5%)
- Normocytic normochormic anemia. Platelets count is increased.
- LAP score is decreased.
- Uric acid is increased
- Vit B12 level is increased (transcobalamin III is released from neutrophils).
- Bone marrow: Hypercellular—myeloid blasts (<5%)
  - Blast crises: Blasts > 30% in the marrow
  - 90% of patients: Philadelphia chromosome BCR ABL positive.

HODGKIN'S LYMPHOMA

Lymphomatous disorder involving predominantly B cells.

Suspect: Hodgkin's disease under following circumstances
If generalized lymphadenopathy:
- Starts in the cervical region
- Firm discrete rubbery lymph nodes
- Presence of B symptoms
- Hepatosplenomegaly

Clinical aspects of Hodgkin's disease
Usual lymph node sites:
- Cervical commonest
- Axillary, mediastinal
- B symptoms:
  - Weight loss
  - Fever
  - Night sweats.
- Fever: PEL Ebstein fever
- Mixed cellularity type presents as PUO (associated with hepatosplenomegaly with abdominal involvement)
- Other features: Alcohol induced pain at site of lymph node after alcohol consumption.

Paraneoplastic manifestations
- Hypercalcemia
- Hemolytic anemia—immune mediated
- Cerebellar degeneration.

Investigations
- ESR is increased
- LDH is increased
- Lymph node biopsy:
  - Giant cell: Reed-Sternberg cell with mirror image nucleoli
  - Markers: CD15, CD30 positive.

 Note

Hodgkin's lymphoma can involve the bone marrow. Lymph node mass can cause compressive effect.

Different Pathological types of Hodgkin's Lymphoma

- Lymphocyte dominant
- Nodular sclerosis
- Mixed cellularity
- Lymphocyte depletion.

Clinical Staging

Staging
1. Involvement of single node region or extra lymphatic site.
2. Two or more lymph node region or extra lymphatic site and lymph node region on the same side of the diaphragm (above or below).
3. Lymph node on both sides of diaphragm with or without extra lymphatic involvement or spleen or both.
4. Diffuse involvement of one or more extra lymphatic tissues.

Extra lymphatic site: Lungs, liver and brain.
Nodular lymphocyte dominant lymphoma: Distinct from classical Hodgkin's.
- It is more closely associated with NHL
- They display CD45 cells
- (Not showing marker of Reed-Sternberg cell: CD15 and CD30)
- Chronic relapses common.

NON-HODGKIN'S LYMPHOMA

- Form of neoplastic disorder associated with lymphocytes.
- It may involve B cell: B cell NHL
- It may involve T cell: T cell NHL

- *Age group*: Usually above 65 years of age
- Possible aetiolgoical factors:
  - HIV infection
  - *H. Pylori* infection—gastric lymphoma
  - Epstein-Barr virus infection: Burkitt's lymphoma
  - T cell lymphoma

Main Types of NHL

- Follicular lymphoma—usually advanced at the time of diagnosis
- Diffuse large cell lymphoma: Most common type of NHL
- Burkitt's lymphoma may occur due to Ebstein-Barr virus
- MALT lymphoma—B cell type—can develop from stomach
- Mantle cell lymphoma affects spleen: Rare
- Adult T cell lymphoma/leukemia—may occur due to HTLV-1 infection

Clinical Features

- Lymphadenopathy
- Can also present with extra nodal involvement
- Fever, weight loss, night sweats, itching, lumps under the skin.

Structures which can be involved

- GIT
- Bone marrow
- Spinal cord
- Skin
- Testis

Can manifest as

- Compression of GIT and spinal cord
- Ascites
- SVC obstruction

Investigations

- CBP: Anemia, thrombocytopenia, lymphocytosis
- ESR is increased
- Coombs' test may be positive
- LDH is increased

- HIV ELISA may be positive
- Chest X-ray, CT chest, abdomen, PET scan for the disease
- Lymph node biopsy and bone marrow biopsy for infiltration by abnormal lymphocytes.
- Immunoglobulin estimation IgM, IgG level.

MULTIPLE MYELOMA

Plasma cells proliferate in a malignant pattern resulting in multiple myeloma.

Suspect myeloma in the following circumstances

- Elderly age
- Severe anemia
- Generalized bony pain
- Spontaneous or pathological fractures
- Organomegaly (rare)

Age group involved—elderly around 70 years.

Clinical Features

Presenting features

- Severe anemia
- Bony pain and pathological fracture: Due to activation of osteoclasts by osteoclast activating factor released by myeloma cells.
- Bone—lytic lesion with release of calcium-resulting in hypercalcemia.
- Can cause collapse compression of vertebra.
- Infection—patients of myeloma are susceptible to infection.
- Renal involvement—can occur in myeloma due to following reasons
  - Hypercalcemia
  - Increase in uric acid
  - Infection
  - Infiltration by myeloma
  - Secondary amyloidosis
- Due to therapy
  - NSAIDs
  - Contrast use
  - Bisphosphonates.

- Hyperviscocity symptoms: Occurs due to macroglobulins—IgM.
- Polyneuropathy—myeloma can present as polyneuropathy.

Lab investigations
- Anemia: Normocytic normochromic
- WBC and platelets—decreased.
- ESR increased (>100 mm/hour)
- Serum calcium is increased
- Serum protein electrophoresis ↑level of IgM, IgA, IgG

Diagnosis
- Bone marrow—plasmocytosis >10% with CD marker 269, 319
- Serum and urine M component—increased
- Estimation of urine—light chain assay.

Symptomatic myeloma
- Patient has clinical symptoms/signs of myeloma
- Bone marrow shows evidence of myeloma
- Urine and serum contain M proteins
- There is evidence of end organ damage.

Asymptomatic myeloma (smoldering myeloma)
- No organ/involvement of tissues.
- Bone marrow plasma cells <10%
- M protein level is more than or equal to 30 g/dl.

Monoclonal gammopathy of unknown significance (MGUS)
- Serum M protein <30 g/L
- Bone marrow plasma cells <10%
- No organ/tissue involvement.

Non-secretory myeloma
- Bony lesion and tissue involvement present
- Marrow plasma cells >10%
- No increase of serum IgM

Solitary plasmacytoma of bone
- There is destruction of single area of bone
- No increase of serum M protein
- There is no bone marrow evidence of myeloma.

WALDENSTROM'S MACROGLOBULINEMIA
- Presents as weakness and fatigue.
- No bony lesion/hypercalcemia
- Lymphadenopathy and hepatosplenomegaly
- Peripheral neuropathy.

Lab features: Serum level of IgM (>30 g/dl)

Bone marrow: 10% lymphoplasmacytoid cells.

Complications:
- Hyperviscocity syndrome
- Peripheral neuropathy
- Recurrent infection

Bleeding/Clotting Disorder
- Clotting of blood/bleeding depends on the interaction between platelets, vessel wall, endothelium, von Willebrand's factor, coagulation system and fibrinolytic systems.
- Bleeding or clotting occurs with abnormality of any of the above factors.

Approach to a Patient of Bleeding or Clotting Disorder

Consider Following Aspects

Sex: Coagulation disorder is more likely to be associated with male sex.

Age: Bleeding tendency from very young age usually suggests hereditary disorder.

Family history: Family history of bleeding disorder suggests hereditary cause of bleeding.

Site of bleed
- Superficial bleed like petechiae, purpura or mucosal bleed is more likely to be associated with bleeding disorder, like abnormality of platelets or abnormality of vessel wall.
- Bleeding into the body cavities, joint bleed is more likely to be associated with clotting disorder.

Precipitating factors for bleeding: Spontaneous bleed, bleeding after minor trauma, after dental extraction, tonsillectomy may be indicative of bleeding/clotting disorder.

History of drug intake

- Intake of NSAIDs, aspirin can cause GI bleed/potentiate bleeding from other causes. Intake of oral anticoagulation is important while approaching bleeding disorders.
- Rule out renal and hepatic cause and hematological malignancy while evaluating a bleeding disorder.

Key Clinical Points in a Patient of Bleeding Disorder

- Menorrhagia and postpartum hemorrhage is common in a patient of bleeding disorder.
- Easy bruisability may not be always due to bleeding disorder. Cushing's syndrome, chronic steroid use, tissue abnormality like Ehlers-Danlos syndrome/senile purpura can cause easy bruisability.
- Hypertension and local nasal can cause spontaneous epistaxis.
- Bleeding into the joint results in severe pain, swelling and later joints become non-functional.
- Airway obstruction can occur due to oral and pharyngeal bleed. Bleeding into the retroperitoneal area and CNS bleed can be life-threatening.
- In a patient of thrombocytopenia spontaneous intracranial bleed can occur if the platelet count is less than 10,000 cells/cmm, and spontaneous bleed can occur with platelet count less than 50,000 cells/cmm. Platelet count above 80,000 cells/cmm is required for surgical procedures.

Examination of a Patient of Bleeding Disorder

Look for

- Severe pallor
  - May indicate massive internal bleed
  - Rule out renal/hepatic disease
  - Rule out hematological malignancy.

- Bleeding spots—look for petechiae, purpura, ecchymosis, subconjunctival bleed, ophthalmic fundal bleed and oral cavity bleed.

 Note

Oral bleed, ophthalmic fundal hemorrhage is more likely to be associated with intracranial bleed.

- Icterus—in a patient of bleeding disorder may be suggestive of liver disease or due to hemolysis of a clot.
- Lymphadenopathy—found in patients with hematological malignancy or systemic disease.
- Bone tenderness—may indicate hematological malignancy.
- Previous healed scars—suggest previous subcutaneous bleeding.
- Hemarthrosis/muscle hematoma—suggests major internal bleed.
- Hemothorax/ascites—due to major bleeding in coagulation disorder.
- Signs of liver/renal disease: Look for evidence of renal/liver disease as they can cause bleeding/clotting abnormality.
- Hepatosplenomegaly: Presence of hepatosplenomegaly may suggest hematological malignancy/liver disease/systemic cause of bleed.

Causes of Bleeding Disorder

Due to platelet abnormalities

Due to decreased survival of platelets

- Hepatitis virus/HIV virus
- ITP
- Systemic lupus erythematosus

Due to marrow abnormalities

- Due to vitamin B12 deficiency.
- Bone marrow aplasia
- Infiltration of the marrow by leukemia, malignancy.

Systemic causes of bleeding

- Acute/chronic liver disease
- Renal disease

- Multiple myeloma and other para proteinemia
- Amyloid deposition, e.g. in the gum.

Investigations for bleeding/clotting disorder

- Complete blood counts:
  - Hb% and total WBC count
  - Differential count
  - Platelet count
  - Platelet functional studies.
- Coagulation parameters:
  - Bleeding time
  - Prothrombin time
  - APTT
  - Fibrinogen levels
  - Peripheral smear
  - Estimation of coagulation factors
  - Estimation of inhibitors of coagulation.

Liver and Renal Function Tests

Bleeding disorders

- Due to decreased platelets:
  - Platelet count is decreased
  - Bleeding time is prolonged
- Due to vascular cause:
  - Normal platelet count
  - Prolonged bleeding time
- Due to platelet function abnormalities:
  - Normal platelet count
  - Platelet aggregation defect
- von Willebrand's disease
  - Prolonged BT and APTT
  - Normal platelet count
  - Decreased VW factor level
  - Restocetin cofactor activity is decreased
- Factor VIII level may be decreased

HESS test

- It is a test for capillary fragility.
- An area of 5 cm in diameter is marked over the skin of the forearm
- Sphygmomanometer cuff is applied to the arm above the area which is marked and cuff is inflated and blood pressure is maintained between systolic and diastolic pressure for 10 minutes.

- Count the number of petechiae in the area marked.
- If the number of petechiae is more than 15—it is abnormal indicating increased capillary fragility.

Coagulation Disorder

Features of congenital coagulation disorder

- Bleeding starts from younger age and will persist throughout life.
- There will be strong family history and male sex preponderance.
- Bleeding can occur spontaneously or following minor trauma.
- They may present as hematoma, hemarthrosis/hemothorax or retroperitoneal bleed.
- Bleeding does not stop spontaneously or by effect of pressure or can have rebleed.

Causes of coagulation disorder

- *Congenital*
  - Hemophilia A.
  - Hemophilia B (Christmas disease)
- *Acquired*:
  - Vitamin K deficiency
  - Liver disease
  - DIC.

Lab evaluation of coagulation disorder

Prolonged prothrombin time—with normal APTT

Due to deficiency of vit K dependent factors:
For example, factor VII deficiency

- Warfarin therapy
- Liver disease
- APLA syndrome
- Vitamin K deficiency

Prolonged APTT with normal PT

- Factor VIII and factor IX deficiency
- Factor XI deficiency
- Coagulation inhibitors
- von Willebrand's disease

Prolonged PT and APTT

- Liver disease

- DIC
- APLA syndrome

PT, APTT prolonged and decreased platelet: DIC.

Thrombosis

Risk factors for venous thrombosis

- Genetic predisposition
- Increase age
- Immobility
- Postsurgical
- Internal malignancy
- Hormonal supplementation
- Obesity
- Procoagulant states

Risk factors for arterial thrombosis

- Genetic predisposition
- Elderly age
- Diabetes mellitus
- Smoking
- Hypertension
- Hyperlipidemia
- Abdominal obesity

SPLENOMEGALY

Functions of Spleen

- Removal of RBCs—which are defective and after 120 days of RBCs life span.
- Clearing the bacteria which are coated with antibodies and also removal of blood cells which are coated with antibodies and clearing parasites.
- May play a role in immune response mechanism.
- Acts as a extramedullary site for hemopoesis.
- Pitting by spleen: Removes
  - Heinz bodies (denatured Hb)
  - Howell-Jolly bodies (nuclear residues and parasites)
- Culling by spleen: Clearing of dead and damaged cells.

Splenomegaly

Symptoms of Splenomegaly

- Fullness and feeling of heaviness in the left hypochondrium.
- Pain in the left hypochondrium
- Splenic pain is due to:
  - Stretch of capsule—acute enlargement of spleen
  - Inflammation of spleen
  - Occlusion of vessels—infarction, e.g. sickle cell anemia
- Rupture of spleen can occur due to trauma and very soft spleen can rupture—resulting in bleeding and shock (e.g. infectious mononucleosis).

Mechanisms of Splenomegaly

- Work hypertrophy
  - Hyperplasia of reticuloendothelial system
  - For example, hemolytic anemia
- Congestive splenomegaly:
  - Portal hypertension
  - CCF
  - Budd-Chiari syndrome.
- Due to infiltration of spleen:
  - Lymphoma
  - Metastasis
  - Bone marrow disorders like myeloproliferation
- Hyperplasia of spleen with immunological mechanism:
  - Connective tissue disorder—SLE
  - Systemic infection
  - Bacterial endocarditis

Disorders which mimic splenomegaly:

- Renal mass
- Pseudocyst of pancreas
- Colonic mass
- Gastric mass

Differential Diagnosis of Splenomegaly

Acute splenomegaly

- Acute attack of malaria
- Enteric fever

- Viral illness: Hepatitis, infectious mono-nucleosis
- Infective endocarditis.

Acute attack of malaria, enteric fever, viral hepatitis—*see* under hepatomegaly.

Infective endocarditis

- Preexisting cardiac lesion.
- Undergone invasive dental or urogenital procedure.
- History of fever
- Signs of infective endocarditis
- Splenomegaly—soft and may be tender
- Presence of cardiac murmur
- Blood culture positive for the organism
- Echo—demonstrates vegetations.

Chronic Splenomegaly

Causes

Moderate to massive splenomegaly

- Chronic malaria
- Chronic myeloid leukemia
- Cirrhosis of liver with portal hypertension
- Kala azar
- Myelofibrosis
- Hemolytic anemia
- Hairy cell leukemia
- Lymphoma—splenic cell

Chronic malaria/tropical splenomegaly syndrome

- Person is from endemic area of malaria (history of fever may not be present)
- Massive splenomegaly
- Increase lever of IgM
- Malarial parasite not detected in the peripheral smear (bone marrow may be positive).
- Sinusoidal lymphocytosis in the liver.

Chronic myeloid leukemia

- 4th to 5th decade of life
- Massive splenomegaly
- Very high WBC count (> 50,000 cells/cm)
- Peripheral smear shows very high WBC count with mature forms with predominant myelocytes and metamyelocytes (blasts are very few <5%).

- Bone marrow—increase myeloid series. Blasts <5%.
- Leucocytes alkaline phosphatase is decreased.
- Philadelphia chromosome (BCR-ABL positive.)

Portal hypertension

- Cirrhotic/non-cirrhotic
- Symptoms of hemetemesis/malena
- Associated symptoms of cirrhosis
- Signs of liver cell failure
- Splenomegaly
- Distended veins over the abdomen
- Ascites—in patients with cirrhosis
- In non-cirrhotic portal fibrosis—massive splenomegaly, dilated tortuous veins over the abdomen, no signs of liver cell failure.
- Ultrasound abdomen—splenomegaly with dilated portal veins.
- Upper GI endoscopy—oesophageal and gastric varices.

📝 *Note*

In extrahepatic portal hypertension like splenic vein thrombosis only gastric varices may be present.

In patients with portal hypertension spleen size can decrease after massive hemetemesis.

- Kala azar
  - From endemic area of leishmaniasis.
  - Fever, chills and rigors of long duration.
  - Massive splenomegaly
  - Lymphadenopathy may be present.
  - Dark pigmentation of skin.
  - Splenic aspiration/bone marrow demonstrates amastigotes of leishmania.

Myelofibrosis

- May not present with specific symptoms—occasionally fatigue.
- Night sweats may be present
- Massive splenomegaly.
- Blood counts—anemia with usually normal WBC and platelets count
- Peripheral smear—tear drop cells and leukoerythroblastic reaction

- Leukocyte—alkaline phosphatase is increased.
- Bone marrow—dry tap: Biopsy—hypercellular, increased marrow reticulins, large mega karyocytes
- JAK-2 mutation is present in the marrow cells.

Hemolytic anemia
- Long standing anemia with recurrent blood transfusions
- Presence of severe pallor and mild icterus: Splenomegaly
- Anemia, anisopoikilocytosis with typical pattern depending on the type of hemolytic anemia.
- Increased reticulocyte counts with increased LDH level
- Abnormal Hb electrophoresis
- Coombs' test positive in autoimmune hemolysis.

Hairy cell leukemia
- More common in males
- Splenomegaly
- Pancytopenia or very high count.
- Malignant cells appear to have hairy projections.
- Bone marrow shows fibrosis and infiltration by malignant cells.

Lymphoma—splenic cell/NHL
- Can present with splenomegaly, associated feature like fever, weight loss.
- Night sweats may or may not be present.
- Bone marrow/splenectomy will show evidence of malignant lymphocytes.

Polycythemia Vera
- Massively splenomegaly
- Evidence of polycythemia
- Hyperviscocity manifestations
- Manifestations with venous or arterial thrombosis
- Aquagenic pruritis
- All cell lines are increased
- JAK2 mutations positive

Causes of Hepatosplenomegaly with Jaundice

Acute
- Viral hepatitis, malaria, infective endocarditis, typhoid fever, etc.
- CCF.
- Acute Budd-Chiari syndrome

Chronic
- Infection: Chronic hepatitis.
- Disseminated TB, fungal infection, brucellosis, HIV infection, etc.
- Cirrhosis of liver with portal hypertension
- Chronic Budd-Chiari syndrome.
- Hepatic veno-occlusive disease.
- Hemolytic anemia
- Lymphomas

Hepatosplenomegaly with lymphadenopathy
- *Infectious disorders*
  - Acute viral hepatitis
  - Infectious mononucleosis
  - Disseminated tuberculosis
  - HIV infection
- *Systemic illness*
  - SLE
  - Sarcoidosis
  - Rheumatoid arthritis
- *Neoplastic disorder*
  - ALL
  - CLL
  - AML
  - Lymphomas
- *Drug induced*: Phenytoin sodium.

Fever with Hepatosplenomegaly

Causes
Acute
- Viral hepatitis
- Acute attack of malaria
- Typhoid fever
- Infective endocarditis
- Acute leukemia

Chronic
- Disseminated tuberculosis
- HIV with opportunistic infections
- Disseminated fungal infection
- Lymphomas

Splenectomy

Indications

- Diagnostic—for staging of lymphoma
- Therapeutic
  - ITP
  - Splenic rupture
  - Hypersplenism
  - Hairy cell leukemia
  - Prolymphocytic leukemia
  - Splenic marginal cell lymphoma
- Hemolytic disease = Hereditary spherocytosis.

Effect of splenectomy: Susceptible to infection with capsulated organisms: *Streptococcus pneumoniae* and *H. Influenzae*.

Hematological findings after splenectomy

- Presence of nucleated RBCs
- WBC and platelet count increase
- Presence of Howell-Jolly bodies (RBC nuclear remnant)
- Presence of Heinz bodies (denatured Hb)
- Before splenectomy—2 weeks before pneumococcal vaccine. Repeat after 5 years (conjugate vaccine). Vaccine against *H. influenzae, N. meningitides*. After splenectomy—person can contract babesiosis.

Indications for splenectomy in thalassemia major

- Patient has got symptoms/signs of hypersplenism.
- Patient has early satiety and effects of massive splenomegaly.
- Transfusion requirement increases by more than 50% compared to previous/or requirement is more than 200 to 220 ml/kg/yr compared to previous requirement.

Hypersplenism: Enlargement of spleen of any cause associated with pancytopenia with active bone marrow and pancytopenia is reversible after splenectomy.

Features

- Splenomegaly
- Pancytopenia
- Normal or active marrow.

Disseminated Intravascular Coagulation

Characteristics

- Formation of blood clots in the vascular system.
- Activation of coagulation process.
- Multi-organ dysfunction.
- Due to activation of coagulation process there will be depletion of clotting factors resulting in severe bleeding.

Conditions which cause DIC

- Infections—sepsis syndrome.
- Polytrauma especially head injury large aneurysms and hemangiomas.
- Pancreatitis and purpura fulminans.
- Severe mismatched transfusions and envenomation.
- Internal malignancy
- APLA syndrome
- Severe liver disease
- *Obstetric complications*
  - Eclampsia, HELLP syndrome, Amniotic fluid embolism, Abruptio
  - Placenta, retained dead fetus syndrome.

Acute DIC: Occurs in sepsis, trauma, envenomation, pancreatitis.

Chronic DIC: Occurs in internal malignancy, giant aneurysms, hemangiomas, chronic liver disease.

Additional factors which occur in DIC

- Fibrinolysis
- Release of inflammatory cytokines.

Clinical features

- Evidence of conditions associated
- Initially multiple sites of clotting
- Multiple sites of bleeding
- Hypotension and shock
- Multi-organ dysfunction.

Investigations

- Complete blood picture
- FDP level, D-dimer level (increased)
- Evacuation for the cause of DIC
- Usually there will be low platelets, abnormal bleeding parameters, schistocytes in the peripheral smear.

Approach to a Patient of Renal Disease

Evidences of Acute Renal Failure

- Acute onset of renal symptoms
- Absence of renal bone disease
- Rapid raise of urea and creatinine.
- Usually normal sized kidneys on ultrasound.

Evidences of Chronic Kidney Disease/ Failure

- Chronic renal symptoms.
- Associated with hypertension.
- Can have isosthenuria—low fixed specific gravity of urine (due to defective concentrating capacity of the kidney).
- Small shrunken kidneys on abdominal ultrasound (associated with thinning of renal cortex).

Evidences for Glomerular Disease

- Presence of proteinuria—usually massive (>1 gm/24 hours)
- Presence of dysmorphic RBCs and RBC casts in the urine.
- Usually associated with edema and hypertension.

Evidence of Nonglomerular
(Tubular Renal Disease)

- Proteinuria is usually not massive (<1 gm/ 24 hours).
- No RBC casts/dysmorphic RBCs in the urine.

- Edema and hypertension is usually less severe compared to glomerular disease.

ACUTE NEPHRITIC SYNDROME
Features

- Pedal edema and puffiness of face.
- Oliguria
- Hematuria
- Hypertension

Nephrotic Syndrome
Features

- Anasarca (generalized edema)
- Massive proteinuria
- 24 hours urine protein excretion >3.5 gm/ sq/m body surface area.
- Hypoalbuminemia.

Markers for Acute Kidney Injury (Failure)
Cystatin C

- Increased blood levels of cystatin C correlates with decrease of GFR.
- It belongs to cystatin protease inhibitors. It is filtered by the glomerulus and not absorbed back by the tubules.

Kidney Injury Molecule I (KIM I)

- Present in the cells of proximal tubules
- It has got phagocytic action.
- In extra renal disorders or without tubular pathology it is not found in the urine.

- Toxin mediated renal injury/or ischemic injury or in patients with cysplatin induced renal damage it is detected in the urine after a short duration.

Neutrophil Gelatinase Associated Lipocalin

- Detected in the urine/plasma after acute kidney injury.
- It is a neutrophilic protein and has got a protective effect on the proximal convoluted tubules.

Other biomarkers for kidney injury:
- Interleukin IL18.

Oliguria/Anuria

Oliguria: Less than 400 ml of urine is excreted/day.

Anuria: Less than 100 ml of urine is excreted/day.

Causes of Oliguria/Anuria

Renal Parenchymal Disease

- Rapidly progressive glomerulonephritis.
- Renal cortical necrosis.
- Acute tubular necrosis.

Renovascular Conditions

- Renal artery occlusion (can have mild proteinuria and hematuria).
- Renal vein occlusion (can have hematuria and massive proteinuria).

Extra renal conditions: Conditions associated with hypotension and shock.

 Note

Rule out urinary tract obstruction in all patients of oliguria/anuria.

POLYURIA

More than 3 liters of urine output per day.

Causes

- *Endocrine disorders*:
  - Diabetes mellitus

- Diabetes insipidus
- Hypercalcemia
- *Renal causes*:
  - Diuretic phase of acute renal failure
  - Long standing hypokalemia with nephropathy
  - Sudden release of urinary obstruction.
- *Drug induced*:
  - Treatment with diuretics
  - Administration of mannitol
- *Central causes*: Hypothalamic disorder.
- *Psychogenic-polydipsia*.

Proteinuria

Physiological

- *Protein excretion*: Normal person—less than 150 mg/day.
- *Urinary excretion of albumin*: Normal <30 mg/day.
- *Normally urine protein contains*: Tamm-Horsfall protein from the renal tubules.

Estimation of Proteinuria

Different Methods

- Early morning sample of urine is preferable.
- 24 hours urinary excretion of protein estimation:
  - There is difficulty in collection of the urine
  - Volume of urine depends on the urine output of the patient
- *Random sample of urine*: Calculate the urine albumin/urine creatinine—albumin/creatinine ratio correlates with micro albuminuria

Normal ratio:

    In females = 2.8 to 28 mg/m Mol
    In males = 2 to 20 mg/m Mol

Microalbuminuria

Microalbuminuria is defined as excretion of protein/24 hours in the urine >30–300 mg/24 hours

Or

Excretion of albumin/minute >20–200 microgram of albumin/minute.

Significance

Indicative of early glomerular disease (important in diabetic nephropathy)

- At this stage it is reversible with treatment with ACE inhibitors or angiotensin receptor blockers.
- There is a high risk of associated coronary artery disease in patients with diabetes mellitus with microalbuminuria.

Conditions associated with microalbuminuria

Physiological: Exercise

Pathological: Early diabetes mellitus with nephropathy

Essential hypertension

Early glomerulonephritis.

Different Types of Proteinuria

Tubular Proteinuria

- Occurs due to disorders of renal tubular system.
- Characteristics—usually less than 2 gm/day.
- Contains predominantly lower molecular weight proteins like beta 2 microglobulins.

Glomerular Proteinuria

- Occurs due to disease of the glomerulus.
- There will be leakage of plasma protein into the urine.

Characteristics of Glomerular Proteinuria

Usually persistent massive proteinuria (if <3.5 gm/24 hours—called massive proteinuria, if >3.5 gm/24 hours—called nephrotic range)

- Associated with hypertension.
- Associated with RBC casts/dysmorphic RBCs in the urine.
- Requires renal biopsy for confirmation of etiology of proteinuria.

 Note

Massive proteinuria causes foamy/frothy urine.

Transient Proteinuria

Characteristics

- Proteinuria is transient. Repeated testing of urine—proteinuria is absent.
- No RBCs, RBC casts or dysmorphic RBC in the urine.
- Proteinuria—minimal (usually less than 1 gm/day)
- Not associated with hypertension.

Causes:

Physiological: Vigorous exercise

Pathological: High grade fever

CCF

Orthostatic proteinuria.

Orthostatic Proteinuria (Only on Standing)

- Proteinuria is present on prolonged standing.
- Usually in the evening hours
- Minimal proteinuria—less than 1 gm/day.
- Hematuria and hypertension are absent with normal kidney function.

Overflow proteinuria: Significant amount of protein leaks into the urine. Tubules are not able to absorb the leaking protein resulting in proteinuria.

Conditions—causing overflow proteinuria:

Rhabdomyolysis: Myoglobin appears in the urine.

Multiple myeloma: Light chains in the urine.

Effect of overflow proteinuria:

- Toxic damage to the kidney
- Can cause acute tubular necrosis.

 Note

The term selective proteinuria is used when there is leakage of only albumin.

For example, minimal change disease causes selective excretion of albumin in the urine. When albumin excretion occurs along with other serum proteins, it is called non-selective proteinuria.

Effect of proteinuria:

- Cytotoxicity due to endothelial damage.
- Inflammatory response due to cytokine release.

Proteinuria can result in:

- Edema and anasarca as a result of hypo-albuminemia.
- Can predispose to bacterial infection including spontaneous bacterial peritonitis.
- Can be a procoagulant state and can result in renal vein thrombosis.
- Diabetes mellitus with microalbuminuria may be a predictor of coronary artery disease.
- Ultimate result of proteinuria—can cause fibrosis and sclerosis of glomerulus.

Evaluation of a patient of proteinuria: To rule out physiological/transient proteinuria and also orthostatic proteinuria.

Urine examination for proteinuria:

24 hours urine protein estimation

Or

Random urine sample for urine albumin/creatinine ratio, and

Detection of microalbuminuria.

Urine microscopy: For RBCs, RBC cast and dysmorphic RBCs—glomerular pathology.

Serum: Creatinine, albumin, cholesterol

ELISA: Hepatitis B, C and HIV infection. ANA, anti-DsDNA, and serum complement levels.

Serum protein electrophoresis.

Anti-GBM antibodies and ANCA titers.

Imaging studies in a patient of proteinuria:

- Ultrasound kidney size—for different renal pathologies.
- Cardiovascular evaluation for associated cardiac disease
- Chest X-ray for chest lesions like vasculitis
- CT abdomen-for different renal pathologies

Renal biopsy—for etiology of proteinuria.

COMMON CAUSES OF PROTEINURIA

Glomerular Causes

- Diabetic nephropathy.
- IgA nephropathy.
- Minimal change disease.
- Focal and segmental glomerulosclerosis
- Membranous glomerulonephritis.
- Amyloidosis

Proteinuria due to light chain excretion: Myeloma, lymphoma and amyloidosis.

HEMATURIA

Normal RBC content of the urine is 1 to 2/HPF.

Significant hematuria

If 3 samples of urine on different occasions show: 3–5 RBCs/HPF in a centrifuged sample of urine.

Or

Presence of frank blood/blood clots in the urine/more than 100 RBCs in the urine/HPF.

Isolated Hematuria

(Not Associated with Proteinuria/RBC Casts)

Causes of Isolated Hematuria

- Urogenital tuberculosis
- Ureteric/renal calculi
- Trauma to the urogenital tract
- Malignancy of the urogenital tract
- Inflammation of prostate.

 Note

Myoglobinuria can cause false positive test for hematuria.

Usually intrinsic disease of the kidney does not produce frank hematuria with blood clots.

Occasionally trauma to the urogenital system or viral infection can cause single attack of hematuria.

There can be gross hematuria in patients with IgA nephropathy/sickle cell disease.

Causes of microscopic hematuria (without glomerular disease)

Common causes	Rarer cause
Ureteric/renal calculi	Injury to renovascular system
Malignancy of urogenital system	Cystic disease of the kidney
Interstitial nephritis	
Papillary necrosis	

Approach to a Patient of Hematuria

Hematuria may be

- Painless/painful
- Transient/persistent
- Isolated/associated with proteinuria

Gross hematuria may manifest as

- Blood in the urine
- Smoky urine or tea-colored urine

Clinical evaluation of hematuria: Rule out menstrual bleed, transient viral illness, trauma and anticoagulant intake before further evaluation of hematuria.

Passage of frank blood/blood clots in the urine is usually of non-glomerular etiology of hematuria—occurs due to renal/ureteric calculus or urinary tract infection.

History of fever, pain while passing urine and frequency of micturition occurs in patients with UTI.

Abdominal trauma or trauma to the back is suggestive of traumatic cause of urogenital bleed.

Sore throat, skin infections prior to hematuria occurs in patients with post-streptococcal glomerulonephritis.

Polyarthritis, rash occurs in SLE/vasculitis/connective tissue disorder with glomerular involvement.

Abdominal mass, hematuria—possibility of polycystic kidney disease/renal malignancy.

IgA: Nephropathy can cause gross hematuria with proteinuria.

All patients with hematuria should be enquired about passing calculi in the urine, Bladder catheterisation, menstrual cycles, pulmonary hemorrhage, systemic bleed should be enquired to rule out respective disorders.

Carcinoma of urinary bladder can present as hematuria.

Enquire the family history of renal disease to rule out:

- Renal stones
- Polycystic kidney disease/collagen disease
- Alport's syndrome.

Investigations: for hematuria

- 3 samples of urine:
  - Urine for proteins—for glomerular disease
  - Urine for dysmorphic RBCs, RBC casts- for glomerular disease
  - Urine culture/sensitivity—for UTI
  - Urine for AFB—for renal tuberculosis
- Platelet count
- Coagulation parameters (BT, PT and APTT)
- Imaging of the kidney
- Cystoscopy
- Occasionally renal biopsy to rule out glomerular cause.

APPROACH TO A PATIENT OF PUFFINESS OF FACE AND PEDAL EDEMA

Disorders which present with puffiness of face with pedal edema.

Common causes

a. *Renal*: Acute glomerulonephritis
   Nephrotic syndrome
   Chronic renal failure.
b. *Cardiac*: Congestive cardiac failure.
c. *Hepatic*: Cirrhosis of liver (including chronic Budd-Chiari syndrome)
d. *Endocrinal*: Hypothyroidism/Cushing's syndrome.
e. Hypoalbuminemia—including nutritional.
f. *Drug induced*: Corticosteroids, NSAIDs, calcium channel blockers.

Note

Allergic angioedema can also present with puffiness of face with pedal edema.

Enquire the following history in a patient of puffiness of face and swelling of feet:

Puffiness of face—usually in the morning hours—characteristic of renal disease.
Swelling of feet—usually in the evening hours: In renal, hepatic and cardiac disorders.

Decrease of urine output—can occur due to:
- CCF
- Acute glomerulonephritis
- Late stages of CRF/cirrhosis.

Associated hematuria/smoky urine: Suggestive of acute glomerulonephritis. Distension of abdomen with jaundice may be suggestive of:
- CCF
- Cirrhosis of liver,
- Acute/chronic Budd-Chiari syndrome

Breathlessness, chest pain and palpitation in a patient of edema: Suggestive of cardiac disease.

Predominant abdominal distension, compared to swelling of feet: Present in cirrhosis of liver, constrictive pericarditis.

History of hemetemesis and malena: Cirrhosis of liver with portal hypertension.

Previous history of TB/pericardial disease: Possible constrictive pericarditis.

Intake of corticosteroids, NSAIDs, and calcium channel blockers—drug-induced edema.

History of constipation, cold intolerance, menstrual irregularities in female: Hypothyroidism.

History of abdominal distension, hirsutism, amenorrhea, hypertension and striae over the abdomen: Cushing's syndrome.

History of diabetes mellitus, hypertension, cardiac/renal disease: Can produce respective complications and edema.

History of alcoholism and previous history of jaundice: Suggestive of chronic liver disease.

History of decrease intake of protein and malabsorption: Suggestive of hypoproteinemia.

Differential Diagnosis of Puffiness of Face and Pedal Edema

Features of renal disease
- Early morning puffiness of face
- Swelling of feet—in the evening
- Hematuria/smoky urine
- Decrease urine output
- Hypertension

On examination
- Periorbital puffiness of face, pitting edema
- Hypertension (acute glomerulonephritis/CKD)
- Anasarca (nephrotic syndrome)
- Severe pallor with hypertension—CRF
- Palpable bilateral enlarged kidney—polycystic disease.

Features of cardiac disease
Breathlessness, PND, orthopnea, palpitation, chest pain and swelling of feet.
Signs
- Pitting pedal edema, later stages—puffiness of face
- Raised JVP (CCF/constrictive pericarditis)
- Pulse abnormalities
- Cardiomegaly, abnormal heart sounds/murmurs.

Features of hepatic disease
- Predominant abdominal distension
- Hematemesis/malena
- Jaundice
- Alcohol intake.
Signs
- Signs of liver cell failure
- Firm enlarged/shrunken liver
- Ascites
- Splenomegaly.

Features of hypothyroidism
- Periorbital puffiness of face
- Non-pitting edema

- Cold intolerance
- Menorrhagia
- Bradycardia
- Presence of goiter
- Delayed relaxing ankle jerk

Features of Cushing's syndrome
- Weight gain
- Moon face
  - Pigmented striae over the abdomen
  - Hirsutism
  - Buffalo hump
  - Abdominal distension
  - Hypertension and hyperglycemia

INVESTIGATIONS IN A PATIENT OF ACUTE RENAL FAILURE

Quantity of Urine

Oliguria
- Urine volume less than 400 ml/24 hours.
- Rule out urinary tract obstruction in all patients with decrease in the volume of urine.

Causes of oliguric renal failure
- Renal cortical necrosis
- Hypotension—septic shock
- Vasculitis syndrome
- Glomerulonephritis—proliferative form

Causes of non-oliguric acute renal failure
- Aminoglycoside nephrotoxicity
- Cisplatin-induced nephrotoxicity
- Acute tubulointerstitial nephritis.

Urine—smoky urine with renal failure
- Acute glomerulonephritis.
- Red-colored urine
  - Intravascular hemolysis
  - Rhabdomyolysis (no RBCs)

Proteinuria in acute kidney injury—usually minimal proteinuria

Massive proteinuria—indicates nephrotic syndrome as the cause for renal failure.

Urine Casts
- RBC casts and dysmorphic RBCs: Acute glomerulonephritis
- Hyaline casts—pre-renal azotemia
- WBC casts—interstitial nephritis
- Granular and epithelial casts—acute tubular necrosis

Large amount of uric acid in the urine: Tumor lysis syndrome.

Eosinophils in urine
- Interstitial nephritis
- Atherothrombotic disease.

Blood Tests

Blood urea and creatinine: Suggestive of acute/chronic renal failure

Blood urea and creatinine: Disproportionate rise of urea compared to creatinine—prerenal azotemia.

Complete blood counts and peripheral smear—severe Hb ↓↓: Hemolysis/hemolytic uremic syndrome

Increased WBC counts: Suggestive of sepsis

Thrombocytopenia: May be due to sepsis/DIC/thrombotic thrombocytopenic purpura (TTP).

Peripheral smear: May show the presence of schistocytes—suggestive of sepsis (microangiopathy).

TTP: Associated with ↓platelets, ↑LDH and schistocytes in the blood smear.

Tubular necrosis: ↑urea, ↑creatinine, ↑potassium↓, calcium and ↑phosphate.

Rhabdomyolysis: ↑CPK, ↑uric acid and ↑phosphate level.

In acute renal failure: There will be metabolic acidosis with increased anion gap.

Low anion gap with renal failure: Due to cationic proteins in myeloma.

In vasculitis: Measure ANA and ANCA titer

Urinary sodium: ↓urinary fractional sodium—prerenal azotemia (rarely it can occur due to early kidney injury in sepsis, muscle injury/due to radiation contrast).

In nephrotoxic/ischemic kidney injury—urinary sodium is ↑.

Imaging Studies

Ultrasound and CT Scan

- For ruling out post-renal obstruction.
- To make out kidney size: Shrunken kidney: In chronic renal disease.
- ARF with increased kidney size—can occur in acute interstitial nephritis.

Kidney Biopsy

Helps to know the underlying pathology—like acute/chronic kidney disease, glomerulo-nephritis, vasculitis and interstitial nephritis.

Biomarkers of Acute Kidney Injury

Cystatin C—correlates with decrease of GFR. KIMI—kidney injury molecule I: Increases in acute tubular injury.

Lipocalin-2 (neutrophil gelatinase associated lipocalin): Increases in acute kidney injury.

Features Favoring Chronic Renal Failure

- Small-sized kidneys
- Evidence of renal bone disease.
- Severe anemia.
- Gross serum calcium and phosphorous abnormality.

Significant Urea Increase without Raise of Creatinine Proportionately in a Patient of Renal Failure

- In prerenal renal failure
- Bleeding into the upper gastrointestinal tract
- Increased protein breakdown
- Corticosteroid administration.

Prerenal Renal Failure

- Urea significant increase without proportionate creatinine increase.
- Urine—no sediment
- Urine osmolality ↑ > 500 mOsm/kg.

Features of Contrast Nephropathy

- Urea and creatinine start increasing after 2–3 days of administrating contrast.
- Level significantly raises up to 5 days and start decreasing after about a week.

Measures to Prevent Contrast Nephropathy

- Adequate hydration—with normal saline
- Administration of N acetylcysteine
- Soda bicarbonate administration.
- Use of less amount of contrast dye.

Features of Renal Failure due to Toxins, e.g.: Aminoglycosides

- Causes non-oliguric renal failure
- Serum creatinine starts raising after about 3–5 days of drug administration and decreases by about 2 weeks.

Some Characteristic Laboratory Abnormalities in Renal Failure

Acute Renal Failure

- Urea and creatinine raised
- Normal size kidneys
- Can have decreased calcium and phosphate and increased potassium levels in the serum.
- Metabolic acidosis with increased anion gap.

Tumor Lysis Syndrome

- Acute renal failure
- Serum uric acid is increased
- Serum phosphate is increased (secondary tumor lysis)
- Serum phosphate is decreased (primary tumor lysis)
- Serum calcium is decreased.

Rhabdomyolysis

- Raised CPK levels.
- Raised phosphate levels.
- Decreased serum calcium levels with raised urea and creatinine.

Multiple Myeloma

- Raised urea, creatinine
- Raised serum calcium and uric acid levels.
- Anion gap is decreased—due to unmeasured cationic ions. Serum protein electrophoresis shows the presence of M band.

Chronic Renal Failure

- Hb%—severely decreased.
- Urea and creatinine is increased.
- Serum calcium is decreased.
- Serum potassium is increased.
- Serum phosphate is increased.
- Metabolic acidosis with increased anion gap.

Imaging Studies in a Patient of Renal Disease

Normal-sized kidney: Usually acute renal failure. Interstitial nephritis—can have increased kidney size.

Normal-sized/increased kidney size with chronic renal failure

- Diabetes mellitus
- Amyloidosis
- HIV nephropathy.
- Polycystic kidney disease.

Unilateral smooth shrunken kidney: Renal artery stenosis.

Bilaterally smooth shrunken kidney: Chronic glomerulonephritis.

Irregularly scarred kidney: Chronic pyelonephritis.

Unilaterally enlarged kidney

- Hydroureteronephrosis
- Renal tumors

ACUTE GLOMERULONEPHRITIS (AGN)

Acute glomerulonephritis results in a clinical condition called acute nephritic syndrome.

Features of Acute Nephritic Syndrome (AGN)

- Puffiness of face/pedal edema
- Oliguria

- Hematuria (smoky urine)
- Hypertension.

Causes of AGN

Common causes: Due to infection or post-infectious:

- Streptococcal infection—post-streptococcal glomerulonephritis.
- Viral infection
- Subacute bacterial endocarditis.
- SLE: Lupus nephritis
- IgA nephropathy.

Less common causes

- Vasculitis syndromes—ANCA mediated.
- Anti-GBM disease.
- Henoch-Schönlein purpura.
- Glomerulonephritis: Membrano proliferative/mesangio proliferative glomerulonephritis.

Other infective causes

- Schistosomiasis
- Malaria
- HIV infection
- Viral hepatitis B and C.

Approach to a patient of acute glomerulonephritis in general

Due to glomerulonephritis and associated fluid retention:

- History of puffiness of face and swelling of feet
- Decreased urine output
- Hematuria/smoky urine

Due to accelerated hypertension:

- Headache
- Convulsions (due to hypertensive encephalopathy)
- Dyspnea (due to left-sided cardiac failure)
- Vague pain in the back: Due to renal involvement.

History of Joint pain and rash: Possible SLE, vasculitis, Henoch-Schönlein purpura.

History of sore throat and skin infection 2–3 weeks before the onset of symptoms: S/O post-streptococcal—glomerulonephritis.

 Note

In patients with IgA nephropathy—symptoms of glomerulonephritis can appear along with strepto-coccal infection (synpharyngitic nephritis).

Past history of similar episodes: Not common in post-streptococcal glomerulonephritis.

On Examination: Observe for
- Puffiness of face
- Pitting pedal edema
- Throat examination for pharyngitis
- Skin examination for pyoderma lesions
- Polyarthritis/rash
- Hypertension
- Vague tenderness—renal angle.

Complications
- Accelerated hypertension with LVF.
- Accelerated hypertension with HT encephalopathy.
- Acute renal failure.
- Can cause chronic renal dysfunction.

Investigations
- Urine color (smoky) and output (decreased)/day.
- Proteinuria (usually <1 gm/day)
- RBCs, RBC casts, dysmorphic RBCs
- Throat swab/skin-culture sensitivity
- ASO titer
- C3, C4 levels
- Renal function tests
- ANA, anti-Ds DNA, ANCA.
- Anti-GBM antibody.
- US abdomen—for location of kidney and kidney size (if biopsy required).

🔑 *Key Points*: Acute glomerulonephritis (PSGN)
- Post-streptococcal glomerulonephritis can have pyuria. PSGN does not recur and usually does not cause renal failure in children.

- In acute glomerulonephritis—serum creatinine may not raise and raise very slowly—due to slow development of inflammation of glomerulus.
- Rapid raise of serum creatinine occurs in rapidly progressive glomerulonephritis which is characterized by glomerular crescent formation.

Post-Streptococcal Glomerulonephritis

🔑 *Key Points*
- Occurs after acute streptococcal infection either due to skin infection or pharyngitis.
- Infection occurs due to nephritogenic streptococci.
- AGN occurs after 2–3 weeks of streptococcal infection.
- Usual nephritogenic Streptococcal strains causing AGN-1, 2, 4, 3, 25, 47, 29, etc.

Pathogenesis and Pathology
Immune complex deposition—IgM, and complements C3, 4 in the glomerulus.

Antistreptococcal antibodies:
Increased titer of anti-streptolysin O antibody, anti-DNAse and anti-hyaluronidase antibody.
There will be infiltration of neutrophils with mesangial and endothelial cell hyper-cellularity.

Clinical Features
- Common in children—5–15 years.
- Can affect adults and elderly.

Symptoms: Puffiness of face and swelling of feet
- Oliguria
- Hematuria/smoky urine
- Headache, dyspnea and convulsions.
- Prior history of streptococcal infection—sore throat/skin infection 2–3 weeks prior to the onset of symptoms.

Signs: Periorbital puffiness
- Pitting pedal edema
- Hypertension.
- Evidence of skin infection (healed/active)
- Evidence of pharyngitis (may not be present).

Note

Pain in the renal angle occurs due to capsule of the kidney being stretched.

Complications: *See* under acute glomerulonephritis.

On investigations:
- Urine volume is decreased.
- Urine color—smoky/hematuria
- 24 hours urine protein excretion—less than 1–2 gm/day
- Presence of—RBCs, RBC casts and dysmorphic RBCs in the urine
- Dysmorphic RBCs: Occurs due to change in the osmolality and change in pH of the renal tubules
- Usually suggestive of glomerular disease. There will be destruction of glycocalyx of the RBCs in the glomerulus and RBCs undergo hemolysis in the tubules with loss of cytoskeletal proteins causing dysmorphic RBCs.
- Blood urea and creatinine may ↑
- Serum potassium may ↑
- Serum complement level C3 is ↓

Evidence of Streptococcal Infection
- ASO titer: >200 IU/ml
- Anti-streptococcal DNA level is raised
- Throat swab culture sensitivity for streptococci
- Skin (pyoderma lesions)—culture sensitivity for streptococci.

Follow-up
- In children—complete recovery within 3–6 weeks.
- Recurrence of PSGN—uncommon.
- Penicillin prophylaxis not required.
- In adults and elderly can develop renal failure and chronic renal disease.

Acute glomerulonephritis secondary to subacute bacterial endocarditis
- Can present as rapidly progressive glomerulonephritis

- Occurs due to immune mediated injury
- Due to emboli from the vegetation on the valves
- Appearance of kidney—flea bitten kidney.

Flea bitten kidney: Petechiae and infarct on the cortical surface of the kidney. Flea bitten kidney can occur in bacterial endocarditis, SLE, leukemia and lymphoma.

SLE Nephritis: Lupus Nephritis
- Features of active SLE and can cause acute renal failure.
- Hypertension, hematuria and massive proteinuria occur
- Urine shows RBCs and RBC casts
- Kidney biopsy diagnostic
- Anti-dsDNA positive.

Pathophysiology
- Cytokine activation with inflammation and cell infiltration.
- Immune complex deposition with activation of complements.
- If associated with APLA—microvascular thrombosis can occur.

Key Points: Treatment
- Active SLE nephritis (stage III and IV) requires corticosteroids and cyclophosphamide
- Stage I, II respond well to treatment
- Stage VI—glomerulosclerosis occur
- ACE inhibitors are indicated for proteinuria and hypertension.
- APLA positivity requires anticoagulation.

Anti-GBM Disease
- Presence of antibodies against glomerular basement membrane.
- If lung hemorrhage is associated: Goodpasture's syndrome.
- Can occur early/late in life.
- Fever, dyspnea and severe hemoptysis can occur.
- Smoking and infection—increases the risk for hemoptysis.

- Oliguria, hematuria and hypertension are the renal manifestations.
- Anti-GBM antibody will be positive and renal biopsy is required for confirmation.

Vasculitis and Renal Involvement

Occurs in patients with ANCA positive vasculitis granulomatosis with polyangiitis (Wegener's granulomatosis).

Features

- Respiratory—URT and LRT involvement
- Renal—massive proteinuria and hematuria
- CNS—mononeuritis multiplex
- ANCA positivity (PR3-ANCA positivity).

CHURG-STRAUSS SYNDROME

- ANCA positive vasculitis: Anti-MPO (anti-myeloperoxide antibodies) positivity
- Eosinophilia
- Asthmatic presentation
- Polyarthritis
- Focal segmental glomerulonephritis
- Small vessel vasculitis.

Microscopic Polyangiitis

- ANCA positive—anti-MPO antibodies
- Respiratory involvement—not significant
- Can have proteinuria and renal involvement
- Nongranulomatous vasculitis.

Membranoproliferative glomerulonephritis (Mesangiocapillary glomerulonephritis).

Features

- Hematuria, proteinuria and pyuria
- Renal biopsy confirmatory
- Types: Type I—idiopathic
- Hepatitis/malignancy related
- Types II and III—idiopathic

Pathology

- Proliferation of mesangium
- Thickening of glomerular basement membrane
- Lower serum C3 level

Mesangioproliferative Glomerulonephritis

- Immunologically mediated
- Occurrence of massive proteinuria resulting in renal failure.
- May be primary or secondary to SLE, falciparum malaria or IgA nephropathy.
- There will be deposit of IgM and C3
- *Treatment*: Steroids/immune suppression.

NEPHROTIC SYNDROME

Causes

Common Causes

- Minimal change glomerulonephritis
- Diabetic nephropathy
- Lupus nephritis
- FSGS
- IgA nephropathy.

Causes of Nephrotic Syndrome

Infective Causes

Malariae Malaria

- Hepatitis B/C
- HIV nephropathy
- Lepromatous leprosy.

Metabolic causes

- Diabetes mellitus
- Amyloidosis

Drug induced: Penicillamine and Gold.

Paraneoplastic: Lymphoma/myeloma

Primary glomerular disease

- Minimal change disease
- Membranous glomerulonephritis
- Membranoprolifetrative glomerulonephritis.
- Focal segmental glumerulosclerosis

Connective tissue disorders

- SLE
- Microscopic polyangiitis

APPROACH TO A PATIENT OF NEPHROTIC SYNDROME (In General)

Ask for the following history: History of puffiness of face, pedal edema, abdominal distension of longer duration with weight gain.

History of secondary causes
- Like diabetes mellitus
- Drug intake (*see* under causes)
- Joint pain, rash (SLE)
- History of fever, weight loss (lymphoma, HIV)
- History of jaundice (hepatitis B, C)

Previous history: Recurrent attacks of puffiness of face and pedal edema (responding to steroids—primary glomerular disease).

On Examination

Evidence of anasarca
- Periorbital edema
- Pedal edema
- Sacral edema
- Limb and abdominal wall edema
- Pleural effusion/ascites

Hypertension (not common in Patients of Minimal Change Glomerulonephritis)

Look for evidence for
- Diabetes mellitus
- SLE
- Other infectious causes including HIV.

Complications of nephrotic syndrome
- Hypercoagulable state and renal vein thrombosis
- Hypertension
- Bacterial infection
- Thyroid function abnormalities
- Hyperlipidemic complications
- End stage renal disease.

Investigations
- Urine examination for 24 hours protein excretion

- Urine—RBCs, RBC casts.
- Serum albumin level—low
- Serum cholesterol and triglycerides—high.
- Serum urea and creatinine.
- *For secondary causes*: Blood sugar, HBsAg, anti-HCV, HIV-ELISA, ANA, anti-dsDNA and ANCA
- Renal biopsy

🔑 *Key Points*: **Nephrotic syndrome**

1. Hypertension is not a feature of minimal change disease. Hypertension in a nephrotic syndrome is suggestive of other causes than minimal change disease.
2. Presence of RBCs, RBC casts suggest other causes of nephrotic syndrome rather than minimal change disease
3. Excellent response to corticosteroids is a feature of minimal change disease.
4. Diabetic nephropathy is a common cause of nephrotic syndrome in adults.
5. Development of renal failure is not a feature of minimal change disease.
6. Minimal change disease which is not responding to steroids—may be FSGS.

Mechanisms of proteinuria in nephrotic syndrome
- Fusion of foot process of glomerulus.
- Intraglomerular pressure increase with increase in pore size.
- Abnormality of basement membrane with alteration and disruption of slit diaphragm.
- Immune complex deposition causing glomerular basement membrane damage.

ANASARCA in nephrotic syndrome occurs due to massive proteinuria causing hypoalbuminemia.

Hyperlipidemia
- Due to loss of lipid regulatory proteins in the urine.
- Change in the hepatic lipid synthesis as a compensation for hypoalbuminemia.
- Decreased level of lipoprotein lipase.

Risk of infection: Due to loss of immunoglobulins in the urine.

Hypercoagulable state: Occurs due to
- Loss of anti-thrombin III in the urine
- Decrease of protein C and S
- Hyperfibrinogenemia
- Due to increased aggregation of platelets.

Minimal change disease
- Idiopathic
- Common in children
- Anasarca, massive proteinuria
- Less likely
  - hypertension
  - Renal failure
  - Microscopic hematuria
- Electron microscopy—kidney biopsy—foot process loss.
- Excellent response to steroids and a few patients may become steroid dependent.

Membranous glomerulonephritis: Common cause of nephrotic syndrome in elderly:
- Can be idiopathic or secondary to drugs, infections, SLE, paraneoplastic—*see* under causes.
- There will be glomerular basement membrane abnormality, immune complex deposition.
- Results in massive proteinuria, hypertension and renal vein thrombosis.
- Renal biopsy confirmatory and responds to immune suppression.

Focal and Segmental Glomerulosclerosis (FSGS)

Can be Primary or Secondary

Secondary causes
- Chronic liver disease
- HIV infection
- Alport's syndrome
- Lymphoma
- Sickle cell disease.
  Scarring of some glomeruli (focal) and part of some glomeruli (segmental).

Clinical Features

- Massive proteinuria
- Hypertension

- Progression to chronic renal failure
- Responds to corticosteroids
- Cyclosporin
- ACE inhibitors

IgA Nephropathy: Berger's Disease

- Commonest glomerular cause of proteinuria.
- Due to IgA deposition in the mesangium and is a form of immune complex nephritis.
- Can have episodes of hematuria.

Clinical Features

- Chronic microscopic hematuria (in all asymptomatic patients)
- Gross hematuria intermittent after URTI
- Associated proteinuria
- Can progress to renal failure
- Renal biopsy—diagnostic
- ACE inhibitors—indicated if proteinuria is present

Other causes of glomerular vascular involvement
- Vasculitis syndrome
- APLA syndrome
- Atherosclerosis with renovascular involvement.

Pulmonary and renal involvement
- *Causes*: Goodpasture's syndrome
- ANCA mediated vasculitis
- Mixed cryoglobulinemia
- Henoch-Schönlein purpura.

RENAL TUBULAR DEFECTS

Bartter Syndrome

Defect: Ascending loop of Henle.

Features
- Polyuria
- Hypokalemia
- Metabolic alkalosis
- Normal or low blood pressure

- Hypercalciuria
- Increased renin and aldasterone level.

Gitelman Syndrome

Defect: Distal convoluting tubule.

Features
- Hypokalemia
- Metabolic alkalosis
- Hypomagnesemia
- Low urinary calcium.
- Increased renin and angiotensin and aldosterone level
- Normal or low blood pressure.

Liddle Syndrome

Features
- Hypokalemia
- Metabolic alkalosis
- High blood pressure
- Low plasma renin and aldosterone level.

TUBULOINTERSTITIAL NEPHRITIS

Disorder of renal tubular structure and interstitium.

It may occur as acute or may be a chronic disorder.

Features of tubulointerstitial nephritis in general:
- Can result in acute/chronic renal failure
- Proteinuria is usually less than 2 gm/day
- Can have sterile pyuria
- No dysmorphic RBC/RBC cast in the urine
- Edema and hypertension is less compared to glomerular disease.

Acute Interstitial Nephritis

Causes

Infective: Bacterial, viral, leptospiral or rickettsial disorder.

Drug induced
- NSAIDs
- Diuretics
- Beta-lactamase inhibitors

Systemic disease
- SLE
- Sjögren's syndrome
- Tubulointerstitial nephritis with uveitis (TINU).
- Secondary to uric acid/light chain precipitation.

Clinical Features
- History of intake of drugs/fever due to infection.
- Symptoms appear after a few days to 1–2 weeks.
- Fever with urticarial rash if drug induced.
- Can have puffiness, pedal edema not as massive as glomerulonephritis.
- Hypertension and hematuria not common
- Results in acute kidney injury.
- Enlarged kidney on ultrasound—due to interstitial edema.

Investigations
- If drug-induced—blood eosinophilia
  Urine: No RBCs, or dysmorphic RBCs
  Sterile pyuria
  Eosinophils (if drug-induced)
  Proteinuria (<1–2 gm/day)
  Serum: Urea, creatinine↑

Ultrasound abdomen: Enlarged kidney—due to interstitial edema.

Chronic Interstitial Nephritis

Results in chronic renal dysfunction and CRF.

May be asymptomatic till late.

Causes

Common
- Chronic NSAID intake
- Chronic urinary tract obstruction
- Vesicoureteric reflux disease.

Less common
- Polycystic kidney disease
- Lithium therapy

- Chronic hypercalcemia and hyperuricemia
- Chronic glomerulonephritis.

Features

- Slowly progressive renal failure
- Polyuria (due to defective concentrating capacity of kidney)
- Proteinuria—usually less than 2 gm/24 hours.
- *Fanconi's syndrome*:
  - Glycosuria.
  - Phosphaturia

Investigations

Isosthenuria—low fixed specific gravity of urine.

- Sterile pyuria
- Serum urea and creatinine is increased
- *Ultrasound abdomen*: Small atrophic and scarred kidney.

ACUTE RENAL FAILURE (Acute Kidney Injury)

Characteristics

- Decrease of glomerular filtration rate occurs in a rapid manner.
- Decrease of GFR occurs when the glomerular perfusion pressure less than 80 mm of Hg systolic.
- There will be retention of salt and water with electrolyte and acid–base abnormalities with accumulation of nitrogenous waste products.

 Note

If ACE inhibitors are administered in a patient of bilateral renal artery stenosis, there will be severe decrease in the renal perfusion and decrease of GFR.

Causes of Acute Renal Failure

Common causes

- Acute gastroenteritis/massive GI bleed causing fluid loss.
- Sepsis and septic shock (malaria, leptospirosis).

- Drugs like NSAIDs/contrast dyes/ACE inhibitors.
- Aminoglycosides.

Less common causes

- Acute pancreatitis
- Rhabdomyolysis
- Burns
- Diuretic therapy
- CCF/cardiogenic shock
- Hepatorenal syndrome.

Mechanism of Acute Renal Failure

Prerenal

Occurs due to volume depletion causing decrease renal blood flow:

- No direct structural damage to the kidney.
- Reversible if the renal perfusion is re-established quickly.

 Note

Prolongation of prerenal state can cause acute tubular necrosis.

Factors which predispose to renal failure

- Elderly age
- Volume depletion
- NSAIDs—block the renal vasodilatory prostaglandins.
- ACE inhibitors/ARBs
  - Causes efferent arteriolar dilatation leading on to decreased GFR.
- Associated renovascular abnormality and atherosclerosis.

Clinical features of acute renal failure

- History and findings suggestive of volume depletion, shock.
- Intake of nephrotoxic drugs.
- Evidence of vasculitis/purpura
- Cardiac failure/cardiogenic shock.
- Evidence of rhabdomyolysis
- Distended bladder, hydronephrosis, mass lesion
  Can have symptoms and signs of:
  - Fluid retention.

- Electrolyte abnormalities—hyperkalemia
- Metabolic acidosis

Acute renal failure
- Early stage—few hours to few days.
  - Oliguria/anuria occurs in 1 to 5 days.
  - Renal injury 1–2 weeks.
- Diuretic phase
  - Significant diuresis
  - Regeneration of renal function occurs.

Conditions associated with anuria in a patient of acute renal failure

Due to cortical necrosis
- Occlusion of renal vessels.
- Shock, severe sepsis and severe ischemia.
- Rapidly progressive glomerulonephritis.

Conditions causing urine output not significantly decreased in acute renal failure
- Diuretic phase of ARF
- Aminoglycoside induced
- Tubulointerstitial damage
- Long standing renal disease causing nephrogenic diabetes insipidus.

Intrinsic renal disease causes acute renal failure due to
- Prolonged ischemia due to decreased renal blood flow
- Sepsis and septic shock
- Drugs and toxins
- Acute post-streptococcal glomerulonephritis and acute interstitial nephritis.

Sepsis
- Causes direct tubular damage.
- Causes hypotension, peripheral vasodilation and shock.

Ischemia causing acute renal failure
- Due to decrease renal perfusion of any cause
- For example, volume depletion of any cause
- Major surgeries

- Microvascular thrombosis: TTP, APLA syndrome.

Drugs and toxins: Concentration of drugs and toxins in the kidney causing parenchymal damage.

Different drugs and toxins causing renal damage

Nephrotoxic drugs	Toxins
• Aminoglycosides	Uric acid
• Vancomycin	Myoglobin
• Amphotericin B	Hemoglobin
• Cisplatin	Light chain
• Contrast agent	precipitation

Postrenal—renal failure
- Obstructive uropathy
- Bladder neck obstruction
- Calculus obstruction
- Papillary necrosis
- Uric acid induced obstruction.

Acute Tubular Necrosis

Occurs due to
- Acute intrinsic disease of the kidney (*see* under renal causes)
- Prolonged ischemia, hypotension
- Drugs and toxins.

There will be damage to the intrinsic renal structures.

Features: See under clinical features and different acute renal failure stages.

Complications of Acute Renal Failure

Due to metabolic abnormality
- Accumulation of urea and creatinine
- Hyperkalemia
- Metabolic acidosis

Due to retention of salt and water
- Sodium and water retention
- CCF

Prone to develop—GI bleed
- Pericarditis
- Systemic infection.

DIABETIC NEPHROPATHY

Clinical Aspects

Uncontrolled blood sugars result in diabetic nephropathy.

Diabetic nephropathy is a leading cause of chronic renal failure.

Type 2 diabetes mellitus can present with nephropathy at the time of diagnosis and can have associated hypertension, hyperlipidemia, obstructive uropathy, infection of the urinary tract as additional factors affecting the renal function.

ACE inhibitors/angiotensin receptor blockers are beneficial in patients with microalbuminuria.

Retinopathy always exists with nephropathy (80%).

Risk factors for the development of diabetic nephropathy

- Uncontrolled hyperglycemia
- Uncontrolled hypertension.
- Family history of diabetic nephropathy
- Hyperlipidemia
- Smoking.

🔑 **Key Points:**

- Diabetic nephropathy can have massive proteinuria even in the range of more than 10–20 gm/day.
- Microalbuminuria can lead to chronic renal failure (ESRD) after about 5–10 years after its development.
- End stage renal disease occurs with uncontrolled diabetes mellitus about 15–20 years after its initial diagnosis.

Pathological changes in the kidney like nodular glomerulosclerosis and Kimmelstiel-Wilson disease are more likely to be associated with nephropathy

- Coronary artery disease and cardiovascular events are likely to be associated with microalbuminuria.
- Smoking causes rapid deterioration in kidney function in patients with diabetic nephropathy.

- Adynamic bone disease is more likely to be associated with diabetic nephropathy.

Pathogenesis

Main factors responsible for changes in the kidney in diabetes mellitus

- Intraglomerular hypertension, hyperfiltration.
- Hyperglycemia
- Angiotensin II
- Lipid abnormalities

Other factors

- Advanced glycation end products
- Growth hormone
- Atrial natriuretic factor
- Insulin-like growth factor

Above factors can result in

- Alteration in the glomerular basement membrane and filtration barrier.
- Changes in the renal mesangial cells and vascular smooth muscle cells with increase in the matrix.
- End result is glomerulosclerosis

Factors which decrease the progress of renal involvement in diabetes mellitus

- Control of hypertension
- Control of lipid abnormality
- Control of hyperglycemia
- Stopping smoking.

Factors which can decrease proteinuria

- Use of ACE inhibitors/ARBs/calcium channel blockers
- Decrease of protein intake.

Factors which are important in treatment of diabetic nephropathy

Renal involvement in adult—diabetes mellitus can also be associated with

- Urinary tract infection
- Obstruction to the urine flow
  - Strictures
  - Calculus
  - BPH
- Nephrotoxic drugs including contrast dyes.

Pathological Changes in Diabetic Nephropathy

- Glomerular basement membrane thickening
- Changes in the electrical charge of filtration barrier (leads on to albuminuria)
- Diffuse and nodular glomerulosclerosis (Kimmelstiel-Wilson bodies)
- Changes in the vascular smooth muscle cells
- Glomerulosclerosis and tubulointerstitial changes
- Normal-sized kidney.

Stages in the Development of Diabetic Nephropathy

Stage 1
- Patient is clinically normal
- Glomerular hyperfiltration with increased GFR
- Increase in the size of the kidney.

Stage II
- Proteinuria can occur due to severe exertion
- Thickening of glomerular basement membrane with mesangial expansion
- Increase in the size of the kidney.

Stage III
- Presence of microalbuminuria
- May be associated with hypertension.

Stage IV
- Deteriorating renal function
- Massive proteinuria
- High blood pressure

Stage V: End stage renal disease.

Renal involvement in a diabetic without nephropathy

Due to:
- Upper or lower UTI
- Obstructive uropathy
- Drug/toxin mediated renal disease
- Vesicoureteric reflux

Therapeutic aspects
Role of ACE inhibitors/ARBs in diabetes mellitus and nephropathy:

- ARBS/ACE inhibitors decrease intraglomerular hypertension (cause efferent arteriolar dilatation)
- Decreases systolic blood pressure
- Decreases proteinuria.

 Note

Combination of ACE inhibitors and ARBs is associated with more renal complications.

ACE inhibitors/ARBS are also helpful in nondiabetic proteinuria.

Other Therapeutic Aspects of Diabetic Nephropathy

- ARBS/ACE inhibitors/diltiazem can decrease proteinuria.
- Maintain blood pressure—around 130/80 mm of Hg.
- Restriction of protein intake to 0.8 gm/kg/day in the presence of proteinuria.
- Patients with diabetic nephropathy can have hyperkalemia due to the development of type IV renal tubular acidosis.

 Note

Associated autonomic neuropathy can result in severe hypotension during dialysis in patients of diabetes mellitus.

- Smoking exacerbates diabetic nephropathy.

Follow-up
- In all diabetes yearly evaluation and testing for microalbuminuria is recommended
- Rule out other causes of proteinuria
- If microalbuminuria is present
  - Repeat the test after 2–3 months
  - Repeat 3 times before establishing proteinuria.

URINARY TRACT INFECTION (UTI)

Common Organisms Causing UTI
Commonest organism: E. coli

Other gram negative organisms:
- Klebsiella
- Pseudomonas

- Proteus
- Acinetobacter
- *Staphylococcus saprophyticus*
- *Candida albicans*
- *Staphylococcus aureus.*

Predisposing Factors for UTI

- Genetic susceptibility
- Urinary tract obstruction:
  - Calculi
  - Stricture
  - BPH
- Vaginal colonization and sexual intercourse
- Anatomical abnormality of the urinary tract
- Vesicoureteric reflux
- Bladder catheterization or foreign body
- Residual urine—neurogenic bladder
- Host factor—like diabetes mellitus.

Clinical features

- Upper UTI: Pyelitis/pyelonephritis.
- Lower UTI: Cystitis, urethritis, prostatitis

Uncomplicated UTI

- In patients without instrumentation of urinary tract
- No anatomical abnormality of the urinary tract.
- Female UTI without pregnancy

Complicated UTI: All UTI except mentioned under uncomplicated UTI.

Clinical features

Asymptomatic bacteriuria:
- No symptoms of UTI
- Bacteriuria is present

Significant bacteriuria: Presence of >10^5 bacteria-colony forming units/ml of urine (midstream sample).

Cystitis

- Infection of the urinary bladder
- Suprapubic pain
- Urinary frequency, urgency and discomfort.
- Fever, hematuria may be present

Urethritis

- Infection of the urethra
- Frequency, dysuria and urgency

Acute pyelitis/pyelonephritis

- Acute infection of the kidney and renal pelvis
- Fever with chills/rigors
- Flank pain
- Vomiting
- Tenderness at renal angle.

Chronic pyelonephritis

- Chronic infection of the kidney
- Common with urinary tract obstruction.

Prostatitis

- Infection of the prostate gland.
- Acute or chronic
- Fever with chills/rigors
- Pain in the pelvic or perineal area.
- Urinary frequency/dysuria

Chronic prostatitis: Presents as chronic pelvic pain.

Investigations

- Urine dip stick test
- Urine—nitrite test (nitrate to nitrite conversion by bacteria)
- Urine—microscopy for pus cells and gram stain
- Urine—culture and sensitivity.

Significant bacteriuria, see above.
Significant bacteriuria for catheterized patient:
- UTI >10^2/ml of urine—colony forming units.
- Patients of UTI require gynecological and urological evaluation and to rule out host factors like diabetes mellitus.

Causes of sterile pyuria (presence of pus cells but urine culture is negative)
- Partially treated UTI.
- Atypical organisms causing UTI (e.g. mycoplasma infection)
- Urogenital tuberculosis
- Papillary necrosis
- Interstitial nephritis
- Rarely tumor/calculi in the urinary bladder

POLYCYSTIC KIDNEY DISEASE

Polycystic kidney occurs due to genetic damage to the tubular growth and development.

2 types of polycystic kidney disease:
- Autosomal dominant type
- Autosomal recessive type

Autosomal Dominant Type

Features

- Positive family history of polycystic renal disease.
- Bilateral enlarged kidneys
- Associated with hypertension in the young.
- Age of presentation 30–50 years.

Associated complications and presentations

- Back pain due to infection of the cyst (gram-negative bacilli)
- Bleeding into the cyst
- Calculi formation
- Secondary hypertension
- Risk for renal cell carcinoma
- Progression to renal failure.

Other systemic involvement

- Hepatic cysts
- Cardiac abnormality
- Hypertension (stimulation of RA axis)
- MVP
- Aortic and tricuspid valve abnormality
- Intracranial aneurysm

Diagnosis

Imaging study

- Ultrasound
- CT scan or
- MRI

Diagnostic criteria for polycystic kidney disease

- 15–29 years of age—at least 2 cysts in one kidney or both kidneys.
- 30–59 years of age: In each kidney at least 2 cysts.
- >60 years age of—4 cysts in each kidney.

Genetic testing—for the gene mutation in PKD1 and PKD2 gene.

Autosomal recessive polycystic kidney disease

- In pediatric age group
- Associated with hepatic fibrosis.

RENAL HYPERTENSION

One of the Common Causes of Secondary Hypertension

Renal Causes of Hypertension

Renal parenchymal disease

- Acute glomerulonephritis
- Chronic glomerulonephritis
- Chronic interstitial nephritis
- Polycystic kidney disease
- Renal tumors—including rennin producing tumors.

Renovascular hypertension
Renal artery disease

- Fibromuscular dysplasia
- Atherosclerosis.

Approach to a Patient of Renal Hypertension

Renal parenchymal disease

Acute and chronic glomerulonephritis: Present as puffiness of face, pedal edema and hypertension-associated with proteinuria, RBC casts and dysmorphic RBCs.

Chronic interstitial nephritis

- History of taking long-term analgesics
- Minimal proteinuria.
- Pyuria
- No RBC casts in the urine.

Polycystic kidney disease

- Positive family history
- Bilateral palpable renal masses.

Renal tumors—can present as hematuria, palpable renal masses.

Renin secreting tumors: Presents as hypertension and high serum rennin level.

RENOVASCULAR HYPERTENSION

Renal artery stenosis can occur with atherosclerosis/fibromuscular dysplasia.

Atherosclerosis

- Elderly age group.
- Can be unilateral or bilateral
- Thickened peripheral arteries.

Fibromuscular Dysplasia

- Bilateral involvement
- Female preponderance with younger age group.

Renin angiotensin mechanism plays a major role in the pathogenesis of renovascular hypertension.

Suspect renal artery disease if:
- There is sudden increase of blood pressure.
- Flash pulmonary edema
- Recent deterioration in renal function.
- If bilateral renal artery disease administration of ACE inhibitors will precipitate renal failure.
- Presence of bruit at renal angle (prolonged bruit suggests significant renal artery stenosis).

Investigations of Renal Artery Disease

- Doppler study of renal artery
- MR angiography
- CT contrast angiography
- Renal vein renin study (renin level is increased on the ischemic kidney side).
- *Captopril renography*: Technitium mercaptoacetyl triglycine scan (MAG3) after captopril: Uptake is reduced on the affected side.

🔑 *Key Points*: **Regarding renal artery stenosis**

- Elderly and patients with atherosclerosis may have some degree of stenosis of renal artery and may not be clinically significant.
- Significant renal insufficiency with non-functioning kidney on the affected side—repair of the renal artery stenosis on the affected side not beneficial.

Renal Bone Disease (Renal Osteodystrophy)

Types

- Osteomalacia

- Osteitis fibrosa cystica
- Adynamic bone disease
- Soft tissue calcification

Pathogenesis of Renal Bone Disease

Occurs usually in chronic renal disease.

Renal disease with decreased GFR → decreased phosphate excretion—hyperphosphatemia.

Hyperphosphatemia results in:
- Synthesis of FGF 23 by the osteophytes.
- Increased PTH production

CKD results in decreased ionic calcium level due to renal failure and FGF-23 causing decreased vitamin D_3 production.

FGF-23 is also a risk for LVH.

Secondary hyperparathyroidism causes osteitis fibrosa cystica.

Adynamic Bone Disease

Occurs due to decreased mineralisation of bone—as a result of suppression of PTH production.

Suppression of PTH can occur due to:
- Administration of phosphate binders containing calcium.
- Vitamin D administration.

Adynamic bone disease causes bone pain, fractures and calcification of blood vessels and heart.

It can also result in soft tissue calcification.

Adynamic bone disease is more likely to be associated with diabetic nephropathy.

Calciphylaxis

What is calciphylaxis: Deposition of calcium in the small blood vessels of the skin tissue and fat.

Conditions associated: CKD, may be on dialysis/transplant.

Manifestations: Painful ulcers—non-healing and secondary infection.

Risk factors: Diabetes mellitus, abnormal calcium metabolism, uremia, warfarin therapy.

Connective Tissue Disorder

APPROACH TO POLYARTHRITIS

Causes of Polyarthritis

- Rheumatic fever
- Rheumatoid arthritis
- Reactive arthritis
- Psoriatic arthritis
- SLE.

Acute onset of Polyarthritis

- Viral arthritis
- Rheumatic fever
- Reactive arthritis

Chronic Polyarthritis

- Rheumatoid arthritis
- Seronegative arthritis
- SLE
- Osteoarthritis.

Asymmetrical Polyarthritis

- Acute onset: Rheumatic fever
- Chronic—occasionally seronegative arthritis
- Sarcoidosis.

Symmetrical Polyarthritis

Acute

- Viral polyarthritis
- Serum sickness syndrome

Chronic

- Rheumatoid arthritis
- Seronegative arthritis
- SLE.

Arthritis Which Presents as Low Back Pain (Involving Axial Skeleton)

- Seronegative spondarthritides
- Tuberculosis of spine
- Brucellosis involving the spine.

Acute Onset of Monoarthritis

- Hemarthrosis: Gouty arthritis
- Rare-psoriatic arthritis: Septic arthritis
- Erythema nodosum: Trauma to the joint

Chronic Monoarthritis

- Osteoarthritis
- Palindromic rheumatism
- Psoriatic arthritis.

Approach to a Patient of Musculoskeletal Pain

Disorders which Present Predominantly as Muscular Pain

Musculoskeletal disorders

- Polymyalgia rheumatica
- Seronegative arthritis
- Polymyositis
- Osteomalacia
- Fibromyalgia

Endocrine disorders

- Hypothyroidism
- Hyperparathyroidism

Drug induced—HMG-CoA reductase inhibitors. Rarely Parkinson's disease.

Approach to a Patient of Polyarthritis

Arthritis—Depending on the Age of Onset

Younger age
- Rheumatic fever
- Viral
- Reactive arthritis

3rd decade to middle age
- Seropositive arthritis (rheumatoid arthritis)
- Evidence of—degenerative arthritis—osteo-arthritis.
- After 50 years: Polymyalgia rheumatica.

Sexual variation with arthritis
- More common in males
  - Ankylosing spondylitis
  - Gout
- More common in females
  - Rheumatoid arthritis
  - SLE

Arthritis with strong family history
- Gouty arthritis
- Ankylosing spondylitis

Joint involvement not due to inflammatory cause
- Acromegaly
- Hemochromatosis
- Hypertrophic osteoarthropathy

Arthritis with predominant upper extremity involvement: Rheumatoid arthritis/osteo-arthritis.

Arthritis with predominant lower extremity involvement: Osteoarthritis, gout, reactive arthritis.

Significance of systemic involvement in a patient of arthritis

Fever
- Infective arthritis
- SLE
- Rheumatoid arthritis
- Vasculitis

Muscle weakness
- Polymyositis
- Mononeuritis multiplex
- Vasculitis

Weight loss: Chronic arthritis

Muscle pain
- Polymyositis
- Statins
- Fibromyalgia

Associated with rash
- SLE
- Dermatomyositis
- Still's disease
- Rheumatic fever
- Psoriasis.

Renal involvement
- SLE
- Rheumatoid arthritis
- Systemic sclerosis
- Gout
- Vasculitis

Carpal tunnel syndrome: Rheumatoid arthritis.

Consider following disorders which may cause severe bony pain mimic joint disease
- Acute leukemia
- Myeloma
- Bony malignancy
- Osteomalacia
- Osteoporosis with fracture
- Scurvy

Musculoskeletal disorder with disturbed night sleep
- Septic arthritis
- Gout
- Fibromyalgia
- Occasionally rheumatic fever/tubercular arthritis.

Approach to a patient of arthritis depending on the joint involvement
- *Proximal interphalangeal joint*
  - Rheumatoid arthritis
  - Reactive arthritis
  - Psoriatic arthritis
- *Distal interphalangeal joint*
  - Reactive arthritis
  - Psoriatic arthritis
  - Osteoarthritis.

- *Wrists predominantly involved*: Possible rheumatoid arthritis.

Arthritis: Involving lower extremity joints
- Seronegative arthritis
- Osteoarthritis.

Arthritis—with metatarsophalangeal joint involvement: Gout.

Arthritis with low back pain with sacroiliitis: Seronegative arthritis.

Causes of Pain in the Back

Intervertebral disc prolapse.

Mechanical causes
- Spondylitis
- Spondylolisthesis
- Fracture of vertebra
- Sacroiliitis

Features of mechanical back pain
- No systemic symptoms
- Sudden onset of pain
- Increases on changing posture like bending
- There is no neurological deficit

Disorders which predominantly present as pain in the hip and knee

Hip pain
- Bursitis of hip—trochanteric bursitis
- Fracture femoral neck
- Avascular necrosis of femur

Pain in the knee
- Prepatellar bursitis
- Popliteal cyst.

Causes of pain in the neck

Common causes
- Cervical spondylosis
- Trauma to the neck
- Intervertebral disc prolapse

Rare causes
- Rheumatoid arthritis
- Osteoporosis

Very rare
- Pharynx pain
- Angina
- Pancoast tumor

Causes of pain in the shoulder
- Supraspinatus tendinitis
- Rotator cuff tendinitis
- Referred pain from gallbladder (right side)
- Referred pain form Pancoast tumor
- Bicepital tendinitis.

Causes of pain in the elbow
- Due to arthritis of elbow joint.
- Pain at the lateral epicondyle: Tennis elbow
- Pain at medial epicondyle: Golfer's elbow.

Wrist involvement
- Rheumatoid arthritis
- C8-T1 radiculopathy
- Juvenile chronic arthritis
- Carpal tunnel syndrome.

Disorders which cause ankle and foot pain
- Plantar fasciitis
- Tendoachilitis
- Subcalcaneal bursitis.

Pain in the back with root pain: Features of root pain—already discussed.

Consider: Neurological involvement in a patient of root pain like cauda equina syndrome.

Features of back pain which suggest dangerous pathology
- Systemic symptoms like fever and weight loss.
- Progressive pain with neurological deficit.
- Extremes of ages.
- Multiple root involvement.
- Spinal tenderness and deformity.

Examination of a Joint

Key Points
- Restriction of joint movement limited to one plane alone is usually suggestive of lesion of periarticular lesion.
- Disorder of the joint usually causes restriction of movement in all directions.
- Increased mobility of the joint may be due to either hypermobility of the joint or joint instability.

Important Clinical Points While Examining the Joint

- Lesion of intraarticular structures produces tenderness over the joint line.
- Lesion of periarticular structures produces tenderness over the periarticular area.
- Swelling of the joint occurs due to:
  - increased synovial fluid accumulation (fluctuating)
  - swelling of soft tissues (not fluctuating)
- Crepitus—coarse sounds produced by damage to the articular cartilage.
- Fine crepitus—occurs due to bursitis.

Pain of musculoskeletal disorders

- Pain of inflammatory arthritis
  - pain is more in the morning/on taking rest
  - relieved by physical activity.
- Mechanical joint pain—increases on movement, decreases by rest.
- Bony pain
  - Rest pain
  - More at night
  - Not related to movement.

Synovial Fluid Analysis

Normal synovial fluid

- Color—clear or straw colored
- Viscocity—high (due to hyaluronic acid)
- Cells—few RBCs and WBCs

Analysis of synovial fluid

- Red colored fluid—presence of blood
- Fluid viscosity is decreased—inflammatory
- Cloudy synovial fluid—presence of bacteria, WBCs, crystals
- Protein in synovial fluid—increased in inflammation.
- Glucose in synovial fluid—very low glucose level in infection and inflammation
- Normal synovial fluid glucose is slightly lower than blood glucose
- Crystals in synovial fluid—due to the presence of uric acid (gouty arthritis) and calcium pyrophosphate arthropathy—pseudogout.
- Cells in the synovial fluid—increased number of WBCs—infection/inflammation. Eosinophils in synovial fluid—parasitic infection.

Synovial fluid in inflammatory arthritis

- Cloudy
- Yellow
- Low viscocity
- Cells—2000 to 50000 cells/cmm

Septic arthritis

- Fluid opaque
- Cells: >50000 cells/cmm
- Neutrophils >70%
- Fluid glucose is markedly decreased.

Hemorrhagic synovial fluid

- Hemophilia
- Trauma
- Malignant disorders
- Synovial fluid in degenerative arthritis is noninflammatory.
- Synovial fluid in crystal-induced arthritis shows presence of monosodium urate crystals.

C-Reactive Protein

- Substance which reflects inflammatory changes.
- Produced by the liver in response to inflammation

Conditions associated with increased CRP

- *Septic conditions*
  - Tuberculosis
  - Pneumonia
  - Osteomyelitis
- Physiological conditions—pregnancy
- Cardiovascular disease—IHD.
- Metabolic disorders: Diabetes mellitus type 2
- Connective tissue disorder—SLE-rheumatoid arthritis.
- Malignant disorders—carcinoma/lymphoma
- CRP—normal 3 to 5 mg/dl

Hs CRP—highly sensitive CRP

Measures the level of CRP up to 0.3 mg/dl. Detects low levels of inflammation.

Importance: Atherosclerosis is a state of inflammation. Detection of Hs CRP is indicative of inflammation. So detection of Hs CRP in addition to lipid profile may predict the future risk of cardiovascular and cerebrovascular disease like myocardial infarction and CVA and peripheral vascular disease.

Conditions associated with increased CPK

- Infections: Myositis/vasculitis
- Drugs and toxins:
  - Statins
  - Alcohol
- Muscle trauma and vigorous exercise.
- Metabolic: Hypothyroidism
- Inflammatory: Polymyositis
- Degenerative: Muscular dystrophy.

RHEUMATOID ARTHRITIS

Features

- Inflammatory polyarthritis
- Chronic disease
- Can have exacerbations and remissions
- Presence of deformities
- Systemic involvement.

Pathophysiology

Following factors may play a role in the pathogenesis of rheumatoid arthritis

- Genetic factor with HLA association (HLA DR4 and DR1)
- Infection with streptococci/Epstein-Barr virus
- Immunoglobulins, cytokines and TNF-α play the role.
- Chronic smoking
- Autoimmune mechanisms involving CD4 cells.
- Interaction between genetic susceptibility and environmental factors play a role in the genesis of rheumatoid arthritis.

Pathology

- Joint with inflammatory infiltration (inflammatory granulation tissue)
- Pannus formation
- Synovitis
- Damage to articular cartilage
- Bone erosion.

Clinical Features

- Female > male.
- Symmetrical polyarthritis starting from smaller joints (proximal interphalangeal joints).
- Morning stiffness for more than 1 hour decreasing with physical activity.
- Most commonly affected joints:
  - Proximal interphalangeal joint
  - Meta carpophalangeal joint
  - Wrist joint
- Knee, ankle and metatarsophalangeal joints also get involved. Knee joint synovitis can cause popliteal cyst (Barker's cyst).
- Less commonly involved: Sacral and thoracic spine.
- Cervical spine involvement: Atlantoaxial joint—can cause cervical myelopathy.
- Chronic disease—produces deformities:
  - Splindling of interphalangeal joints
  - Ulnar deviation of wrist
  - Swan neck deformity of finger

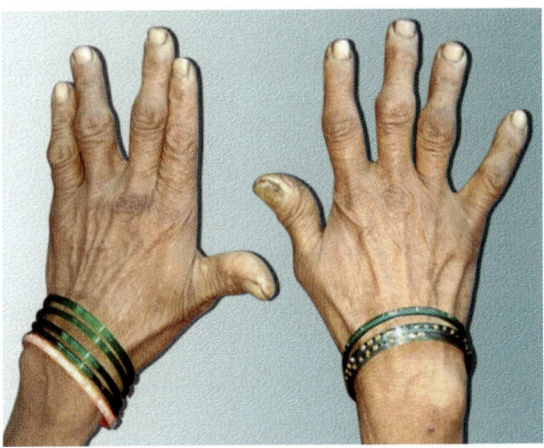

Fig. 7.1: Spindle-shaped deformity in RA

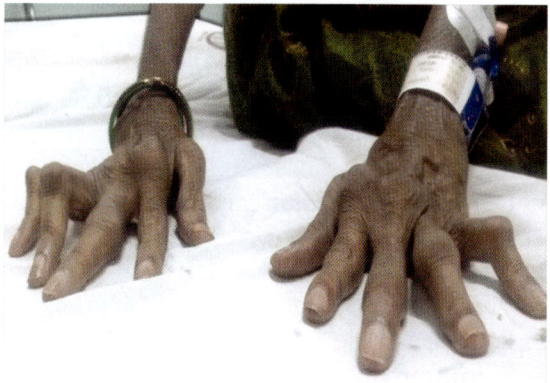

Fig. 7.2: Swan neck and boutonnieres deformity in rheumatoid arthritis

– Boutonnieres deformity of fingers
– Z-like deformity of thumb and wrist.

Extra-articular involvement

General manifestations

- Fever
- Weight loss
- Fatigue
- Generalised lymphadenopathy

Subcutaneous nodules

- Nodules of around 1 cm
- Firm
- Non-tender

Sites of involvement—areas prone for daily trauma

- Elbow
- Heel
- Sacrum

Presence of subcutaneous nodules indicates more aggressive disease and higher level of rheumatoid factor.

Can be present over the serosal surfaces.

 Note

Compared to rheumatic nodules (<1 cm), rheumatoid nodules are bigger in size (1.5 to 2 cm), usually present at the elbow and persist for a longer duration (months to years) and associated with active disease.

Rheumatic nodules usually persist for 1 to 2 weeks and associated with carditis.

Cardiac

- Pericarditis and effusion
- Cardiomyopathy
- AR and MR

Pulmonary

- Pleuritis and pleural effusion
- Pulmonary infiltration and fibrosis

Caplan's syndrome: Rheumatoid nodules and cavity in the lung with rheumatoid factor +ve with pneumoconiosis (silicosis).

Hematological

- Normocytic normochromic anemia
- Thrombocytopenia
- Leucopenia, Felty's syndrome.

Other manifestations

- Entrapment neuropathy
- Mononeuritis multiplex
- Vasculitis
- Coronary artery disease
- Glomerulonephritis

Laboratory evaluation

- High ESR and CRP
- Presence of anti-CCP antibody
- Presence of rheumatoid factor (IgM in 70–80% of patients)
- Synovial fluid analysis: Inflammatory pattern
- Joint X-ray:
  – Swelling of soft tissues
  – Erosion of cartilage
  – Loss of joint space
  – Osteopenia
  – Destruction of the joint
  – Ultrasound and MRI of the joint is helpful in the diagnosis.

Variants of rheumatoid arthritis

- Felty's syndrome
- Sjögren's syndrome

Investigations in rheumatoid arthritis

- Complete blood picture
  – Severe anemia
  – Thrombocytopenia.

- Evidence of active disease
  - ↑ ESR
  - ↑ CRP
- Evidence for the disease
  - Anti-CCP positive
  - Rheumatoid factor positive
- X-ray of the joint
  - Early part of the disease
    - Swelling of soft tissues
    - Osteoporosis of periarticular structure
    - Inflammation of the periosteum.
  - Late stage of the disease
    - Decrease of joint space
    - Erosion of articular surface
    - Ankylosis
    - Secondary osteoarthritis
- Rheumatoid pleural effusion
  - Glucose level is very low
  - LDH level is high.
- Synovial fluid analysis
  - Inflammatory pattern
  - Color opaque/yellow
  - Viscocity low
  - Cells count 40,000–50,000 cells/cmm

Complications of rheumatoid arthritis
Acute
- Atlantoaxial subluxation
- Cricoarytenoid subluxation
- Acute myocardial infection.
Chronic
- Deformities
- Entrapment neuropathy
- Rheumatoid lung
- Glomerulonephritis
- Amyloidosis

Rheumatoid factor
- Antibody detected in 70–80% of patients of rheumatoid arthritis.
- It is usually an IgM antibody (can also be IgG) against IgG antibody produced by lymphocytes and plasma cells and is an autoantibody.

Tests performed for detection of rheumatoid factor
- Rose-Waaler test
- Latex agglutination test.

Significance of rheumatoid factor
- If level less than 40 IU—test negative.
- If more than 60 IU or titer more than 1:80: Significant for rheumatoid arthritis.

High levels of rheumatoid factor suggests
- More aggressive disease
- More likely to be associated with extra articular involvement
- More chance of presence of rheumatoid nodules
- More likely to have rheumatoid lung disease.

Disorder which can be associated with false positive rheumatoid factor
- Elderly (5%)
- Chronic infection
- SLE
- Sjögren's syndrome
- Primary biliary cirrhosis.

Anti-CCP antibody (antibodies to cyclic citrullinated peptide)
- Found in patients with rheumatoid arthritis.
- Suggestive of inflammation of synovium
- Has got specificity of >95%
- Can be detected early and even in asymptomatic patients before the diagnosis of rheumatoid arthritis.

FELTY'S SYNDROME

- Variant of rheumatoid arthritis
- Seropositive arthritis
- F >M

Features

- More common in females
- Polyarthritis with deformities
- Splenomegaly and lymphadenopathy
- Pancytopenia (predominant neutropenia)
- Recurrent infection

Extra-articular Features

Special features
- Pancytopenia due to sequestration of cells in the spleen with destruction.
- Antibodies were coating the granulocytes.

Lab investigations
- High ESR
- Granulocytopenia and pancytopenia
- Rheumatoid factor positive.

Complications: Sepsis, respiratory and skin infection.

SJÖGREN'S SYNDROME

- Autoimmune disease
- Considered as a variant of rheumatoid arthritis.
- Structures involved mainly salivary and lacrimal glands.
- Age and sex
  - F > M
  - Middle-aged
- Consequence—may progress to malignant lymphoma.

Types of Sjögren's Syndrome

- Primary—not associated with other auto-immune disorder
- Secondary—associated with other auto-immune disorder.
- *Pathophysiology*
  - Associated with HLA DQA1
  - Formation of autoantibodies (IgM) against immunoglobulins
  - T and B lymphocyte activation leading to cytokine production and inflammation
  - Infiltration of B and T lymphocytes in salivary and lacrimal glands.

Clinical Features

- Chronic progressive disease
- Dry mouth (xerostomia) with salivary gland enlargement (especially in primary)
- Dry eye—keratoconjunctivitis sicca.

- Can have involvement of exocrine gland of respiratory, gastrointestinal tract.

Extraglandular involvement
- Common with primary Sjögren's syndrome.
- Similar to extraglandular manifestations of rheumatoid arthritis.

Differential diagnosis
1. Hepatitis C
2. HIV infection
3. Diabetes mellitus
4. Sarcoidosis.

Lab investigations
- High ESR
- Schirmer's test for dry eye.
- Lip biopsy for lymphocytic infiltration of salivary glands.
- Additional tests: Rheumatoid factor
- Ultrasound and MRI of salivary glands.

STILL'S DISEASE

Considered as a form of juvenile chronic (rheumatoid) arthritis.

Aetiology
- Not known.
- May be a form of autoimmune disorder.

Clinical features
- High grade spiking fever.
- Transient (evanescent) salmon colored rash—nonitchy
- Generalised lymphadenopathy.
- Hepatosplenomegaly
- Respiratory symptoms: URT symptoms
- Pleuritis/effusion
- Pericarditis
- Polyarticular arthritis

Lab evaluation
- High WBC count with neutrophilia.
- High ESR and CRP.
- Very high serum ferritin level (>2000 nano grams/ml)
- Negative investigations for infection
- Rheumatoid factor negative
- ANA and ANCA are negative.

SERONEGATIVE ARTHRITIS

Features of Seronegative Arthritis

- Rheumatoid factor negative.
- Present as back pain and sacroiliitis
- Involves predominantly lower extremity joints.
- Presence of enthesitis
- No subcutaneous nodules

Other features
- Anterior uveitis
- Positive family history
- HLA B27 positivity
- High ESR and CRP
- Very good response to NSAIDs.

ANKYLOSING SPONDYLITIS

Suspect ankylosing spondylitis under the following circumstances
- Presence of back pain
- Less than 45 years of age
- Evidence for sacroiliitis
- Enthesitis
- Extra-articular features
- Elevated inflammatory markers
- HLA B27 positivity

Features
- Seronegative arthritis
- Sacroiliitis with low back pain
- Associated with HLA B27 positivity

Age and sex group involved
- Male > female
- Starts at 2nd to 3rd decade of life.
Presentation—low back pain with sacroiliitis.

Clinical features
- Sacroiliitis
- Low back pain—improves with activity and increases with rest.
- Other joints can be involved.
- General symptoms like fever/weight loss.

Extra-articular manifestations
- Anterior uveitis
- Aortic regurgitation

- Apical pulmonary fibrosis
- Decrease of chest expansion.

Disease progression leads to
- Decreased movement of spine (positive Schober's test)
- Patient's height is decreased due to exaggerated thoracic kyphosis and forward neck flexion.
- Restrictive lung disease.

Complications
Due to spine abnormality
- Quadriplegia and cauda equina syndrome
- Pulmonary upper lobe fibrosis
- Respiratory failure type I
- Cardiac: Aortic regurgitation/conduction defect.

PSORIATIC ARTHRITIS

- A form of seronegative arthritis
- Inflammatory arthritis causes erosive arthritis and enthesitis.

Characteristic features
- Joint involvement
- Nail changes
- Skin changes of psoriasis.

Joint involvement
- Asymmetrical involvement of joint with involvement of 2 or 3 joints (oligoarthritis)
- Low back pain: Sarcoiliitis
- Destructive form of arthritis called arthritis mutilans.
- Arthritis of distal interphalangeal joint.
- Symmetrical joint involvement can occur
- Can have spine and sacroiliac joint involvement.

Nail involvement
- Pitting and horizontal ridging of nail.
- Destruction of nail (onycholysis)
- Hyperkeratosis of subungual region
- Nail discoloration occurs with yellowish discoloration.

Skin changes: Scaly lesion over extensor surfaces.

Note

In patients with psoriatic arthritis there may be only past history of psoriasis/family history of psoriasis/ family history of psoriasis without present evidence of skin lesions. More severe arthritis occurs with pustular psoriasis and HIV infection.

Extra-articular features

- Eye—conjuctivitis, iridocyclitis
- Cardiac involvement in the form of aortic regurgitation.
- Peripheral neuropathy.

Investigations

- Increased ESR.
- Normocytic normochromic anemia
- Rheumatoid factor negative.
- HLA B27 positivity
- X-ray evidence of inflammatory joint involvement.
- Synovial fluid analysis—evidence of inflammation.

SYSTEMIC SCLEROSIS

- Autoimmune disease
- Multisystem involvement.

Typical features of the disease: Inflammation, fibrosis with diffuse microangiopathy.

Aetiopathogenesis

- Genetic susceptibility and histocompatible antigens make the person susceptible.
- Infection with Epstein-Barr virus may be a precipitating factor.
- Exposure to silica, drugs like cocaine and bleomycin may contribute to the development of systemic sclerosis.
- Altered cellular and humoral immune mechanism play a major role in the pathogenesis.
- Fibrosis and microvascular involvement involving skin, respiratory, cardiac and renal and gastrointestinal tract.

Type of disease

Diffuse cutaneous type:

Diffuse skin involvement with lung and renal involvement.
- Limited cutaneous—skin involvement— trunk is spared.

Initial presentation of systemic sclerosis
- Raynaud's phenomenon
- Thickening of skin.

Consequence and complications
- Progressive renal failure
- Accelerated hypertension
- Restrictive lung disease
- Development of internal malignancy (GIT/ lungs, etc.).

Clinical features

- Thickening of skin especially digits with fibrosis including face.
- Raynaud's phenomenon.
- Pulmonary fibrosis and pulmonary hypertension.
- Esophageal motility disturbance and malabsorption
- Constipation
- Progressive renal insufficiency, accelerated hypertension, scleroderma renal crisis.

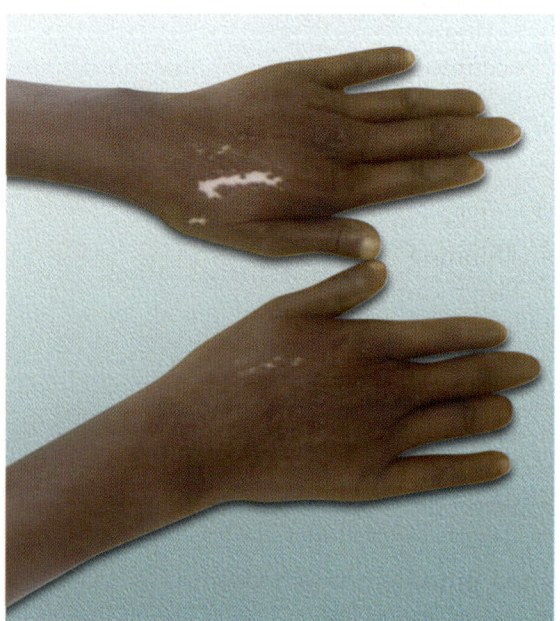

Fig. 7.3: Fingers in systemic sclerosis

- Constrictive pericarditis, myocardial ischemia, abnormalities of the cardiac conduction system.
- Arthralgia, polyarthritis, myopathy.

Hand involvement in systemic sclerosis
- Digital ulcers
- Raynaud's phenomenon
- Thickening of skin
- Edema (puffiness of fingers)
- Contractures (can produce clawhand appearance)
- Calcinosis

Lab investigations
- High ESR
- Anemia: Normocytic, normochromic (chronic disease)
  - Microcytic hypochromic
  - Macrocytic (B12 malabsorption)
  - Microangiopathic hemolytic anemia.
- Presence of autoantibodies
  - Anti-topoisomerase I (Scleral-70)
  - Anti-centromere
- Other antibodies like antiU1 RnP antiU3 RnP may be present.
- Skin biopsy for evidence of: Thickening of collagen, T cell infiltration, increased accumulation of extracellular matrix.

Special features
- Face: Mauskopf face
- Expressionless face
- Thickened shiny skin over the face
- Thinning of lips
- Fish mouth appearance—due to difficulty in opening
- Loss of wrinkles over the face

Skin
- Thickened
- Vitiligo can be present
- Fixed flexion contracture of fingers.

CREST syndrome: Combination of calcinosis cutis, Raynaud's phenomenon, oesophageal dysmotility, sclerodactyly and telangiectasia.

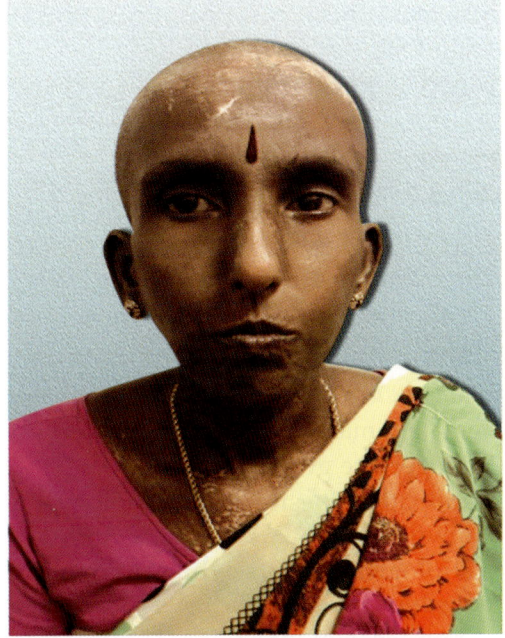

Fig. 7.4: Mauskopf face in systemic sclerosis

Morphea: Localised involvement of skin pertaining to particular parts of the body.

MICROSCOPIC POLYANGIITIS

Type of Disease—Necrotising Vasculitis

Type of Vessel Involved

Arteries—small and medium sized
- Venules
- Capillaries

Clinical Features

Non-specific symptoms:
- Myalgia and arthralgia
- Fever
- Weight loss

Most important abnormality: Glomerulonephritis.

Other structures involved
- Pulmonary vessel
- Alveolar hemorrhage with vasculitis
- Involvement of gastrointestinal tract
- Vasculitis of skin
- Mononueritis multiplex

Investigations
- High ESR
- p-ANCA positivity.

TAKAYASU'S ARTERITIS
Disease Entity—A Type of Vasculitis
Type of Vessel Involved
- Large and medium-sized vessels
- Predilection for: Aorta and its major branches.

Age and sex involved
- Female > male
- Younger age group.
- Aetiopathogenesis—exact aetiology—unknown
- Aetiological factors which may be responsible:
  - Spirochaetal infection
  - Mycobacterium tuberculosis
  - Autoimmunity and autoantibodies.

Pathophysiology: Inflammation of aorta and its branches—pan vasculitis with granulomatous inflammation.

Types of Takayasu's Arteritis
Depending on the branches involved
- *Type I*: Aortic arch branches
- *Type IIa*: Aortic arch, its branches and ascending aorta
- *Type IIb*: Thoracic aorta and type IIa
- *Type III*: Thoracic aorta, abdominal aorta with or without renal artery involvement
- *Type IV*: Abdominal aorta with or without renal involvement
- *Type V*: Combination of type IIb and IV.

Clinical features
Non-specific symptoms
- Fever
- Weight loss
- Joint pain.
Cardiac involvement
- Upper limb pulses feeble or absent
- Hypertension

- Aortic regurgitation
- Bruit at carotid and abdominal aorta.

Neurologic involvement: TIA, CVA, seizures.

Characteristic involvement of retina
- Retinal ischemia and hemorrhage
- Microaneurysms and cotton wool exudates.

Complications
Cardiac: Hypertension—due to narrowing of renal arteries and narrowing of aorta above renal arteries.
- Myocardial infarction
- Aortic aneurysm
- Pulmonary hypertension
- CCF due to pulmonary hypertension
- Dilated cardiomyopathy

Cerebrovascular complications
- CVA
- Seizures

Toxemia of pregnancy can occur in Takayasu's arteritis

Investigations
- High ESR
- Mantoux test (may be positive)
- Angiogram

Differential diagnosis of Takayasu's arteritis
- Atherosclerotic vascular disease
- Primary vasculitis syndrome
- Coarctation of aorta
- SLE
- TAO

Investigations
- High ESR
- Raised globulin
- Echocardiography
- Arteriography
- Vessel biopsy.

Vessel biopsy
- Evidence of vasculitis
- Infiltration with lymphocytes and granuloma formation with giant cells.

Treatment
- Corticosteroids
- Disease—modifying agents—methotrexate

- Anti-TNF alpha agents
- Angioplasty/surgical correction.

OVERLAP SYNDROME

Term given to the presence of clinical features and lab features of two different autoimmune diseases at the same time in a patient.

Examples of overlap syndromes
- Mixed connective tissue disease—presence of antiU1-RNP antibody.
- Polymyositis and scleroderma overlap—presence of anti-PM/SSc antibody.

MIXED CONNECTIVE TISSUE DISEASE (MCTD)

What is MCTD?

Disease entity characterised by combined manifestations of rheumatoid arthritis, SLE, polymyositis and systemic sclerosis.

Clinical Features

- Arthralgia/polyarthritis (erosive)
- Rash of SLE
- Raynaud's phenomenon (usually the presenting feature)
- Heliotroph rash of dermatomyositis
- Manifestations of systemic sclerosis.

 Note

Features of one of the disorders like either rheumatoid in MCTD/SLE may predominate

Complications
- Membranous glomerulonephritis.
- Pulmonary fibrosis and pulmonary artery hypertension.
- Pericarditis/oesophageal dysmotility.

Lab investigations
- High ESR
- High titer of U1-RNP antibodies
- Autoantibodies specific for systemic sclerosis are negative.

Treatment: Corticosteroids.

HENOCH-SCHÖNLEIN PURPURA (Anaphylactoid Purpura)

What is Henoch-Schönlein purpura?

- It is a form of IgA mediated vasculitis (allergic vasculitis).
- Vessel involved—small vessels of skin.

Precipitating event
- Viral infection of URT or Shigella or Yersinia infection.
- May be drug induced.
- Age group involved—common in pediatric age, rare in adults.

Presenting features
- Rash or purpura over the legs
- Abdominal pain and vomiting
- Knee and ankle joint pain.
- Passing blood in the stools.

Investigations: Platelet count normal. Proteinuria, ↑ ESR.

Skin biopsy: Leucocytoclastic vasculitis with IgA deposition.

Clinical features
- Skin—ecchymotic patches—lower extremities and buttocks.
- GIT-colicky abdominal pain (submucosal bleed). Bleed in the stools and malena.
- Renal—glomerulonephritis and nephritic syndrome. Adult can have more severe involvement.
- Joint involvement—polyarthritis/arthralgia.
- *Treatment*: Corticosteroids, plasma exchange, cytotoxic therapy.

Conditions associated with increased CPK
- Infections: Myositis/vasculitis
- Drugs and toxins:
  - Statins
  - Alcohol
- Muscle trauma and vigorous exercise.
- *Metabolic*: Hypothyroidism
- *Inflammatory*: Polymyositis
- *Degenerative*: Muscular dystrophy.

Systemic Lupus Erythematosus (SLE)

Connective tissue disorder. Autoantibodies and immune complexes damage the connective tissues.

Structures involved
- Connective tissues and joints
- Vascular system—blood vessels
- Involves especially renal, CNS and cardiac system.

Age and sex predilection
- Female > male ratio, 11:1
- Age: 3rd to 5th decade (child bearing age)

Aetiopathogenesis
Exact aetiology unknown. Following factors may be responsible:
- HLA B8 and DR3 correlation—genetic factors may be responsible forming auto-antibodies.
- Exposure to sunlight: UV light
- Precipitated by infective agents like Epstein-Barr virus.
- Autoantibodies and immune complexes damage the tissues which occur due to activation of B cells and T cells.
- Drugs can induce SLE:
  - Hydralazine, quinine, oestrogen and oral contraceptive pills
  - Phenytoin and methyldopa can induce SLE

Clinical features
- Nonspecific features—fever, weight loss, muscular and joint pain.
- Ocular—retinal ischemia, optic neuritis.
- Skin—photosensitive butterfly rash.
- Renal—glomerulonephritis.
- Musculoskeletal
  - Non-erosive polyarthritis
  - Occasionally features of rheumatoid and lupus coexist (Rhupus).
- CNS: Headache, seizures, neuropathy, vascular occlusion
- Cardiac: Myocardial infarction, pericarditis, Libman-Sacks endocarditis, myocarditis, CCF, cardiac arrhythmias

- *Pulmonary*: Pleuritis, pleural effusion, pulmonary fibrosis, alveolar hemorrhage, pulmonary hypertension.
- Hematologic—anemia, hemolysis, pancytopenia.
- *GIT*: Peritonitis, intestinal vasculitis.

Diagnostic Criteria

Required for diagnosis—minimal of 4 (minimal of 1 clinical and minimal of 1 lab criteria).

Clinical criteria	Lab criteria
Renal involvement	Anti-dsDNA positive
Nervous system involvement	Anti-SM positive
Oral ulcers, hair loss	APLA positive
Cutaneous lupus erythematosis	Complement levels ↓
Evidence of hemolysis	Coombs' test positive
Pancytopenia	ANA positivity
Synovitis	

Pregnancy and SLE
- SLE can have secondary APLA syndrome.
- SLE becomes more severe during pregnancy.
- Recurrent abortions and toxemia can occur.
- Multiple infarction of placenta can occur.
- Newborn can have complete heart block due to anti-Ro antibodies from the mother transmitted across the placenta.

Drug-induced Lupus
- Drugs responsible: *See* above.
- Characteristic antibody—antihistone antibody
- Genetic factors may be responsible.
- Withdrawal of the drug can reverse the situation.

Anti-Sm (anti-Smith) antibody
- Antibodies against small nuclear ribonuclear protein particles.
- Specific for SLE

Anti-Ro (SS-A) antibody: Antibody associated with Sicca syndrome. Associated with congenital heart block and neonatal lupus.

Anti-La (SS-B) antibody: Antibody associated with anti-Ro antibody.

Significance of antinuclear antibody
- ANA global is used for screening test for SLE.
- ANA test repeatedly negative almost rules out SLE.

Other autoantibodies which can be present: Antiphospholipid, antierythrocyte, antiplatelet antibodies.

Antibodies for neuronal antigen in SLE
- For CNS involvement: Anti-neuronal antibody.
- For depression and psychosis: Anti-ribosomal P antibody

Antinuclear antibody
- Present in patients who are having antibodies (autoantibodies) against their own tissues.
- These antibodies have the capacity to bind and react with nuclear structures of the cell (anti-nuclear antibodies).

They are expressed as titers
- Like—less than 1: 50 negative
- Less than 1:80—not clinically significant
- More than 1:160—clinically significant.

Antinuclear antibody in SLE
- Antibodies—specific for SLE: High titer of antibody against double stranded DNA.
- Antibody specific for drug-induced SLE: Antihistone antibody.

POLYARTERITIS NODOSA (PAN)

Type of disease: PAN is a form of vasculitis resulting in necrotizing vasculitis.

Type of vessel involved: Medium and small-sized arteries—necrotising vasculitis.

Vessel involvement
- Bifurcation and branches of arteries
- Aneurysmal dilatation of arteries
- Pulmonary arteries not involved

Clinical features
Presents as
- Hypertension
- Arthralgia/arthritis
- Renal failure.
Systemic involvement:
Cardiac
- Hypertension
- Myocardial infarction
- CCF
- Pericarditis
Nervous system
- Seizures
- CVA
- Mononeuropathy multiplex
Gastrointestinal tract
- Pain abdomen
- Infarction of bowel
- Abdominal visceral infarction
Skin involvement
- Purpura
- Raynaud's phenomenon
Genitourinary system and eye also can be involved.

INVESTIGATIONS

- High ESR
- Anemia of chronic disease
- 30% of patients: HbsAg positive.
- P-ANCA positive.
- Angiography—dilatation and aneurysm formation of small and medium-sized arteries.
- Biopsy of the vessel: For evidence of vasculitis.

Churg-Strauss Syndrome (Eosinophilic Granulomatosis with Polyangiitis)

Disease entity: It is a form of granulomatous vasculitis with eosinophilia.
- Predominant organ involvement—lungs.

- Types of pathology—granulomatous vasculitis.
- Vasculitis—pan vasculitis with involvement of capillaries, veins and vessels.

Pathology: Infiltration with eosinophils with granuloma formation in the tissues and organs.

Clinical features
- Presents like bronchial asthma
- Will have polyarthritis
- Fever, weight loss
- Glomerulonephritis and mononeuritis multiplex.

Diagnosis
- Eosinophilia >1000 cells/cmm
- High ESR
- P-ANCA positivity
- Chest X-ray—pulmonary infiltration
- Biopsy—granulomatous vasculitis.

Reactive Arthritis (Reiter's Syndrome)

Combination of
- Arthritis
- Conjunctivitis
- Urethritis

Arthritis
- May have monoarthritis with knee involvement
- Lower extremity joint involvement
- Interphalangeal joint involvement
- Can have plantar fasciitis/Achilles' tendonitis.

Eye: Conjunctivitis/uveitis

Urethritis: *Will have symptoms and signs of urethritis*

Other features
Circinate balanitis
- Glans penis is involved due to vesicles
- Vesicles can rupture and form erosions
- Will have features of urethritis, prostatitis, cervicitis or salphingitis.

Skin lesion
- Macular rash, can have vesicles and pustules.

- Keratoderma blenorrhagica—vesicles and pustules becoming hyperkeratotic forming crust.
- Infective organisms which can cause reactive arthritis by infecting gastrointestinal/urinary tract
  - Shigella
  - Salmonella
  - Campylobacter
  - Yersinia
  - Chlamydia.

Key points of reactive arthritis
- Evidence of preceding gastrointestinal or urethral infection (1–4 weeks)
- Triad of urethritis, conjunctivitis and arthritis
- Associated with HLA B27 positivity
- Presence of skin lesions
- Features of fever, weight loss, fatigue.
- Pleuropulmonary involvement, cardiac conduction defect and aortic regurgitation.

Lab evaluation
- High ESR and increased CRP
- Positivity of HLA B27
- Evidence of infection may not be present
- X-ray of joint:
  - Erosive arthritis
  - Sacroiliitis and spondylitis.

VASCULITIS

Types of the disease: Inflammation of blood vessel.

Consequence of the disease: Narrowing of the blood vessel with ischemia to the end organ.

Pathophysiology: Exact aetiology unknown.

Following factors together may predispose to vasculitis
- Abnormal immune regulating mechanisms
- Genetic factors.
- Environmental agents.

Mechanisms of blood vessel damage
- Antibody mediated cell damage due to immune complex formation with damage to blood vessel.
- Cytokine release due to cytotoxic T cells causing damage to blood vessels.
- Formation of granuloma in and around the blood vessel.
- Microbial agent infiltration of vessel wall is also considered.

Classification of vasculitis—depending on the type of vessel involvement

Vasculitis involving large vessel
- Giant cell arteritis
- Takayasu's arteritis

Vasculitis involving medium-sized vessel
- Polyarteritis nodosa
- Kawasaki's disease.

Vasculitis involving small-sized vessel

ANCA mediated
- Wegener's granulomatosis: Granulomatosis with polyangiitis
- Churg-Strauss (eosinophilic granulomatosis).
- Microscopic polyangiitis

Vasculitis depending on the underlying disorder
- Primary: Involvement of vessel is the only manifestation of the disease.
- Secondary: Vasculitis is a manifestation of a secondary disease.

Consider following disorders which mimic vasculitis
- APLA syndrome
- Infective endocarditis
- Atrial myxoma
- Atherosclerotic vascular disease
- Disseminated fungal infection
- Internal malignancy
- Syphilis

Types of vessel involvement in vasculitis
- Small vessel vasculitis
- Microscopic polyangiitis

Anti-Nuclear Cytoplasmic Antibody (ANCA)
- Mainly associated with vasculitis syndrome.
- Autoantibodies of IgG subtype.

Antibodies against
- Antigens in the cytoplasm of neutrophil granulocytes
- Detected by ELISA technique

Types of main ANCA antibodies

Cytoplasmic: ANCA-C ANCA

Perinuclear: ANCA-P ANCA
- C-ANCA: Antibody against proteinase-3 cytoplasma of neutrophil and monocytes.
- Mainly found in patient with (80–90%) of:
  - Granulomatosis with polyangiitis (Wegener's granulomatosis)
  - Other conditions: Inflammatory bowel disease
  - Rheumatoid arthritis.
- P-ANCA—antibody against myeloperoxidase
- Mainly found in
  - Polyarteritis nodosa
  - Microscopic polyangiitis

OSTEOARTHRITIS
- Degenerative disease of the joint
- Age group involved—elderly age
- Joint involved—usually weight-bearing joint

Common joints involved
- Knee
- Hip
- Spine—lumbar and cervical spine.

Joints which are less involved
- Interphalangeal joints—distal and proximal
- Shoulder and wrist and elbow.

Pathology
- Chronic inflammation of the synovium
- Additional factors like inflammatory joint diseases may add to the disease.
- Destruction and degeneration of articular cartilage and formation of new bone.
- Mild synovitis.

Features
- Pain in the joints
- Pain is more on physical activities and decreases at rest
- Can have evidence of inflammation.

Clinical features
- Involvement of weight bearing joints with pain
- Restriction of joint movement
- Presence of crepitus and bony enlargement
- Inflammatory signs are absent but mild to moderate effusions can occur
- Wasting of muscles and deformity of the joint can occur at later stages

Investigations
- Synovial fluid—noninflammatory
- X-ray of the joint
- Reduction of the joint space.
- Formation of nodes: Heberden's nodes at the distal interphalangeal joints.

Osteoarthritis is common in following type of patients
- Elderly age
- Obese patients
- Hereditary factor play a role
- Trauma to the joint
- Overuse/work of the joint.

 Note

If synovial fluid shows inflammatory pattern in osteoarthritis, suspect gout/inflammatory arthritis.

BEHÇET'S SYNDROME

Features
- Oral aphthous ulcers
- Genital ulcers
- Skin involvement—vasculitis and erythema nodosum
- Eye involvement = Iridocyclitis

Pathology: Vasculitis of autoimmune origin.

Associated features
- Arthralgia/arthritis
- Deep vein thrombosis

- Can have cortical venous sinus thrombosis, brainstem involvement.
- Can have involvement of gastrointestinal tract.

Investigations
- High ESR and high CRP
- Biopsy

Pathergy: Occurs in patients with Behçet's syndrome. Unusual response to trauma. Minor trauma will result in skin lesions with ulcers which are difficult to heal.

Treatment:
- Local/systemic corticosteroids
- Azathioprine
- ANT, TNF-α agents

POLYMYOSITIS

Form of disease: Inflammatory myopathy.

Clinical Features

General Features
- Fever
- Weight loss

Muscle weakness
- Acute/chronic and can be progressive
- Muscle pain and muscle tenderness
- Dysphagia—due to pharyngeal muscle weakness
- Neck muscle weakness
- Wasting of muscles
- DTR are preserved till late.

Structures—spared
- Ocular and facial muscles
- No sensory involvement.

Other features
- Not usually associated with rash.
- Presence of other connective tissue disease.

Complications
- Respiratory muscle paralysis
- Cardiac conduction defect
- Cardiomyopathy

- Associated internal malignancy less likely compared to dermatomyositis

Differential diagnosis: Exclude other causes of acute/chronic muscle weakness.

Lab investigations
- Increased CPK level
- EMG: Myopathic pattern
- Muscle biopsy—inflammatory myopathy.

DERMATOMYOSITIS

Type of disease: Inflammatory disorder with involvement of skin and muscle.

Clinical features
- Rash: Heliotroph rash.
  - Upper eyelid: Blue purple discoloration
  - Edema of eyelid
  - Erythematous rash—face and upper trunk.

Gottron's papules
- Over the knuckles
  - Raised rash with scaly eruptions
  - V sign—rash over the anterior chest.
  - Shawl sign—rash over the back and shoulder
- Rash is photosensitive
  - Muscle involvement: Proximal muscle weakness.
  - Can present in combination with MCTD/scleroderma
  - Usually associated with malignancy like:
    - Carcinoma breast
    - Melanoma
    - Oat cell carcinoma lung
    - Carcinoma colon.

Investigations and management: Same as polymyositis.

Inclusion Body Myositis

Type of Disorder
- Inflammatory myopathy
- Age group involved: Above the age of 50 years

- Muscle involvement
  - Distal muscle weakness and atrophy
  - Weakness of quadriceps: Knee weakness (Buckling of knees)
- Weakness of dorsiflexors of foot
- Weakness of small muscles
- Hand and diaphragm and pharyngeal muscles weakness.

Associated features: Other connective tissue disorders.

FIBROMYALGIA

Main features
- Musculoskeletal pain of long duration.
- Associated with neuropsychiatric disturbance.

Age and sex prediction: F > M
- Generalised body pain with tender points by pressure.
- Anxiety, depression, fatigue and sleep disturbance, cognitive dysfunction.
- Can be associated with inflammatory, degenerative/musculoskeletal disorder
- Usually associated with psychological stress.

Pathophysiology
- Genetic factor play a role
- Abnormal central pain processing mechanism.

Laboratory evaluation
- Lab tests are within normal limits.
- Rule out—other connective tissue disorder.

Differential diagnosis
Common
- Thyroid dysfunction
- Endocrine: Hypercalcemic disorder
- Connective tissue disorder
- Infection: HIV infection
- Psychiatric: Depressive disease
- Drug induced: Statins
Less common
- Infective: Hepatitis C
- Demyelinating—multiple sclerosis
- Joint disorder—osteoarthritis

ANTIPHOSPHOLIPID ANTIBODY (APLA) SYNDROME

- Autoimmune disorder
- Tendency for venous or arterial thrombosis. Occasionally bleed.
- Can have fetal loss
- Types:
  - Primary—without any evidence of associated disorder.
  - Secondary—associated with other connective tissue disease

Criteria for diagnosis (verify): There should be minimal of one clinical and one lab criteria.

Clinical criteria

- At least one episode of vascular occlusion (arterial/venous)
- Recurrent pregnancy loss:
  - 3 or more recurrent, consecutive spontaneous first trimester abortions
  - Unexplained fetal loss before 34th week of pregnancy due to toxemia of pregnancy.
  - Unexplained death of normal fetus after 10th week of pregnancy

Lab criteria

- Detection of lupus anticoagulant or anticardiolipin antibody or
- Antibody against beta2 glycoprotein—2 times with an interval of 3 months.

Features

- Recurrent thrombosis (TIA, DVT, CVA, pulmonary embolism)
- Recurrent pregnancy loss/premature birth
- Renal—small vessel occlusion—nephropathy
- Cardiac: Endocarditis (Libman sacks)
- Pulmonary hypertension
- Hemolytic anemia
- Thrombocytopenia

Mechanism of thrombosis

- Complement activation
- Platelets become activated and gets adhered to the endothelium.
- Endothelial activation.
- Formation of procoagulant state due to antibodies against protein C and S and prothrombin.

Conditions—associated with secondary APLA

- SLE
- Hepatitis C
- HIV infection.
- Syphilis

Lab abnormalities

Presence of antibodies (*see* above for lab criteria), thrombocytopenia, prolonged PT and APTT

- ANA and increased ESR
- ANCA positivity
- Evidence of hemolysis

Differential diagnosis of APLA syndrome

- Infection: Retroviral illness.
- Drugs—oral contraceptive pills
- Vasculitis—primary or secondary vasculitis
- Hypercoagulable state—protein C and S deficiency
  - Internal malignancy.
  - Factor V Leiden mutation
  - Anti-thrombin antibody.
- Metabolic: Hyperhomocystinemia
- Diffuse atherosclerosis.

GOUT AND PSEUDOGOUT

Gout and pseudogout are forms of crystal-induced arthritis.

Monosodium urate: Can cause acute gout and chronic tophaceous gout.

Calcium pyrophosphate dehydrate: Can cause: Acute pseudogout and chondrocalcinosis and chronic pyrophosphate arthropathy.

Deposition of monosodium urate crystals

- Can occur in connective tissue—called tophi
- Can form uric acid stones
- Can get deposited in the interstitium of the kidney.

Acute gouty arthritis
- Monoarthritis—involving metatarsophalangeal joint
- Can be intermittent
- Causes nocturnal attack
- Acute attack of severe pain, warmth, tenderness and redness
- Mimics cellulitis.

Precipitating factors for acute gout
Medical disorders
- Myocardial infarction
- CVA
- Trauma to the joints
- Surgery
- Dietary excess—containing purines; alcohol, sea foods, shell fish and meat.
- Alcohol intake

Chronic gouty arthritis
- Mimics rheumatoid arthritis
- Can have chronic tophaceous gout
- Associated with hypertension and renal failure.

Chronic hyperuricemia occurs due to decreased renal excretion
For example,
- Renal failure
- Renal tubular defect.

Other causes of chronic hyperuricemia: Hypertension, obesity, alcoholism, thiazides insulin resistance, hypothyroidism.
- Pyrazinamide
- Cyclosporin

Increased turnover of purines
For example,
- Chronic myeloproliferative disorder
- HGPRT synthase deficiency.

Crystal-induced arthritis can cause
- Deposition of tophi
- Bursitis
- Tendonitis
- Enthesitis
- Mono/polyarthritis.

Lab investigations
- Serum uric acid level.
- Synovial fluid—for monosodium urate crystals.
- 24 hours—urine: Uric acid excretion and for crystals.

Pseudogout

Type of the disease
- A form of crystal-induced arthritis
- Occurs due to
  - Deposition of calcium pyrophosphate in the articular cartilage.
  - Crystals are released into the synovial fluid.

Clinical features
- Acute attack—mimics gout
- May be acute/subacute/chronic disease.
- Can have recurrent attack
- Acute attack is also called pseudogout
- Common joint involved—knee joint.
- Features may mimic rheumatoid/osteoarthritis
- Diagnosed by synovial fluid examination for calcium pyrophosphate crystals.

Endocrinology

ENDOCRINE DISORDERS

THYROID GLAND

Anatomy

Location: Anterior to the trachea.

Extent
- Below—up to the suprasternal notch
- Above—up to the cricoid cartilage

Parts
- Larger right lobe
- Smaller left lobe
- Connecting between the lobes—isthmus of the gland.

Consistency: Soft

Vascular supply
- Superior and inferior thyroid artery
- Arteria thyroidea ima

Posterior to the thyroid: Parathyroid glands.

Lateral border of thyroid: Recurrent laryngeal nerve.

Cells of thyroid
- Follicular cells secrete thyroxine (mainly T4 and smaller amount of T3)
- Parafollicular C cells: Secrete calcitonin.

THYROID DISORDERS

Clinical Aspects of Thyroid Examination

- Always look for cervical lymphadenopathy whenever the thyroid is examined.

- Look for a previous scar of thyroid surgery.
- Look for distended neck veins—in a patient of thyroid swelling. Distended neck veins indicate underlying superior vena caval obstruction (retrosternal goiter).
- Lingual thyroid and presence of thyroglossal cyst can be made out by inspecting protrusion of the tongue.
- Thrill and bruit over the thyroid is located in the upper or lower lateral part of the thyroid in patients with Graves' disease.

Clinical Examination of Thyroid

Inspection of Neck
- Minimum extension of neck is helpful for inspecting the thyroid.
- Inspect the neck in the region of thyroid from suprasternal notch up to the cricoid cartilage.

Palpation
- Thyroid can be palpated from either anteriorly or posteriorly.
- Patient can be either seated or standing.

Palpation of the Thyroid

Anterior approach
- Minimal flexion of the neck—beneficial
- Identify: Cricoid cartilage
- Palpate the isthmus of thyroid (in front of the Cricoid cartilage)

- Sternomastoid can be retracted and lateral lobes can be palpated with the thumb.
- Patient is asked to swallow and palpate for the lower border.
- Look for size and consistency of the thyroid.
- Look for previous surgical scars and distension of neck veins.

Palpation from posterior aspect from behind
- Patient is seated and palpate the thyroid from behind.
- Identify the isthmus and hand (thumb) is moved laterally for lateral lobes under the sternomastoid.

Important Aspects of Examination of Thyroid

Thyroid bruit: Usually auscultated over the lateral poles of thyroid—superior or inferior lateral.

Berry's sign
- Examine the carotid pulsation while examining the thyroid.
- Absence of carotid pulsation in a patient of thyromegaly is more likely to be associated with malignancy of the thyroid (Berry's sign).

Thyroid ophthalmopathy (eye involvement in Graves' disease): Eye involvement in Graves' disease can occur before or some time after the other clinical manifestations. It is mediated through antibodies.

Eye involvement in Graves' disease
- Increased sympathetic activity leads to the retraction of the lid.
- Inferior rectus is the most common muscle affected early followed by medial rectus.
- Diplopia can occur due to muscle involvement with muscle swelling.
- Papilledema can occur due to compression of the optic nerve at the apex of the orbit and there will be permanent loss of vision.

Method to look for proptosis
- Patient is asked to sit and look straight.
- Stand behind the patient.

- Examiner is asked to look downwards from the level of forehead towards the chin of the patient.
- Cornea appears to be protruding outside the orbital margin.

Other methods for looking for proptosis: Keep the eye in the primary position. There will be appearance of sclera in between the lower limbus and lid margin.

Naffziger's method (sign)
- Examiner is looking from above standing behind the patient.
- Eyeballs appears to be protruded outside the rim of the orbit.

Effects of Graves' disease on the eye
- Proptosis
- Lid retraction
- Diplopia
- Chemosis
- Corneal damage and loss of vision.

Thyrotoxicosis

Thyrotoxicosis: General term for any cause which results in excess level of circulating thyroxine with its action.

Hyperthyroidism: Excess level of thyroxine is due to the primary disorder of thyroid itself.

Causes of Thyrotoxicosis

Due to the disease of the thyroid (primary hyperthyroidism)
- Graves' disease
- Toxic multinodular goiter
- Solitary adenoma (becoming toxic)
- Carcinoma of thyroid

Due to excess of thyroid hormone release (hyperthyroidism is not actually present)
- Thyroiditis—subacute/silent
- Amiodarone therapy
- Radiation

Other causes (secondary)
Due to excessive intake of thyroxine
- Factitious

- Struma ovarii
- Drugs—excess intake of iodine/iodine containing substances

Due to the overaction of the pituitary.

Clinical Manifestations

General Features

- Excess appetite
- Loss of weight—due to very high metabolic rate.
- Alopecia
- Intolerance to heat
- Diarrhea/hyperdefecation

Eye Signs in Hyperthyroidism

von Graefe's sign: Lid lag

Dalrymple's sign
- Widened palpebral fissure
- Upper eye lid retraction.

Stellwag's sign: Infrequent blinking.

Joffroy's sign: On looking upward creases on the forehead are absent.

Mobius sign: Lacking of convergence.

Lid Lag: Ask the patient to look downwards. There will be appearance of sclera between the corneal limbus and upper eyelid margin.

Lid retraction

- Ask the patient to look straightforward. There will be starring appearance of eyes due to palpabral fissure widening.
- This is due to the higher positioning of upper eyelid. Sclera is seen between the superior corneal limbus and upper lid margin.
- Lid retraction and lid lag are due to excess activity of Müller muscle due to increased sympathetic activity due to hyperthyroidism.

📝 *Note*

Normally upper eyelid covers 2 mm of upper cornea and the lower eyelid is at the level of lower limbus of cornea.

Wolff-Chaikoff effect

- Ingestion of large amount of iodine causes decrease in thyroid hormone synthesis.
- This is due to inhibition of thyroid paroxidase RNA and protein synthesis.
- This can occur in normal individuals and also in patients with Graves' disease.
- In normal individuals the effect persists for shorter duration and then normal hormone synthesis occurs.
- In patients with Graves' disease the effect can persist for a prolonged time.

Systemic Features of Thyrotoxicosis

Cardiovascular

- Palpitation—due to tachycardia
- Can cause atrial fibrillation/supraventricular tachycardia.
- High volume pulse
- Ejection systolic murmur—pulmonary or aortic area
- High output cardiac failure
- Deterioration of underlying coronary artery disease.

Means-Lerman's Scratch

- Heard in patients with hyperthyroidism
- It is a mid-systolic sound
- Over the 3rd intercostal space over the precordium
- Due to rubbing of pericardium with pleural layers (due to cardiac overactivity).

Thyrocardiac

- Involvement of cardiovascular system in thyrotoxicosis.
- Due to increased sympathetic discharge.
- Manifestations
  - Tachycardia
  - Atrial fibrillation
  - High output cardiac failure.
- Common in elderly with toxic adenoma/toxic multinodular goiter.

Nervous System Manifestations of Thyrotoxicosis

- Anxiety symptoms
- Sleeplessness
- Fine tremors of hands
- Proximal muscle weakness
- Rarely chorea may be a manifestation
- Periodic paralysis associated with hypokalemia and bulbar palsy.

Manifestations: Particular to Graves' Disease

Goiter

- Diffuse, firm and enlarged thyroid.
- Presence of thrill/bruit over the thyroid.

Ophthalmopathy—already described.

Dermopathy: Pretibial myxedema (indurated pink/purple colored plaque over the lower part of the leg).

Thyroid acropachy

- Clubbing occurring in a patient of Graves' disease.
- Acropachy is always associated with other manifestations of dermopathy.

Other manifestations of thyrotoxicosis:

- Generalized pruritis
- Hair loss
- Palmar erythema and hyperpigmentation
- Women—oligomenorrhea
- Men—gynaecomastia
- Sexual dysfunction.

Apathetic thyrotoxicosis

- Form of thyrotoxicosis found in elderly persons.
- Presents as significant weight loss and easy fatigability.
- Other manifestations of thyrotoxicosis-may not be evident.

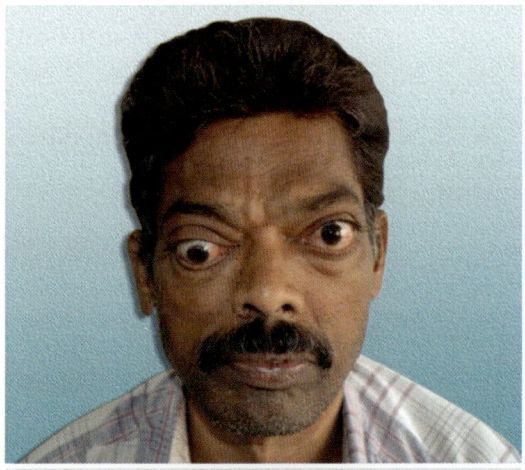

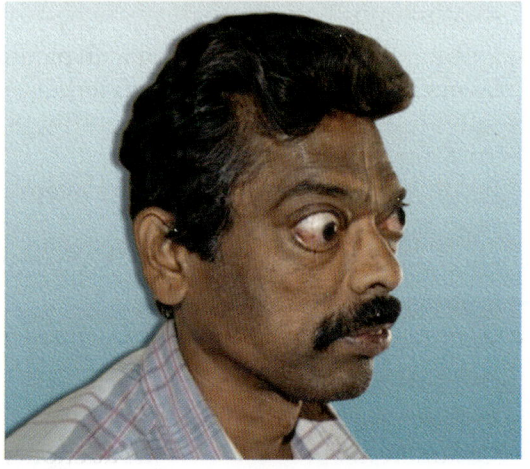

Fig. 8.1: Ophthalmopathy of Graves' disease

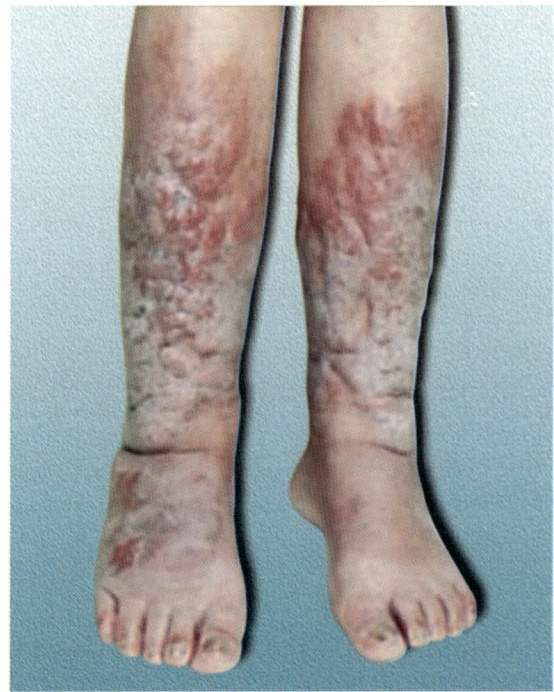

Fig. 8.2: Pretibial myxedema in Graves' disease

Apathetic Thyrotoxicosis

Features	Features which are not present
• Older patients • Prolonged disease • Significant weight loss • Depressive symptoms (apathy) • Cardiac failure and atrial fibrillation • Proximal muscle weakness	No features of tremors/hyperactivity No eye signs

Hypothyroidism

- Hypothyroidism occurs due to decreased thyroid hormone function.
- It may be due to the disease of thyroid or due to pituitary dysfunction.

Causes of Hypothyroidism

Common causes

- Deficiency of iodine
- Autoimmune: Hashimoto's thyroiditis
- Iodine 131 therapy
- Post-thyroid surgery

Other causes

- Pituitary/hypothalamic disease
- Congenital.

Manifestations of hypothyroidism: Decrease of thyroxine leads to accumulations of glycosaminoglycans which trap water leading to manifestations of hypothyroidism.

General Features

- Constipation
- Decreased appetite
- Weight gain
- Menorrhagia
- Edema of feet

Signs

- Severe pallor
- Periorbital edema
- Non-pitting edema
- Outer one-third of eyebrow loss (madarosis)

- Skin—coarse, dry with hair loss.
- Goiter—in patients with Hashimoto's thyroiditis
- Slow relaxing ankle jerk (hung-up reflex)
- Enlargement of calf muscle—Hoffmann's syndrome.

Systemic Manifestations

Cardiovascular

- Bradycardia
- Diastolic hypertension (due to increased peripheral resistance)
- Cardiomyopathy
- Pericardial effusion

Respiratory

- Pleural effusion
- Obstructive sleep apnea

Nervous system

- Reversible dementia
- Myxedema madness/coma
- Delayed relaxing ankle jerk: Hung-up reflex—pseudomyotonia
- Carpal tunnel syndrome
- Enlargement of calf muscle: Hoffmann's syndrome.
- Cerebellar disturbance

Due to accumulation of fluid

- Middle ear—deafness
- Vocal cord—hoarseness of voice
- Autoimmune hypothyroidism can be associated with other autoimmune diseases.

Cretinism: Congenital hypothyroidism—usually due to iodine deficiency and hypothyroidism in the mother.

Features

- Dwarfism
- Mental retardation
- Defective bone maturation
- Skin thickening
- Macroglossia
- Protruded abdomen.

Secondary hypothyroidism

- Less common than primary hypothyroidism

- There will be features of other hormone deficiency
- Gross features of myxedema are less common

Differential Diagnosis of Pain Over the Thyroid

1. *Thyroiditis:*
   - Acute
   - Subacute
   - Chronic
2. Malignant neoplasm of the thyroid and lymphoma of thyroid.
3. Bleeding into the cyst of thyroid.

Acute Thyroiditis

Cause: Bacterial infection of the thyroid.

Features
- Fever
- Pain in the region of thyroid
- Referred pain to ears and throat.

Signs
- Tender enlarged thyroid
- Local lymphadenopathy.

Subacute thyroiditis (*de Quervain's/granulomatous*)

- Present with symptoms and signs of thyroiditis
- Can be due to viral infection and can have preceding URTI.
- Can pass through phases of hyperthyroid to hypothyroid to normal thyroid status.

Chronic (*autoimmune thyroiditis*)

- Presence of anti-TPO (thyroid peroxidase) antibodies
- For example, Hashimoto's thyroiditis
- Slowly progressive disease
- Can progress to hypothyroidism
- Presence of goiter—firm to hard

Riedel's thyroiditis

- Slowly progressive disease
- Firm to hard nontender goiter
- Can cause pressure symptoms

- Result in fibrosis of the thyroid
- Normal thyroid function

GOITER

Enlargement of the thyroid gland is called goiter.

Goiter
- Smooth and diffuse, e.g. Graves' disease
- Nodular: Solitary
  - Multiple
  - Toxic/non-toxic

Pathogenesis of goiter

Any defect in the thyroid function

↓

Hypothyroidism

Primary hypothyroidism → ↑ TSH—excessive growth of thyroid → Goiter

For example, iodine deficiency

Biosynthetic defect of thyroxine synthesis

Thyroid growth can also be due to
- Lymphocyte infiltration like in autoimmune thyroiditis
- TSH receptor induced in Graves' disease. Growth of the gland becomes disordered and can cause nodularity and fibrosis.

Solitary nodule of the thyroid
- Single thyroid nodule
- Can become toxic autonomous nodule
- Symptoms and signs of thyrotoxicosis
- Atrial fibrillation—common

Diffuse goiter—non-toxic
- Due to iodine deficiency in endemic area
- Dietary goitrogen, e.g. thiocyanates containing consumption of cabbage and cauliflower.
- Also called colloid goiter due to thyroid follicles are filled with colloid
- Diffuse enlargement of thyroid without toxicity symptoms/signs.

 Note

Goiters are more common in females.

- May be because of autoimmune disorder—more common in females.
- Also due to iodine is required in larger amounts due to pregnancy.

Diffuse toxic goiter: Occurs in Graves' disease.

Multinodular goiter: Nontoxic
- Multiple nodules over the thyroid.
- Can compress the neighbouring structures.
- Cytokines, growth factors and TSH are responsible
- Can contribute to hyperplastic response.
- Can become toxic multinodular goiter.

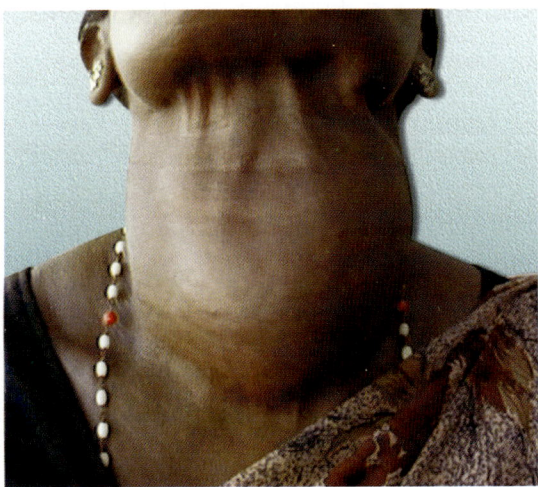

Fig. 8.3: Uniformly enlarged Goiter in Graves' disease

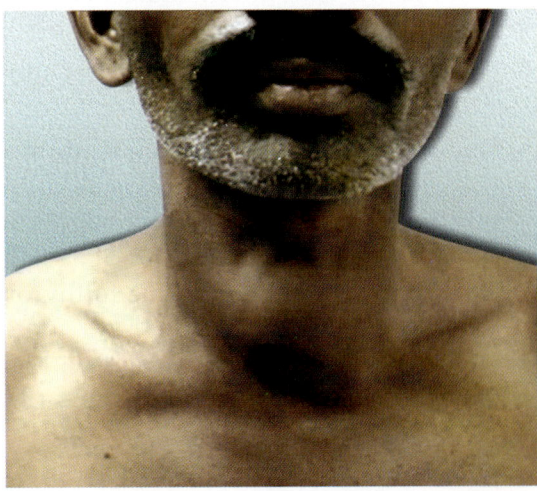

Fig. 8.4: Nodular goiter

THYROID STORM
What is Thyroid Storm?
Medical emergency due to the excess release of thyroid hormone due to inadequately treated or inadequately controlled hyperthyroidism. It is a life-threatening hypermetabolic state.

Characteristics
- Patient is restless
- Vomiting
- Convulsions
- Coma
- Tachycardia
- Cardiac failure

Precipitating Factors
- Cerebrovascular accident
- Stress and infection in a patient of thyrotoxicosis
- Iodine therapy in hyperthyroidism
- Surgery/trauma/CCF in a patient of thyrotoxicosis
- Preparation inadequate prior to surgery in hyperthyroidism.

Complications of Thyrotoxicosis
General
- Weight loss
- Severe sweating
- Hyperpyrexia

CVS
- Sinus tachycardia
- Atrial fibrillation
- High output cardiac failure.

Nervous system
- Myopathy
- Periodic paralysis
- Bulbar palsy

Jod-Basedow effect
Due to administration of iodine exogenously.

Usual sources of iodine
- Radiological contrast agents

- Oral supplementation of iodine
- Amiodarone

Effect is common in patients with iodine deficiency goiter or autonomous nodules/toxic multinodular goiter—results in hyperthyroidism.

Subclinical hypothyroidism
- No clinical features of hypothyroidism
- Biochemical evidence of hypothyroidism

Indications for thyroxine supplementation in subclinical hypothyroidism
- If TSH level is more than 10 without symptoms
- In pregnancy status
- In psychiatric disturbance
- Obesity
- Dyslipidemia
- Heart failure
- Associated IHD
- Infertility

Thyroid swelling may press on the following structures and results in manifestations
Trachea
- May cause shift of trachea.
- Pressing on trachea-scabbard trachea (minimal pressure on lateral lobes of thyroid results in stridor.)

Kocher's test: This is the test for evidence of tracheal compression by the thyroid swelling-usually in patients with large multinodular goiter or carcinoma of thyroid. Compression of the goiter by the fingers causes further narrowing of trachea causing stridor.

Oesophagus—can cause dysphagia.

Carotid pulsations may be absent suggestive of malignancy (Berry's sign).

Recurrent laryngeal nerve: Results in hoarseness of voice.

Can also press on the sympathetic trunk and larynx.

Retrosternal extension of Goiter (Pembeton's sign)
- Ask the patient to raise the arms above the shoulders and keeping them in that position for a while with the arms touching the ears.
- Observe for facial congestion, cyanosis, venous distension.

Myxedema Coma
- In a known patient of hypothyroidism
- Develops severe manifestations of myxedema.

Features
- Decrease in the conscious level
- Convulsions
- Bradycardia
- Hypothermia
- Respiratory depression

Precipitating factors
- Sedative hypnotics
- Anesthetic administration
- Pneumonia
- Congestive cardiac failure
- Sepsis
- Myocardial infarction.

Complications of Hypothyroidism
Metabolic
- Weight gain
- Hyperlipidemia
- Hyponatremia
- Hypothermia

Cardiovascular
- Diastolic hypertension
- Pericardial effusion
- Myocardial dysfunction

Hematological: Severe anemia.

Respiratory
- Pleural effusion
- Respiratory depression

Gynaecological
- Menorrhagia
- Infertility

Nervous system
- Depression
- Coma

- Entrapment neuropathy
- Proximal muscle weakness
- Cerebellar dysfunction
- Hoffman's syndrome

OBESITY

Body mass index

Calculated by $\dfrac{\text{Weight in kg}}{(\text{Height in meter}^2)}$

Obesity is characterised by increase in the body mass index (BMI)

Body mass index and obesity (BMI)

BMI < 18.5 kg/m²   Underweight
18.5–24.9   Normal
25–29.9   Overweight
>30   Obese
>35   Morbid obesity

BMI and Asian and Indian population

<18.5   Underweight
18.5–24.9   Overweight
> 25   Obesity

 Note

Cardiovascular risk is more with BMI of 23 and above in Indian/Asian population.

Waist circumference

- Measure the waist circumference with the measuring tape which is held between lower ribs and the top of hip bone (iliac crest).
- It usually corresponds at the level of umbilicus.

 Note

Waist circumference of >102 cm in males and 88 cm in females represent visceral fat excess and is more risk of development of metabolic syndrome diabetes mellitus and IHD.

Waist/hip ratio: Measure the waist circumference as above.

Measurement of hip: At the level of widest part of hips and calculate waist/hip ratio.

Clinical significance
- Normal waist/hip ratio in men < 0.9
- In women < 0.85

Waist/hip ratio
- If ratio is less than 0.8: Prognosis better (typical of pear-shaped obesity).
- If the ratio is more than 0.8: Typical of apple-shaped obesity.

Significant of waist/hip ratio
If ratio is > 0.9
- Associated with abnormal lipid profile
- Insulin resistance is more common
- Development of diabetes mellitus type 2
- Increased risk of coronary artery disease.

Different types of obesity
- Pear shaped (already described)
- Apple shaped (already described)
- Cushingoid—deposits of fat over the neck, face and upper part of the body
- Limbs are thin.
- Male pattern—android type—fat distribution—over the waist
- Female pattern—gynaecoid type—fat distribution—over the hips.

Approach to a patient of obesity
- Enquire the dietary history and physical activity of the individual and family—history of obesity.
- Rule out secondary causes like:
  - Hypothyroidism
  - Acromegaly
  - Cushing's syndrome
  - Polycystic ovary syndrome
  - Drug induced:
    - Corticosteroids
    - Tricyclic antidepressants
    - Valoproate carbamezepine
    - Sulfonylureas, pioglitazone including insulin
- Measure the body height, weight, waist/hip ratio
- Measure the blood pressure, examine the cardiovascular, respiratory, GIT, CNS and

musculoskeletal systems for complications.
- Also look for secondary causes of obesity.

Complications of obesity

Cardiovascular
- IHD
- Hypertension
- CCF
- Pulmonary embolism
- Varicose veins

Endocrinal
- Dyslipidemia
- Metabolic syndrome
- Diabetes mellitus
- Polycystic ovary syndrome

Respiratory
- Obesity and hypoventilation
- Obstructive sleep apnea
- Pickwickian syndrome

Musculoskeletal
- Gouty arthritis
- Osteoarthritis
- Carpal tunnel syndrome

Gastrointestinal tract: Non-alcoholic steato-hepatopathy.

Dermatological
- Cellulitis/carbuncle
- Striae/scar due to repeated stretching of skin

Psychosocial: Endogenous depression.

Hyperprolactinemia

Normal serum prolactin level

Males
- Less than 20 ng/ml
- Non-pregnant females: 15 to 40 ng/ml
- Pregnant females: 80 to 400 ng/ml

Causes

Physiological conditions
- Lactation
- Pregnancy
- Sleep
- Chest wall stimulation

Drug induced
- Metaclopramide
- Reserpine
- Alpha methyldopa
- Amitryptaline

Pituitary disorders: Prolactinoma, acromegaly.

Due to damage to pituitary stalk
- Pituitary mass pressure on the pituitary stalk
- Surgery and irradiation of pituitary.

Systemic disorders
- Epileptic seizures
- CRF
- Hypothyroidism.

Clinical features

Women
- Amenorrhea
- Galactorrhea
- Weight gain
- Decreased libido

Men
- Lack libido
- Impotence

There can be visual loss due to compression on the optic chiasma.

PROLACTINOMA

Prolactin producing tumors from lactotroph cells
- Produces excess prolactin
- Can occur both in men and women
- May not become symptomatic for long duration.

Manifestations
- Microadenoma <1 cm does not cause involvement of surrounding structures.
- Macroadenoma >1 cm can involve surrounding structures.

Manifestations

In males
- Loss of libido and impotence.
- Infertility

In females
- Galactorrhea
- Amenorrhea
- Infertility

Features due to pressure effect
- Headache
- Compression of optic chiasma
- In microadenoma prolactin level may be <100 µg/Lit
- In macroadenoma prolactin level >200 µg/Lit
- MRI brain—diagnostic.

ACROMEGALY

Enlargement of parts of body like hands, feet and jaw due to increased secretion of growth hormone by the pituitary occuring in adults.

Causes
- Adenoma of the pituitary: Somatotroph—acidophil adenoma
- Part of MEN syndrome

Ectopic secretion of growth hormone
Causes
- Bronchogenic carcinoma
- Hypothalmic tumors

Other causes: Pancreatic islet tumors.

Pathophysiology
Clinical manifestations are due to
- Increase in the level of growth hormone.
- It is also due to increased action of insulin like growth factor-I action.
- *In children*: It produces increase in growth resulting in pituitary gigantism.
- *In adults*: Increase in the size of body parts (especially terminal body parts) resulting in acromegaly.

Clinical features: Slowly progressive manifestations.

Features due to pituitary mass/tumors
- Severe headache

- Bitemporal hemianopia—due to pressure effect on optic chiasma
- Hyperprolactinemia.

Gigantism: Standard height above the 2.5 standard deviation above the height of corresponding age and sex.

Features of Gigantism and Acromegaly
Height—tall stature.

Facial features
- Coarse exaggerated skin folds
- Frontal bossing
- Prognathism—mandibular enlargement
- Incisor teeth—widely placed.

Upper limbs
- Increase size of hands
- Carpal tunnel syndrome
- Tightening of rings
- Increased size of gloves

Skin
- Thick and greasy
- Pigmentation
- Acanthosis nigricans.
- Excess skin tags

Joints and muscle involvement
- Proximal muscle weakness
- Kyphosis
- Osteoarthritis

Cardiovascular
- Hypertension
- LVH
- IHD and cardiomyopathy

Respiratory
- Hoarseness of voice
- Sleep apnea—due to upper airway obstruction

General features
- Weight gain
- Hyperglycemia
- Hirsutism
- Colonic polyp

Feet
- Enlarged
- Increase in the size of shoes

 Note

Gigantism—all features of acromegaly along with tall stature. Hands, feet and head are large.

Complications of acromegaly
Cardiovascular and cerebrovascular:
- Hypertension
- IHD
- Cardiac arrhythmias
- Cardiomyopathy
- CCF
- CVA

Endocrinal: Diabetes mellitus.
Respiratory: Obstructive sleep apnea due to upper airway obstruction.
GIT: Increased incidence of colonic polyps and malignancy.
Due to pressure effect of the tumor on the surrounding structures.

Lab investigations
- Measurement of growth hormone (single level not reliable).
- Measurement of IGF-1 level
- In ectopic causes: GHRH level
- Due to compression of pituitary stalk—increased prolactin level
- Measurement of TSH, ACTH, gonadotropine level.
- Oral GTT: There is no suppression of growth.

Hormone level after glucose administration.

Imaging studies
X-ray for heel pad thickness: On the lateral X-ray of foot: >21 mm thickness is abnormal.

Causes of increased heel pad thickness
- Acromegaly
- Myxedema
- Pedal edema states
- Obesity.

Other X-ray findings
- Increased size of sinuses
- Thickening of skull bones
- Mandibular enlargement.

CT/MRI for
- Pituitary enlargement
- Microadenoma <10 mm
- Macroadenoma >10 mm
- For structures surrounding pituitary.

HYPOPITUITARISM
Decrease in the production of hormones from the anterior pituitary.

Causes
Disorders of Pituitary
- Autoimmune hypophysitis
- Granulomas
  - Tuberculosis
  - Sarcoidosis
  - Fungal infection
  - Histiocytosis
- Sheehan's syndrome
- Tumors of the pituitary
  - Adenoma
  - Secondary deposits
  - Craniopharyngioma
- Decreased production of hormone—genetic causes.

Disorders of hypothalamus
- Granulomatous disorder
  - Tuberculosis
  - Sarcoidosis
  - Fungal infection
  - Histiocytosis
- Neoplasms—gliomas
- Head trauma
- Resection of pituitary stalk
- Genetic defect: Kallmann's syndrome

Features of hypopituitarism
- Depends on the etiology and type of hormone deficiency.

- Earliest loss will be growth hormone deficiency—may not present with clinical abnormalities in adults.
- Leutinizing hormone will decrease after the occurrence of growth hormone deficiency.
- ACTH and TSH—decrease late to occur.

Effect of hormone deficiencies
- GH deficiency—in children—growth retardation
- In adults: Decreased muscle mass
- Increased body fat
- Decreased bone mineralisation
- Depression

Decreased gonadotropins
Males: Decrease/loss of secondary sexual character
- Infertility
- Loss of libido
Females
- Menstrual irregularity
- Infertility

Decrease of ACTH/corticotrophin releasing hormone
- Decreased cortisol effect
- With normal mineralocorticoid activity.

Decreased TRH/TSH deficiency
- Children—decreased growth
- Adults—hypothyroidism
Prolactin decrease:
- Decreased lactation.

Long standing pituitary deficiency
- Increased cardiovascular and cerebrovascular mortality.
- If the posterior pituitary is involved—diabetes insipidus.

Laboratory evaluation
Measurement of hormone levels
- Growth hormone deficiency
- Prolactin decrease
- Cortisol decrease
- T4 ↓ and TSH ↓
- FSH ↓ LH ↓

Stimulation tests
- For thyroid deficiency: TSH stimulation
- For growth hormone deficiency:
  - Insulin-induced hypoglycemia and growth hormone response
- For LH and FSH: GNRH administration tests.
- For cortisol response: CRH stimulation and cortisol response and ACTH stimulation.

Evaluation for aetiology: Blood tests, imaging of pituitary, serological tests.

Hirsutisim: Male Pattern Growth of Hair in a Female
Causes
Endocrinal
Ovarian
- Polycystic ovary
- Ovarian tumors

Adrenal
- Adrenal tumors
- Congenital adrenal hyperplasia
  - Acromegaly
  - Cushing's syndrome
  - Hyperprolactinemia

Drug induced
- Cyclosporin
- Phenytoin sodium
- Minoxidil
- Androgens preparation

Other causes
- Idiopathic
- True hermaphroditism
- Pregnancy-related.

Virilism
- Development of feature of a male in a female patient
- Due to excess androgen level
- Commonly occurs with adrenal or ovarian tumors

Features
- Male pattern baldness
- Decreased breast size

- Male pattern voice—deepening of voice
- Increased muscle mass
- Enlargement of clitoris
- Development of acne
- Excessive libido

DIABETES INSIPIDUS

Occurs due to deficiency of vasopressin.

Causes

- Central (pituitary) induced diabetes insipidus
- Posthead injury (to the pituitary)
- Tumors of the pituitary
- Meningitis/encephalitis
- Granulomas of the pituitary: TB/sarcoidosis
- Genetically determined
- Autoimmune hypophysitis
- Sheehan's syndrome

Nephrogenic (Arginine vasopressin does not act at the renal level)

- Genetic disorder involving vasopressin receptor gene
- Drug-induced: Lithium/Demeclocycline
- Hypercalcemia
- Hypokalemia
- Idiopathic.

Clinical features

- Polyuria—large amount of urine >10 liters/day
  - Nocturia
  - Low osmolality of urine
- Polydipsia: Excessive thirst due to increase plasma concentration
- Elderly—decreased fluid intake—can have dehydration.
- Drowsiness.

Differential diagnosis

Central diabetes insipidus

- Urine volume is increased
- Urine osmolality less than 300 mOsm/day
- Serum osmolality >300 mOsm/day

- Low arginine vasopressin level.
- MRI brain—detects hypothalamic pituitary disease.

Nephrogenic diabetes insipidus

- Urine volume is increased
- Urine osmolality is decreased
- No action of arginine vasopressin
- Serum arginine vasopressin level—normal

Psychogenic polydipsia

Features

- Chronic excess intake of water
- Evidence of psychiatric illness
- No evidence of water intoxication or hyponatremia.

Mass Lesions of Pituitary/Hypothalamus

Effect of Pituitary/Hypothalamic Mass Lesions

- Headache: Dura gets stretched due to pituitary enlargement
- Pressure effect: Optic chiasma—bitemporal hemianopia
- On cavernous sinus
  - 3rd, 4th, 6th cranial nerve palsy
  - Vth nerve involvement
  - Facial sensory loss

Following structures can be involved/invaded

- Invasion of optic nerve/optic chiasma
- Involvement of pituitary stalk—causes hyperprolactinemia
- Extension into the sphenoidal sinus—obstruction to the nasopharynx
- CSF rhinorrhea.

Involvement of hypothalamus

- Abnormal temperature regulation
- Diabetes insipidus
- Disturbed sleep and appetite
- Precocious puberty/hypogonadism

Involvement of frontal and temporal lobe

- Convulsions, change of personality
- Smell abnormality.

Causes of pituitary mass lesion
Adenoma of pituitary
- Gliomas
- Meningiomas
- Craniopharyngioma.

ENDOCRINE HYPERTENSION

Common causes
- Corticosteroid administration
- Diabetes mellitus
- Obesity induced
- Thyrotoxicosis
- Hypothyroidism.

Other causes
- Cushing's syndrome
- Pheochromocytoma
- Acromegaly
- Primary hyperparathyroidism.

Aldosterone related
- Primary aldosteronism
- Bilateral adrenal hyperplasia
- Primary adrenal hyperplasia
- Glucocorticoid remediable hypertension—genetic mutation
- Familial hyperaldosteronism.

Other rarer causes
- Renin secreting tumors
- Liddle syndrome
- Licorice ingestion

Renin and Hypertension
- Juxtaglomerular apparatus produces renin.
- Renin acts on the angiotensinogen which is produced in the liver and converts it into angiotensin I. In the lung angiotensin I will be converted to angiotensin II in the presence of converting enzyme. Angiotensin II is a very powerful vasoconstrictor causes hypertension.

Features of Low Renin Hypertension
- Common in black race and elderly population.
- Lesser cardiovascular risk
- Low plasma renin activity
- Increased angiotensin II activity in vascular endothelium and kidney
- ACE inhibitors are effective. Diuretics are the drug of choice. Spironolactone and eplerenone are effective.

Causes of low renin hypertension
- Primary hyperaldosteronism
- Congenital adrenal hyperplasia
- Liddle syndrome
- Some cases of essential hypertension

DIABETES MELLITUS

General Examination in a Diabetic Patient
- Measure the BMI
- Measure the waist circumference
- Measure the waist/hip ratio

Look for
Pallor
- Represent chronic kidney disease in a diabetic
- Associated B12 deficiency (metformin induced)
- Autoimmune: Pernicious anemia (in type 1 DM)

Icterus: Diabetes with liver disease due to NASH.
Edema: Diabetes with nephropathy, CCF, autonomic neuropathy, pioglitazone induced.

Pulse
- Evidence for thickening of vessel wall—atherosclerosis.
- Peripheral pulse for evidence of peripheral vascular disease
- Carotid bruit.

Blood pressure
- On lying down and also on standing
- On standing—for postural hypotension.
- Postural hypotension: Autonomic neuropathy
- Drug induced (antihypertensives)

Eye examination
- For refractory errors
- Diabetic retinopathy
- Cataract
- Laser scars
- Xanthelasma

Look for ptosis
- 3rd nerve palsy
  - Ophthalmoplegia
  - 4th and 6th nerve palsy
  - 7th cranial nerve palsy

Skin examination including mucus membranes
Look for
- Acanthosis nigricans—axilla
- Vitiligo—type I diabetes mellitus
- Skin/Shin spots
- Cutaneous infections
- Furuncle/carbuncle/herpes zoster
- Oral candidiasis
- Bullous lesions
- Necrobiosis lipoidica diabeticorum

Examination of hand
- Dupuytren's contracture
- Carpal tunnel syndrome
- Wasting of small muscles of hands—due to motor neuropathy
- Can have sensory loss—sensory neuropathy

Prayer's sign
- Difficulty in straightening of fingers.
- Extension of metacarpophalangeal joint is affected in both hands.

Lower limb examination in a diabetic
- Pulse—peripheral pulse for vascular disease, record ankle brachial index.
- Signs of ischemia—blackening of limbs
- *Sensory neuropathy*
  - Sensory loss
  - Painless trophic ulcers
  - Infection between toes and nails (fungal infection)
- *Motor neuropathy*
  - Deformity—clawing of toes
  - Loss of ankle jerk

- Muscle wasting
- Charcot's joints.

Systemic examination
CVS
- Cardiomegaly
- Murmur due to ischemic MR
- CCF

Abdominal examination: Fatty liver—hepatomegaly.
CNS
- Cranial nerve palsy
- Sensory and motor neuropathy
- Autonomic neuropathy

Other important clinical signs to look for in diabetes mellitus
- Oral candidiasis
- Dehydration: Diabetic ketoacidosis/hyperosmolar state
- Thyroid enlargement (type 1 diabetes mellitus and thyroiditis)
- Emaciation: Type 1 diabetes mellitus
- Obesity: Type 2 diabetes mellitus
- Kussmaul's breathing—diabetes ketoacidosis.

Insulin injection sites
- Look for evidence of infection
- Look also for lipoatrophy/hypertrophy.

ADRENAL GLANDS

General Aspects
Location
- Above the kidney
- Has got its own blood supply
- Has got outer cortex and inner medulla.

Cortex—3 parts
- Zona glomerulosa—outermost—secretes aldosterone
- Zona fasciculata—secretes sex steroids
- Zona reticularis—secretes glucocorticoids.

Cushing's Syndrome
Clinical condition occurs due to excess of corticosteroids.

Causes

Iatrogenic: Corticosteroid administration.

Due to excess ACTH
ACTH dependent: Adenoma of the pituitary—called Cushing's disease.
Due to ectopic ACTH—paraneoplastic: Oat cell bronchogenic carcinoma.
Not dependent on ACTH
- Adrenal adenoma
- Adrenal carcinoma
- Adrenal hyperplasia

Manifestations of Cushing's Syndrome

General features
- Weight gain
- Moon face and buffalo hump
- Hypertension—diastolic
- Hyperglycemia.

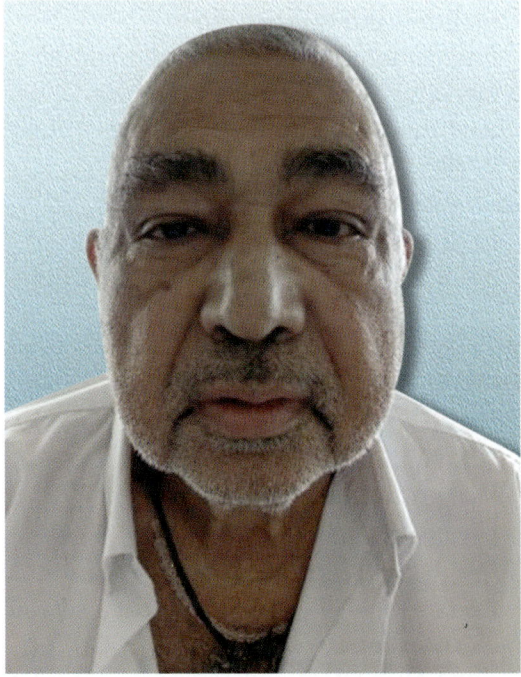

Fig. 8.5: Cushingoid facies (steroid therapy)

Dermatological
- Striae—purplish color over the abdomen
- Easy bruisability
- Pigmentation of knuckle

Gynaecological
- Amenorrhea (hypogonadotropism)
- Hirsutism

Neuropsychiatric manifestations: Depression and anxiety.

Cardiovascular: Hypertension

Musculoskeletal
- Pathological fracture
- Proximal myopathy

Face in Cushing's syndrome: Rounded and plethoric (moon face).

Adrenal Insufficiency

Primary adrenal insufficiency: Addison's disease—due to defect in the adrenal gland.

Causes
- Autoimmune adrenalitis
- Tuberculosis/fungal infection of the adrenal.
- Bleeding into the adrenal, e.g. meningococcal sepsis
- Lymphoma, metastasis involving adrenal glands.
- Drugs like aminoglutethimide, ketaconazole
- Bilateral adrenalectomy.

Secondary Causes
- Prolonged glucorticoid therapy—due to suppression of hypothalamo-pituitary axis.
- Pituitary/hypothalamic disease
  - Autoimmune hypophysitis
  - Mass lesion
  - Irradiation
  - Hemorrhage into the pituitary
  - Tuberculosis/fungal infection.
  - Sarcoidosis.

Features: In general
- Pallor
- Pigmentation of scars, creases—due to excess proopiomelanocortin (POMC) production.

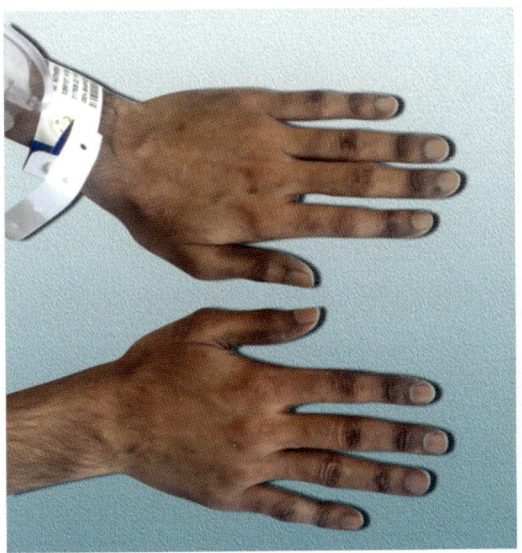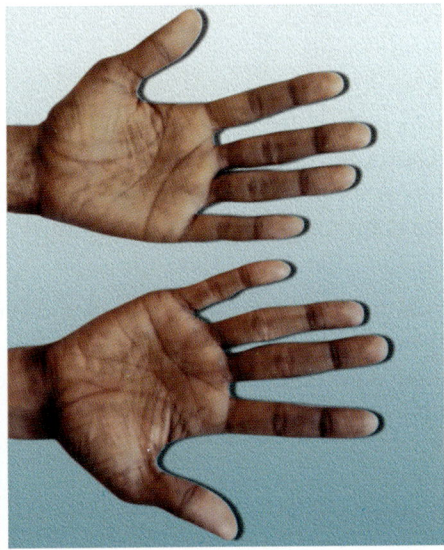

Fig. 8.6: Pigmentation of knuckles and palmar creases in Addison's disease

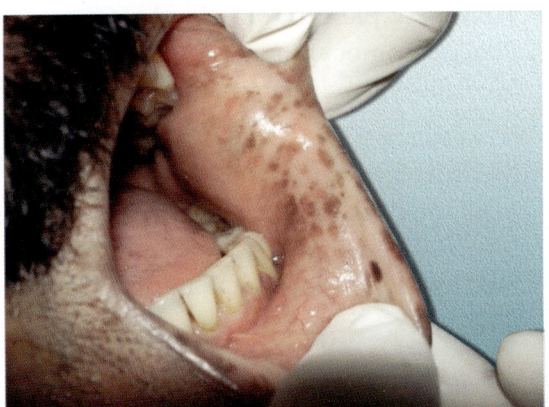

Fig. 8.7: Oral mucosal pigmentation in Addison's disease

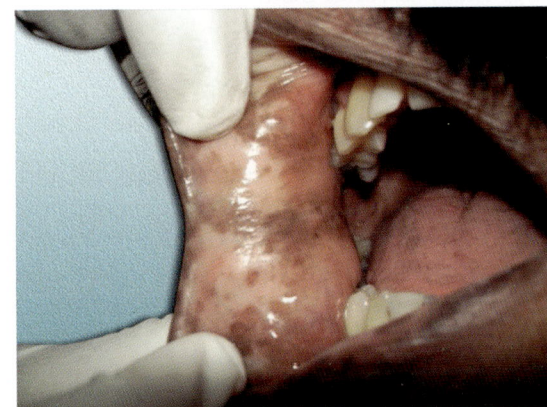

Fig. 8.8: Oral mucosal pigmentation in Addison's disease

Due to decreased level of adrenal androgens
- Fatigue
- Decreased libido and decrease of pubic hairs (in women)

Due to decrease level of mineralocortocids (in primary deficiency):
- Hyponatremia
- Hyperkalemia
- Postural hypotension.

Due to decreased level of glucocorticoids
- Hyponatremia, hypoglycaemia and fatigue.

- Low blood pressure
- Loss of appetite and weight
- Anemia with high eosinophil count.

ACUTE ADRENAL INSUFFICIENCY

Adrenal Crises/Addisonian Crises

Medical Emergency
- It may occur in a patient of: Chronic adrenal insufficiency.
- On long-term corticosteroid therapy with abrupt stoppage
- Patients with pituitary insufficiency

Participating factors

- Infection/sepsis
- Stress
- Surgical procedure
- Development of hyperthyroidism
- Sudden stoppage of corticosteroids if the patient is on long-term steroid therapy.

Clinical features

- Postural hypotension with development of hypovolemic shock.
- Nausea, vomiting, abdominal pain and tenderness.
- Fever
- Altered sensorium and coma
- Hypoglycemia.

Other features

In primary adrenal insufficiency:

- Pigmentation
- Hyponatremia
- Hyperkalemia
- Acidosis and dehydration.
- Hypercalcemia (due to decreased GFR and increased tubular calcium reabsorption and also due to increased calcium mobilization from the bone).

Primary Hyperaldosteronism

Causes

Adrenal adenoma

- Conn's syndrome
- Adrenal hyperplasia
- Idiopathic
- Aldosterone producing carcinoma

Features

- Due to hypokalemia: Fatigue and muscle weakness
- Hypertension—diastolic
- Absence of edema
- Metabolic alkalosis.

Secondary Hyperaldosteronism

Due to conditions causing increased renin and aldosterone.

Causes

- Cirrhosis of liver
- CCF
- Nephritic/nephrotic syndrome
- Renin secreting tumor
- Renal artery stenosis
- Accelerated hypertension
- Bartter's and Gitelman's syndrome

Multiple Endocrine Neoplasia Syndrome (MEN Syndrome)

Type 1

- Tumors of anterior pituitary
- Tumors of islets of pancreas
- Tumors of parathyroid gland

Type 2

- Tumors of parathyroid glands
- Phaeochromocytoma
- Medullary carcinoma of thyroid

Type 3 (Type 2 B)

- Medullary carcinoma of thyroid
- Marfanoid features
- Mucosal neuromas
- Dysfunction of intestinal autonomic ganglia

Mineralocorticoid Excess

Causes

- Unilateral adrenal cortical adenoma: Primary hyperaldosteronism
- Bilateral adrenal hyperplasia
- Carcinoma of adrenal cortex
- Genetic defect causing hyperaldosteronism responding to glucocorticoids
- Cushing's syndrome
- Congenital adrenal hyperplasia
- Apparent mineralocorticoid excess syndrome

Phaeochromocytoma

Benign tumor producing sympathetic amines
Common site: Adrenal medulla

Extra adrenal site

- Sympathetic ganglia in the abdomen and chest.
- *Secrete*: Epinephrine.
- *Most tumors secrete*: Epinephrine ocassionally norepinephrine and dopamine.
- Age group involved: 20 to 50 years
- Cells responsible: Chromaffin cells
- May be a part of MEN syndrome

Triggering factors for manifestations

- Anxiety
- Emotional upsets
- Induction of anesthesia and surgery
- Change of body position
- Labor and delivery
- Consumption of food containing tyramine-like cheese

Clinical features

- Headache, sweating, palpitation
- Weight loss, nausea, vomiting
- Chest pain, fear of death
- Can have postural hypotension
- Can present with accelerated hypertension
- Predominantly systolic hypertension and blood pressure is difficult to control.

Complications

- Hypertensive crises
- Using beta blocker alone worsens hypertension
- CCF
- Cerebrovascular accident
- Renal failure

Parathyroid Glands

There are two pairs of parathyroid glands (total 4) which are situated posterior to the thyroid gland.

Hormone secreted: Parathyroid hormone (PTH)—peptide hormone

Secreted by: Chief cells of the parathyroid glands.

Actions of parathyroid hormone

At renal tubular level

- Increase reabsorption of calcium, magnesium
- Enhances excretion of phosphorous and bicarbonate

At intestinal level: Increases absorption of calcium from the intestine.

At renal level: Facilitates formation of 1–25 $(OH)_2$ vitamin D = D3 from the kidney.

At the bone level: Facilitates movement of calcium from the bone.

Normally serum calcium and phosphorous are under the influence of:

- Parathyroid hormone
- Calcitonin
- Vitamin D_3

Calcitonin

Secreted by—para follicular—C cells of thyroid.

Actions: Decreases serum calcium level.

At renal tubular level: Decreases absorption of calcium and increases its excretion.

At bone level

- Increases osteoblastic activity.
- Decreases osteoclastic activity.

Action of vitamin D_3: Facilitates increased calcium absorption from the gut.

PRIMARY HYPERPARATHYROIDISM

- Due to primary disease of parathyroid glands.
- Causes hypercalcemia and its manifestations.
- One of the most common causes of hypercalcemia.

Causes

- Common: Adenoma of parathyroid gland
- Rare: Parathyroid hyperplasia
- Parathyroid carcinoma

Manifestations: Triad of symptoms:

- Moans: Psychiatric manifestations

- Groans—bony pain
- Abdominal pain—due to renal calculi
- Neuropsychiatric
  - Fatigue
  - Neuromuscular weakness
  - Muscle atrophy
  - Memory loss
  - Coma
- Metabolic
  - Hyponatremia
  - Hypercalcemia
  - Hypoglycemia
  - Renal: Polyuria
  - Nephrocalcinosis
  - Skeletal: Bony pain
  - Fractures
  - Osteitis fibrosa cystic
  - GIT: Peptic ulcer disease
  - Pancreatitis
  - Cardiovascular: Hypertension
  - Vascular calcification
  - Arrhythmias
  - Ocular: Cataract

Laboratory Evaluation

- Main features
  - Serum calcium is raised
  - Serum phosphorus is low
- Serum PTH is increased
- Other features—24 hours—urinary calcium is increased
- Short QT interval
- X-ray skull: Pepper pot appearance of skull
- Osteitis fibrosa cystica
- Localisation of lesion: CT scan, MRI scan and ultrasound scan of the neck.

Secondary Hyperparathyroidism

- Due to prolonged hypocalcemia
- There will be hyperplasia of parathyroid gland.

Causes

- Chronic renal failure

- Gastrointestinal loss of calcium
- Decrease of vitamin D

Tertiary Hyperparathyroidism

Due to prolonged hypocalcemia
↓
Prolonged secondary hyperparathyroidism
↓
Autonomous change in the parathyroid gland
↓
Causes increase secretion of parathyroid hormone

HYPERCALCEMIA

- Normal level of serum calcium: 8.5 to 10.5 mg/dl
- Normal level of ionised calcium level: 4.4 mg/dl
- Degree of hypercalcemia:
  - Mild: 10.5 to 12 mg/dl
  - Moderate: 12 to 14 mg/dl
  - Severe: >14 mg/dl (medical emergency)
- 90% of cases of hypercalcemia are either due to primary hyperparathyroidism or internal malignancy. Primary hyperparathyroidism produces mild to moderate hypercalcemia.
- Severe hypercalcemia is invariably secondary to internal malignancy.

Causes

Common

- Primary hyperparathyroidism
- Hypercalcemia of malignancy
- Due to paraneoplastic manifestations, e.g. carcinoma of lung
- Secondary to hematological malignancies: Lymphoma.
  - Myeloma
- Visceral malignancy with metastasis.
- Excess vitamin D/calcium administration.

Drug induced:
- Lithium therapy
- Thiazide therapy

Rare causes
- Milk alkali syndrome
- Sarcoidosis
- Thyrotoxicosis
- Long-term immobilisation

Clinical aspects of hypercalcemia

Drug induced

Lithium: Long-term lithium intake can cause increase in the parathormone level and can cause parathyroid adenoma.

Thiazides: There will be increased calcium absorption from proximal convoluted tubule.

Malignancy related hypercalcemia

Paraneoplastic—due to PTH-like peptide: For example, squamous cell carcinoma—lung.

Hematological malignancy: Cytokine and lymphokine-mediated (osteoclast activating factor).

Lymphoreticular malignancy—due to increased level of (1–25 $(OH)_2$) vitamin D.

Vitamin D related
- Due to increased intake of vitamin D and vitamin D intoxication.
- Excess vitamin D intake causes increased absorption of calcium from the gut.

Granulomatous disorders: Sarcoidosis, tuberculosis—occurs due to increased (1–25 $(OH)_2$) vitamin D from macrophages.

William's syndrome: Due to abnormal sensitivity to vitamin D.

Hyperthyroidism: Thyroxine-induced—increased turnover of bone and bone resorption.

Immobilization: Long-term immobilization causes increased mobilization of calcium from the bones.

Hypocalcemia

Hypocalcemia occurs when the serum calcium level is below 8.5 mg/dl.

Causes of Hypocalcemia

Hypoparathyroidism
- Primary
- Postoperative

- Pseudohypoparathyroidism
- Vitamin D deficiency
- Chronic phenytoin/phenobarbitone therapy
- Hypomagnesemia
- Hyperphosphatemia
- Severe sepsis
- Renal failure
- Bisphosphonate therapy
- Massive blood transfusion (chelation of calcium due to EDTA).

📝 *Note*

- *Normal level of ionic calcium is 4.40 mg/dl.*
- *Alkalosis decreases the ionic calcium levels.*
- *Acidosis decreases binding of calcium to proteins and increases the free calcium levels.*

Manifestations of Hypocalcemia

Can Present with

Musculoskeletal features
- Fatigue
- Muscle cramps
- Spasm of laryngeal muscles
- Convulsions
- Respiratory depression and arrest.

Neuropsychiatric features
- Psychosis
- Irritability
- Depressive episodes

Cardiac
- Decreased effect of digitalis
- QT prolongation
- Cardiac arrhythmias

Gastrointestinal: Intestinal cramps.

Signs
- Chvostek's sign
- Trousseau's sign.

Transient Hypocalcemia Occurs in

Blood transfusion recurrently: Due to chelation of calcium with EDTA.

Severe burns: Decreased level of ionized calcium.

Acute severe sepsis: Due to protein binding of calcium.

Metabolic alkalosis: Impaired secretion and action of PTH.

Acute pancreatitis
- Release of pancreatic enzymes results in autodigestion of mesenteric fat with releasing of free fatty acids and calcium forms salt with free fatty acids. Additional factors like sepsis also play a role.
- Drug induced: Heparin therapy causes decreased calcium.

Pseudohypoparathyroidism
- Condition characterized by resistance to the action of parathyroid hormone
- Features of hypocalcemia will be present
- Parathyroid hormone level is normal

Features
- Skeletal—short 4th and 5th metacarpals
- Rounded face.
- Mental retardation
- Subcutaneous calcification
- Obesity.

Pseudopseudohypoparathyroidism
- Only morphological features of pseudo-hypoparathyroidism
- Serum calcium is normal.

SHORT STATURE (Dwarfism)

There is decrease in the total body height.

Definition: Standing height is 2 standard deviation below the mean for corresponding age and sex.

In general the short stature or dwarfism is due to:
- Disorders of hormone controlling the growth.
- Either constitutional or growth defect which is intrinsic in nature.

- Chronic systemic disease can also cause short stature.
- Occasionally it may be due to genetic disorder or disorder of growth plate.

Causes of Short Stature/Dwarfism

Endocrine disorders
- Growth hormone deficiency
- Hypothyroidism
- Panhypopituitarism
- Adrenal insufficiency
- Diabetes insipidus/mellitus

Genetic disorders
- Down's syndrome
- Turner's syndrome
- Achondroplasia
- Constitutional disorders
- Familial

Chronic systemic disease
- Chronic cardiac disease including CCF
- Chronic pulmonary disease
- For example, cystic fibrosis, severe asthma
- Chronic renal disease
  - CRF
  - Renal tubular defect
- Chronic GIT disease: Inflammatory bowel disease.

Nutritional
- Malnutrition
- Calorie deprivation

Metabolic
- Glycogen storage disease
- Mucopolysaccharidoses

Psychosocial
- Starvation
- Emotional and social deprivation.

Short stature may be

Proportionate
- All body parts are small
- For example, deficiency of growth hormone/parents are short

Disproportionate
- Some parts of the body are short/other parts above average
- For example, short limbs/normal trunk as in achondroplasia.

Approach to a Patient of Short Stature

History in a Patient of Short Stature
- Dietary intake for malnutrition
- History of systemic diseases like renal GIT, respiratory and cardiac disease.
- History of recurrent hypoglycemia: In GH deficiency.
- History of chronic diarrhoea possible—malabsorption, chronic inflammatory bowel disease.
- History of polyuria—CRF/renal tubular defect/diabetes mellitus
- History of constipation and weight gain, fatigue
  - Hypothyroidism
  - Cushing's syndrome
- Headache, vomiting and visual disturbance: ICSOL.

Enquire also the following details in the history
- Child birth weight and height
- Growth pattern of the child
- Parents and grandparents final height and weight
- Age at which menarche attained by the mother
- Father's age at which final weight was attained.

Clinical Examination in a Patient of short Stature

Measure
- Total height and body weight
- Upper segment and lower segment
- Normal ratio is 1:1
- Upper segment > lower segment in patients with short stature—achondroplasia.
- Severe pallor
  - Malnutrition

- Chronic disease
- CRF
- Obesity
  - Hypothyroidism
  - Cushing's syndrome (abdominal striae may be present)
- Hypertension: CRF
- Thick coarse skin with goiter—hypothyroidism
- Disproportionate bones—skeletal dysplasia—severe rickets.
- Midline abnormalities:
  - Frothy bossing, flat nasal bridge and crowded teeth: Growth hormone deficiency
- Dysmorphic feature: Genetic syndrome—Down's/Turner's syndrome
- Examine also for development of secondary sexual characters

Short trunk compared to limbs
- Mucopolysaccharidoses
- TB spine

Shorter limbs—
- Achondroplasia/other bone dysplasia
- Refractory rickets
- Osteogenesis imperfecta.

Prediction of child's height
For boys
Paternal height (in cm) + 13 cm } divided
Maternal height in cm } by 2

For girls
Paternal height (in cm) – 13 cm } total divi-
Maternal height in cm } ded by 2

Look for features of
- Rickets
- Achondroplasia
- Mucopolysaccharidoses.

Look for
- Evidence of GIT/respiratory and cardiac disease.
- Evidence of malnutrition/hypothalamic defect.

Look for

- Endocrine abnormalities
- For example, hypothyroidism/panhypo-pituitarism
- Presence of goiter (hypothyroidism, Hashimoto's thyroiditis)
- Short 4th metacarpal/metatarsals: Pseudo-hypoparathyroidism.

Investigations in a patient of short stature: CBP, ESR, FBS, urine analysis, stool analysis, RFT, LFT.

Special tests

- Thyroid function test
- GH stimulation tests
- Bone age estimation
- Coeliac serology
- Karyotyping
- Duodenal biopsy

Bone age: Estimated by performing X-ray of hand and wrist—looking for epiphyseal fusion.

🔑 **Key Points:**

In all cases of short stature secondary to pathological cause bone age is delayed compared to chronological age.

Delayed bone age compared to chronological age

- Decreased growth hormone.
- Hypothyroidism
- Cushing's syndrome
- Chronic system illness.

Bone age is equal to chronological age

- Familial
- Genetic syndromes

Significance of dental age in deciding skeletal age

- Eruption of primary and secondary teeth
- Delayed
  - Growth hormone deficiency
  - Hypothyroidism
- Evaluate also for renal, cardiovascular and pulmonary disorder and bone dysplasias.

Differential diagnosis of short stature

Common causes

- Idiopathic
- Constitutional delay
- Familial

If dysmorphic feature present: Consider genetic syndromes, e.g. Down's syndrome.

If symptoms and signs of endocrine/GIT disorders

- Hypothyroidism
- Cushing's syndrome
- Coeliac disease
- Inflammatory bowel disease

If evidence of malnutrition and severe anemia

- Decreased nutritional intake
- Coeliac disease

If history of drug intake—like chronic steroid intake—consider drug induced.

If symptoms of chronic illness, consider: Cardiac, renal, pulmonary/GIT cause.

If history of deprived socioeconomic support—consider psychological cause.

General Physical Examination

Temperature Abnormalities

Different Types of Fevers

Saddleback fever

- Sudden onset of high grade fever which persists for 1–2 days and then afebrile period for 1–2 days and then again appears as high grade fever. 2 peaks of high grade fever with an afebrile period in between.
- For example, dengue fever.

Camel hump fever

- There are two fever spikes in 24 hours (double quotidian fever)
- For example, kala azar.

Hyperpyrexia: Temperature recording above 106.7°F or 41.5°C.

Causes

- Falciparum malaria
- Heat hyperpyrexia
- Pontine hemorrhage
- Malignant hyperthermia
- Thyrotoxic crisis
- Atropine datura poisoning

Drug fever

- Usual offending drugs: Antibiotics, anticonvulsants
- Appearance of fever—usually after 7–10 days after starting the offending drugs.

Features

- No signs of toxaemia

- No associated tachycardia
- May have drug rash
- Previous history of drug fever may be present

Lab features

- No raised ESR or leucocytosis
- Eosinophilia may be associated.

Treatment

- Stopping the drug
- Disappears usually within 24 to 48 hours after stopping the drug
- Responds to corticosteroids.

Fever with relative bradycardia

Causes

- Typhoid fever
- Dengue fever
- Leptospirosis
- Legionnaires' disease
- Chlamydial infection.

Fever with relative tachycardia

- Rheumatic carditis
- Diphtheria myocarditis
- Sepsis syndrome

Fever decreasing by lysis: Decrease of temperature after starting the treatment occurs slowly in a step ladder pattern, e.g. typhoid.

 Note

In a patient of typhoid if the temperature decreases by crisis (sudden) suspect intestinal hemorrhage/perforation.

Fever decreasing by crisis

- Sudden decrease of temperature after starting the treatment associated with severe sweating.
- For example, lobar pneumonia.

Facial Abnormalities of Clinical Significance

Puffiness of face

- Acute nephritic syndrome
- Nephrotic syndrome
- SVC obstruction
- Late stages of cardiac failure
- Cirrhosis of liver
- Cushing's syndrome/steroid therapy
- Hypothyroidism
- Angioneurotic edema (may be unilateral).

Face in Systemic Disorders

- Face in systemic sclerosis: *See* the chapter on connective tissue disorders
- Myotonic dystrophy: Hatchet face—*see* the chapter on neurology.
- Elfin face—*see* cardiovascular system.
- Face in COPD:
  - Bluish discoloration of lip and tongue
  - Pursed lip breathing
  - Facial puffiness
  - Prominent eyes
  - Suffused conjunctiva
- *Leonine face*
  - Saddle nose
  - Madarosis
  - Thickening of skin of the face with thickening of ear lobes
  - Seen in lepromatous leprosy
- *Parkinsonism*
  - Dull expression less face
  - Monotonous speech
  - Blinking—less frequent
  - Oculogyric crises (in postencephalitis parkinsonism).
- Mitral facies: *See* under mitral stenosis.
- Thalassemic facies: *See* under thalassemia.

Eye abnormalities

- Prominent eyes—proptosis/exophthalmos
- Yellowish discoloration over the lids or near the inner canthus; xanthelasma palpebrum, e.g. hyperlipidemia.
- Ptosis—unilateral/bilateral
  - Neurogenic: 3rd nerve palsy/Horner's syndrome
  - Myogenic—myasthenia
  - Mechanical—tumors/mass over the upper lid
- Subconjunctival hemorrhage
  - Leptospirosis
  - Bleeding disorder
  - Whooping cough
- Lens dislocation with iridodonesis (tremulousness of iris)
  - Marfan's syndrome (upwards and temporal)
  - Homocystinuria (down and medially)
- Bitot's spots: In vitamin A deficiency
- Phlycten: In tuberculosis
- Corneal ulcers
  - Exposure keratitis—7th nerve palsy
  - Due to lack of sensation—5th nerve palsy
  - Due to Herpes zoster.
- Enlargement of lacrimal glands
  - For example, Sjögren's syndrome
  - Mikulicz disease
- Blue sclera: Osteogenesis imperfecta
- K.F Ring: Wilson's disease
- Ophthalmic fundus—examination
  - Retinopathy: Hypertension
  - Diabetes mellitus
  - Papilledema
  - Optic atrophy
  - Roth's spot
  - Choroid tubercles
  - Cytoid body: In SLE/neuroretinitis
  - Macular star: Hard exudates in a star pattern near/around the macula
  - For example, neuroretinitis.

Abnormalities of the tongue

- Small stiff tongue with fasciculations: Bulbar palsy.
- Flabby tongue with fasciculations: Bulbar palsy.
- Enlarged tongue
  - Myxedema
  - Acromegaly
  - Amyloidosis
  - Tumors of the tongue
  - Angioneurotic edema

Multiple white lesions over the tongue

- Oral candidiasis
- Lichen planus
- Leukoplakia
- Hairy leukoplakia
- Excessive dryness of tongue.

Multiple ulcers over the tongue

- Aphthous ulcers
- Herpes simplex infection
- B12 deficiency
- Behçet's syndrome/SLE
- Pemphigus vulgaris

Discoloration of tongue

- Bluish discoloration—central cyanosis
- Red appearance—glossitis/polycythemia
- Black hairy tongue: Candidiasis

Pigmentation of the tongue:

- Multiple polyposis of colon (Peutz-Jeghers syndrome)
- Addison's disease

Skin abnormalities

- Pigmentation: Generalised hyperpigmentation
  - B12 deficiency
  - Addison's disease
  - Ectopic ACTH production (paraneoplastic)
  - Hemachromatosis
  - Drug induced: Chloroquine
  - Clofazemine therapy
- Pigmentation of exposed parts—pellagra

- Photosensitive rash over the face—SLE/dermatomyositis
- Localied or patchy area of pigmentation
  - Acanthosis nigricans
  - Drug reaction
  - Chloasma
  - Café-au-lait spots.
- Hypopigmentation of the skin: Generalised albinism
- Patchy area of hypopigmentation with surrounding hyperpigmentation

General physical examination

- Fungal: Tinea versicolor
- Leprosy
- Vitiligo

Causes of multiple nodular lesion in the skin

- Neurofibromatosis
- Lipomas
- Erythema nodosum
- Cyscticercosis (usually muscles)
- Vasculitis lesions
- Secondary deposits
- Xanthomas

Abnormalities in the Nail

- Ridging and pitting of nail—psoriasis
- Koilonychia and platonychia (iron deficiency anemia)

Beau's lines over the nail

- Presence of transverse ridges over the nail
- Rate of growth of the nail is affected due to illness
- For example
  - Febrile illness
  - Measles
  - Mumps
  - Malnourishment.
- Lindsay nail: Nail is proximally white with distal part of the nail is red, it is also called half and half nail. Usually found in patients with CRF
- Onycholysis separation of the nail occurs from the nail bed
  - For example, thyrotoxicosis.

- Mees' lines: Horizontal white lines occurs over the nail
- For example, arsenic poisoning
- Terry's nail: White nail with ground glass appearance with distal part of the nail is pink.
- For example, cirrhosis, CRF, CCF

Abnormalities of height and weight

Short stature: Child weight is 2 standard deviation or more—below the mean for that children of that same age and sex.

Body Habitus

- *Ectomorphic*
  - Tall in height
  - Thin long limbs
  - Waist and thorax are narrow
- Mesomorphic—well built, muscular with normal stature.
- Endomorphic: Quick gainer of weight, short built, arms and legs are thick.

Arm span > height

Causes
- Marfan's syndrome
- Homocystinuria
- Eunuchoidism
- Hypogonadism
- Klinefelter's syndrome

Lower segment > upper segment

Causes: Same as above.

Hand abnormalities in medical disorders

- Thick spade like hand—acromegaly
- Arachnoldactyly: Long and thin figures
  - Marfan's syndrome
  - Homocystinuria
  - Hypogonadism
- *Short 4th and 5th metacarpals*: Pseudo-hypoparathyrodism
- *Hypoplastic thumb*: Holt-Oram syndrome.
- Multiple fingers (polydactyly:) Laurence-Moon-Biedl syndrome
- *Single palmar crease*: Down's syndrome.

Abnormalities of the feet in medical disorders

- Pes cavs: Syringomyelia
  - Friedreich's ataxia
  - Hereditary sensory motor neuropathy
- Rocker bottom feet: Flat foot with protuberant heel.
- For example, trisomy 18 (Edwards syndrome)
- Associated with PDA

Cervical Lymph Nodes

Outer Waldeyer's ring *(horizontal)*

- Occipital
- Postauricular (mastoid)
- Preauricular (parotid)
- Submandibular
- Submental

Facial nodes: Infraorbital, buccinator, etc.

Superficial cervical

- Anterior cervical: Anterior to jugular vein.
- Posterior cervical: Posterior to jugular vein.
- Deep cervical
  - Jugulodigastric (tonsillar)
  - Prelaryngeal
  - Pretracheal, paratracheal
  - Infrahyoid, omohyoid
  - Supraclavicular and scalene

INTERNAL WALDEYER'S RING

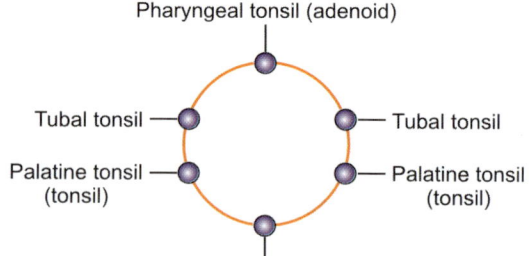

Fig. 9.1: Internal Waldeyer's ring

Axillary Lymph Nodes

Pectoral *(anterior)*

- Situated along the lower border of pectoralis minor behind pectoralis major.

- Drains lateral quadrant of the breast and superficial, anterior and lateral abdominal wall.

Subscapular (posterior)
- In front of subscapularis muscle.
- Drains superficial vessels from the back up to the iliac crest.

Lateral
- Along the medial aspect of brachial vessels
- Drains most of the vessels from upper limb.

Central group
- Center of the axilla in the axillary fat.
- Drains from anterior groups.

Apical
- Apex of the axillary fat
- Drain from all other axillary nodes.

Infraxillary/deltopectoral: Not strictly axillary. In the groove between deltoid and pectoralis major.

Chapter

10

Miscellaneous

RADIOLOGY

Causes of Multiple White Matter Lesions in the Brain MRI

Periventricular Lesions

Common causes
- Aging process
- Small vessel ischemia
- Multiple sclerosis

Rare causes
- ADEM
- Progressive multifocal leucoencephalopathy
- Vasculitis
- HIV encephalopathy
- Osmotic myelinolysis
- Posterior reversible ischemic encephalopathy
- CADASIL syndrome
- CNS lymphoma
- Wernicke's encephalopathy
- Tropical regions: Tuberculosis.

Hot cross bun—sign in the MRI brain
- This is the appearance of pons in patients with multisystem atrophy.
- It is due to selective degeneration of pontocerebellar junction.

Humming bird sign in MRI brain
- Seen in sagittal view of MRI.
- Found in patients with progressive supranuclear palsy (PSP).
- It is due to preservation of pons with midbrain atrophy.
- It is also called penguin sign
- Body of the bird is formed by the normal pons.
- Head of the bird with beak extending towards the optic chiasma—formed by atrophied mid-brain.

MRI—features of multiple sclerosis
- Thinning of corpus callosum—in T1 image
- Multiple white matter lesions—asymmetric-hyperintense in T2
- Dawson's fingers—perpendicular to the lateral ventricles (triangular shaped with outward extension): In images in the flair sequence.

Intracranial Calcifications in the CT/MRI

Causes of normal intracranial calcifications
- Pineal gland
- Choroid plexus
- Basal ganglia

Rarely
- Dura mater
- Superior sagittal sinus
- Dentate nucleus of cerebellum

Pathological causes of intracranial calcifications
- Age related and arterial atherosclerosis
- Infective causes
  - Calcified granulomas

- Cysticercosis
- Toxoplasmosis
- Vascular—vasculitis
- AV malformations/aneurysms
- Previous disorders: Infarct/hemorrhage/abscess
- Tumors
  - Craniopharyngioma
  - Oligodendroglioma
  - Meningiomas
  - Pituitary adenoma
- If calcification is >1 cm, it is called brain stones.

Causes of ring enhancing lesions in the brain in the CT scan

- Tuberculoma
- Abscess
- Neurocysticercosis
- Metastasis
- Lymphoma
- Glioblastoma multiformae
- Thin regular walled lesions—s/o—abscess
- Thin walled with calcified foci about 1–2 cm: Neurocysticercosis
- Mass lesions: Irregular with adjacent secondary lesions with surrounding edema:

- Glioblastoma
- Lesions: at gray and white matter: Junctions—abscess/metastasis.

CT appearance of toxoplasmosis of brain

- Sites: Basal ganglia region.
- Corticomedullary junction
- Size 1–3 cm
- Can cause—mass effect.
- Contrast appearance: Ring enhancing lesions
- Calcification—dot-like appearance
- MRI: Hyperintense lesions with surrounding edema
- MR spectroscopy
  - ↑Lactate peak
  - ↓Choline peak

Radiological differences between lymphoma vs toxoplasmosis in MRI brain

Lymphoma	Toxoplasmosis
Single lesion	Multiple lesions
Site: Subependymal	Basal ganglia
Hemorrhage: Rare	Hemorrhage can occur
Contrast: Solid enhancement	? cystic/nodular enhancement
MRI—spectroscopy ↑Choline peak	Decreased choline peak

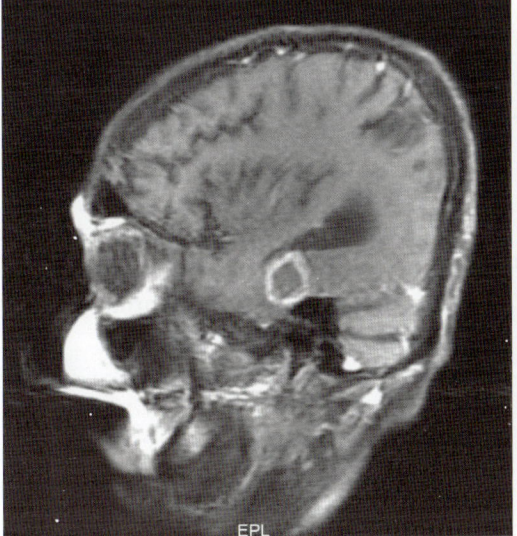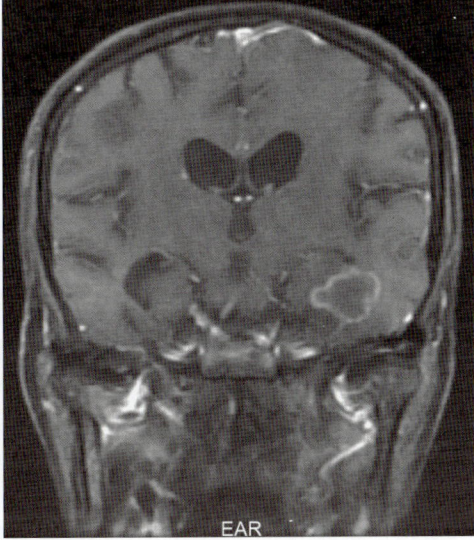

Fig. 10.1: Ring enhancing lesion in the brain

Cryptococcomas in Brain

- Radiologically—can form hydrocephalus
- Involvement of perivascular space with pseudocyst of basal ganglia.

CNS Tuberculosis

CT Appearance

Features

- Enhancement of leptomeninges
- There will be thick exudate formation at the base of the brain.
- Extension of the exudates over the cortical surface is not common (common in bacterial meningitis)

Tuberculoma

- Ring enhancing lesions with edema of the surrounding space.
- Extensive surrounding meningeal enhancement.

CT/MRI Images of Cerebrovascular Disorders

Chronic infarct (cerebral)

- CT scan: Hypodense equal to CSF density.
- No mass effect (negative mass effect)
- Presence of gliosis
- Sulci are widened
- Ipsilateral ventricle is dilated.

Feature of cardioembolic CVA

Features

- Multiple sites of embolization with infarction in the brain.
- Common to cause MCA infarct
- Next common: PCA infarct
- Hemorrhagic transformation can occur (due to vessel injury and reperfusion)
- Features less likely—lacunar infarction.

Radiological appearance of different intracranial vascular lesions.

Cerebral infarct

Acute infarct

- Embolus/thrombus inside the vessel can be directly visualized.

- For example, inside the middle cerebral artery—hyperdense MCA sign or MCA cord sign.

Early hyperacute phase

- Loss of insular ribbon sign:
- There will be loss of differentiation between grey and white water in the lateral margin of the insular cortex (insular ribbon)

Why insula is susceptible?

- Insula has got least collaterals from anterior cerebral and posterior cerebral arteries.
- More susceptible to ischemia of MCA occlusion.

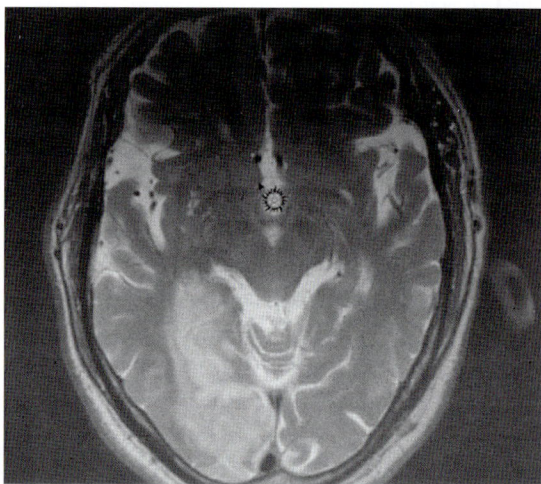

Fig. 10.2: MRI appearance of acute cerebral infarction

Subdural Hematoma

- Usually unilateral
- Site of occurrence—convexities at the fronto-parietal junction.
- Occasionally middle cranial fossa.
- Acute
  - Hyperdense in occurrence compared to cortex.
  - Crescent shaped.
- Chronic
  - Hypodense lesion
  - Mimics subdural hygroma

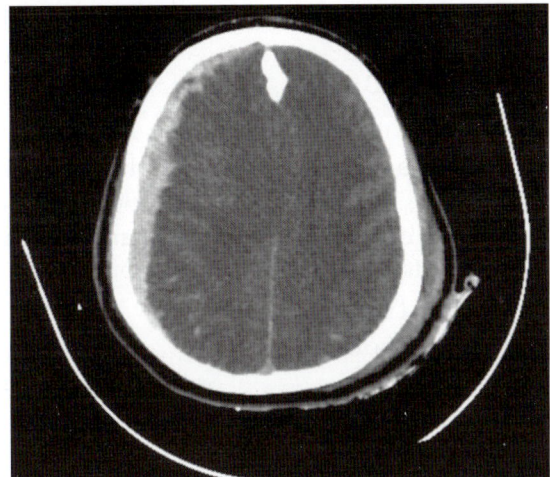

Fig. 10.3: Subdural hematoma

Extradural hematoma

- Lens-shaped biconvex in appearance
- It does not cross the suture lines

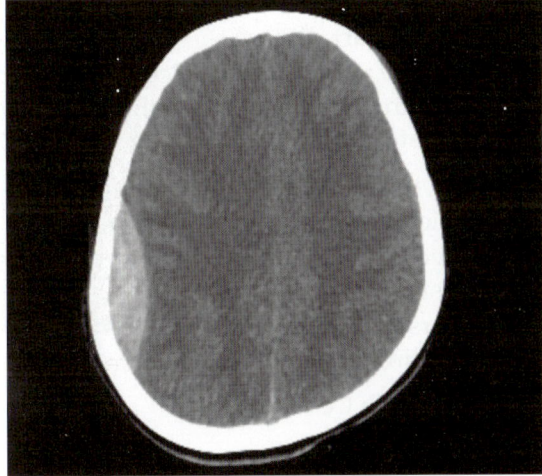

Fig. 10.4: Extradural hematoma

Subarachnoid hemorrhage

- Hyperdense material—filling the subarachnoid space
- Usual site—around the circle of Willis.
- This is the usual site of berry aneurysms.

Intracerebral hemorrhage—CT appearance

- Due to hypertension—common sites: Basal ganglia, putamen
- Thalamus

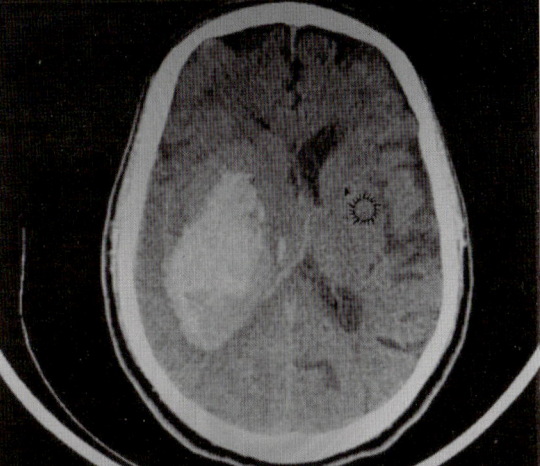

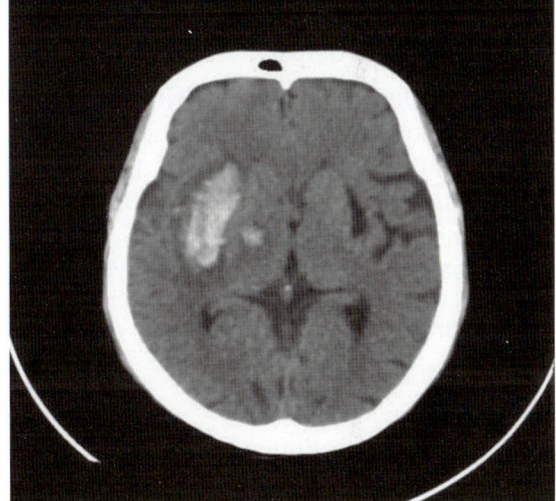

Fig. 10.5: CT (non-contrast) hypertensive intra-cerebral hemorrhage

- Pons
- Cerebellum
- At putamen—terminal branches of middle cerebral arteries—form aneurysms called Charcot-Bouchard aneurysms.
- CT shows hyperdense lesion in the brain parenchyma

Cortical Venous Sinus Thrombosis

CT without contrast: Hyperdensity of the sinus—cord sign:

- Thrombosed venous sinus appears as homogenous and hyperattenuated.

- This is called cord sign
- This is due to increased attenuation of thrombosed material in the venous sinus
- This sign is common in patients with thrombosis of transverse sinus.

Supersagittal sinus (postcontrast)
- Empty delta sign—due to filling defect.
- Hemorrhage into the infarct can occur

Empty delta sign
- Contrast CT—surrounding area of contrast enhancement with lower density in the center—due to thrombosed superior sagittal sinus.
- Surrounding density—due to venous dural collaterals.
- Central lower density: Thrombosed sinus.

Moyamoya appearance in the MRI
- Moyamoya means puff of smoke.
- This is the name given to the appearance of basal telangiectasias in the MRI
- It consists of collateral branches of lenti-culostriate and thalamostriate arteries.

Important ECG Abnormalities

ST Segment Elevation

Causes
- Early repolarisation syndrome
- Transmural MI
- Prinzmetal's angina
- Acute pericarditis.

ST elevation of acute MI; ST/J point elevation of 0.1 mV in corresponding leads. In V2 and V3 leads:

(>0.2 mV) men > 40 years
Men <40 years → 0.25 mV
Women → 0.15 mV

ST segment depression
- Non-Q wave MI
- Sub-endocardial ischemia
- Reciprocal changes in acute MI

Nonischemic ST segment depression
- RVH
- Digitalis effect

- Hypokalemia
- MVP
- RBBB, LBBB

Prominent U wave in the ECG
- U wave is usually in the same direction of T wave.
- U wave can occur with bradycardia with heart rate less than 45/min.

Prominent U wave
- Severe hypokalaemia
- Bradycardia

Occasionally
- Hypothermia
- Hypomagnesemia
- Hypocalcemia
- Digitalis induced

Inverted U wave
- Severe IHD
- Hypertensive heart disease
- Valvular heart disease
- Inverted U wave may predict left anterior descending/LMCA (left main coronary artery) stenosis.

Wellens syndrome (sign)
- In patients with unstable angina.
- T waves in V2-V3—deeply inverted or biphasic.
- It occurs in critical stenosis of left anterior descending coronary artery.

ECG changes in COPD
- P pulmonale
- P wave axis—right shift
- RS right axis deviation
- Low voltage QRS—V4–V6
- Clockwise rotation of the heart—prominent S wave in V6.

Low voltage criteria: Less than 5 mm of QRS voltage in limb leads and less than 10 mm of QRS voltage in precordial leads.

Lead I sign: In emphysema
Lead I shows isoelectric complexes. P, QRS and T waves are not visible.

Other ECG changes in emphysema—S1, S2, S3 pattern and low voltage complexes.

Acute pericarditis

- Diffuse ST segment elevation with concavity upwards.
- PR segment elevation in lead aVR.
- Depression of PR segment in all other leads (atrial injury)
- Increased heart rate
- No reciprocal ST depression.

Early repolarisation syndrome: Benign condition occurring in young healthy individuals.

Characteristics

- Elevation of J point/ST segment of 0.1 mm in 2 contiguous leads
- ST elevation is less than 25% of T wave amplitude.
- ST elevation is with concavity upwards.
- ST elevation is predominantly in inferior and lateral leads.
- No reciprocal changes
- QRS <120 milliseconds.

Digitalis effect and toxicity
Digitalis effect
- Short QT interval
- ST segment downsloping (reverse tick or hockey stick appearance)
- Mild PR prolongation
- Can cause prominent U wave
- T wave flattened/inverted

Digitalis toxicity: Frequent VPCs, all types of arrhythmias except Mobitz type I.

Digitalis effect ST	Ischemic ST
ST depression—down-sloping—reverse Tick mark	ST depression—horizontal or downsloping
T wave flat or inverted	Inverted
In all the leads	Only corresponding leads
PR prolonged	PR not prolonged
Prominent U wave	ECG changes are dynamic (changes with time)

Himalayan P wave

- Prominent P waves lead II, III and AVF and V1
- Prominent in lead II may become even taller than QRS
- Due to gross enlargement of right atrium, e.g. Ebstein's anomaly
  - Tricuspid stenosis.
  - Tricuspid stenosis + pulmonary stenosis

Complete heart block

- P waves are not related to QRS.
- Atrial rate is more than ventricular rate
- Ventricular rate usually <40/especially in acquired complete heart block
- QRS narrow or wide
- QRS narrow: Junctional escape focus in the AV node.
- Wide QRS—ventricular focus—idioventricular rhythm.

AV dissociation

- Independent rhythm in atrium and ventricles.
- One of the causes of third degree heart block
- Complete AV dissociation—atria and ventricles are always independent of each other.
- Incomplete AV dissociation: There will be intermittent capture of atrium and ventricular focus.

ECG-VT vs SVT with Aberrancy
ECG Changes Favoring VT
Positive or negative concordance in the chest leads

- From V1 to V6—complexes are either positive or all complexes are negative.
- RS complexes are not seen.
- Negative concordance more significant

QRS axis: Extreme axis—north west axis.

Broad QRS complexes: >160 milliseconds.

Presence of a fusion beat: Fusion of sinus beat with ventricular beat.

Presence of a capture beat: SA mode captures the ventricle in the presence of AV dissociation to produce a QRS complex of normal duration.

rsr' complex
- With taller left rabbit ear—Rsr'—s/o—VT
- With taller right rabbit ear–rsR'—s/o—RBBB.

Additional factors favoring VT
- Presence of IHD/structural heart disease
- Previous history of MI
- Cardiomyopathy/CCF
- Age> 35–40 years
- Family history of sudden cardiac death.

Causes of sudden cardiac death in the family
- HOCM
- Congenital QT prolongation
- Brugada syndrome
- Arrhythmogenic RV dysplasia

Ectopics—Extrasystoles

Types

Unifocal
- Ectopics arise from single focus which is active.
- Each VPC is identical.

Multifocal: Ectopics arise from 2 or more ectopic foci. They are of multiple QRS morphology.

RV ectopic: In lead V_1: There is LBBB morphology dominant S wave in V_1.

LV ectopic: RBBB pattern in V_1 with dominant R wave in V_1.

VPCs couplets: Two consecutive VPCs.

Triplets: Three consecutive VPCs.

Bigeminy: VPCs are alternating with sinus beat.

Trigeminy: Every 3rd beat is a VPC.

Quadrigeminy: Every 4th beat is a VPC.

Malignant ventricular ectopic
- Those result in dangerous ventricular tachyarrhythmias
- In acute MI > 10/hour after 10 to 16 days.

- Ectopics appearing on R on T phenomenon
- Outflow tract ectopics.

Causes of Dominant R Wave in Lead V_1
- Normal physiological variant
- Misplaced precordial leads
- Mirror image dextrocardia.

Pathological
Common causes
- RVH
- RBBB
- Pulmonary embolism
- Septum secundum ASD

Rarer causes
- True posterior wall MI
- LV ectopic
- Duchenne muscular dystrophy
- WPW syndrome (type-A)

Left anterior hemiblock
- QRS axis—left axis deviation (usually between 45° and 90°)
- Lead I and aVL-qR pattern (small q and tall R wave)
- Lead II, III and aVF-rS pattern (small r and deep S wave)

Other features
- Increased QRS voltage in limb leads
- QRS duration—normal or slightly prolonged.

Left posterior hemiblock
- QRS axis right axis deviation > + 90°
- Lead I and aVL-rS pattern (small r wave and deep S wave)
- Lead II, III and aVF-qR pattern (small Q wave with tall R wave)

Other features
- QRS—normal or slightly prolonged
- No RVH or any other cause for right axis deviation.

Atrial fibrillation
- Varying R-R interval
- Absence of P wave
- Undulating base line—fibrillary waves.

Regular R-R interval in AF: AV junctional tachycardia.

R on T phenomenon
- Ventricular ectopic beat occurs on the T wave of the previous beat.
- It is likely to initiate sustained VT.

VPCs associated with risk of mortality
- Frequent ventricular ectopic…of 2 or more VPCs
- Multimorphic VPCs
- Post MI >10 VPCs/hour
- R on T phenomenon

Pulmonary embolism
- Right axis deviation
- Sinus tachycardia
- Dominant R wave in lead V_1
- T wave inversion in leads V_1 to V_4
- Right atrial enlargement
- Incomplete or complete RBBB
- S1 Q3 T3 pattern
- Clockwise rotation of the heart
- Atrial tachyarrhythmias

Osborn (J) wave
- Positive deflection of the J point
- Most prominent in precordial leads
- Found in patients with hypothermia.

Ashman phenomenon
- Occurs due to change in the QRS cycle length resulting in physiological aberrancy of ventricular conduction with wide QRS complex.
- Commonly occurs in patients with AF with a longer cycle is followed by a shorter QRS cycle.
- Can also occur in supraventricular tachyarrhythmias.
- When a supraventricular beat reaches HIS bundle and Purkinje fibers, one of the branches is still refractory to the conduction. This causes slowness of conduction resulting in bundle branch block pattern without actual block. Usually it is RBBB pattern as right bundle has got a longer refractory period.

Wenckebach's phenomenon: In which a pulse from the atrium do not reach the ventricle which is characterised by progressive prolongation of the P-R interval till when a pulse (conduction) is dropped.

BRUGADA SYNDROME
- Genetic disorder
- Form of channelopathy
- Affects RV outflow tract
- Cardiac muscle sodium channel becomes abnormal with local blockage in the conduction.

Clinical features
- Life-threatening ventricular arrhythmias.
- Can have sudden nocturnal death
- Abnormal breathing pattern at night

ECG features: ECG features are present in one of the leads from V_1 to V_3.

Characteristic features
- ST elevation of more than 2 mm in lead V_1 with T wave inversion (J point elevation of at least 2 mm).
- Can have RBBB pattern.

Brugada sign: ST elevation of more than at least 2 mm in at least 2 leads out of V_1 to V_3 lead.

Right Ventricular Hypertrophy
Type A
ECG features
- Tall R wave in lead V_1 with prominent S wave in V_5, V_6
- *Causes*: Severe pulmonary hypertension. Severe pulmonary stenosis.

Type B
- "R" wave in V_1 > 0.5 mV with R/S ratio > 1, rsr¹ pattern
- No S wave in V_5 V_6
- For example, volume overload of right ventricle. For example, ASD.

Type C
- No definite evidence of RVH in the ECG.
- Indirectly made out by the RA enlargement reflecting RVH (except in severe tricuspid stenosis).

- For example, COPD, acute pulmonary embolism.
- Prominent R wave is not made out in V_1— may be due to vertical position of the heart, lung hyperinflation and low and flat diaphragm in COPD.

ECG criteria for RVH
- R/S ratio is more than one in V_1
- Right axis deviation
- R in V_1 > 0.7 m volts.

Diagnosis of LVH in the presence of LBBB
Points favoring LVH
- Presence of left atrial enlargement
- If voltage of QRS in precorodial leads satisfying LVH criteria
- QRS duration > 160 ms.

COMMON DERMATOLOGICAL AND INFECTIVE DISORDERS

Psoriasis

- Common dermatologial condition.
- Part involved
  - Scalp
  - Trauma prone areas (Koebner's pheno-menon)
  - Elbow
  - Knee
  - Gluteal region.
- Features
  - Plaque-like and popular lesions
  - Red erythematous lesions covered by silvery scales.
- Type
  - Plaque-like psoriasis
  - Guttate psoriasis
    - Papular lesions
    - Occurs in younger age groups
  - Pustular psoriasis
    - Scaling of skin with erythema
    - Lesions will be pustular
    - Associated with fever
- Involvement of other structures
  - Nail

  - Pitting and thickening of nail
  - Destruction of nail can occur.
- Joint involvement
  - Can mimic rheumatoid arthritis
  - Can cause oligo and polyarthritis with destruction of joint (arthritis mutilans)
- Cardiovascualr involvement: Increased associations with cardiovascular events and psoriatic lesions and also increased association with metabolic syndrome.

Treatment
- Topical steroids
- Topical retinoids
- UV light
- Methotrexate
- Cyclosporin

Malaria

Causative Organism

Protozoal disease
- *Plasmodium vivax*
- *Plasmodium ovale*
- *Plasmodium falciparum*
- *Plasmodium malariae*
- *Plasmodium knowlesi.*
- Transmitted by bite of female anopheles mosquitoes.

Life cycle
Mosquito cycle

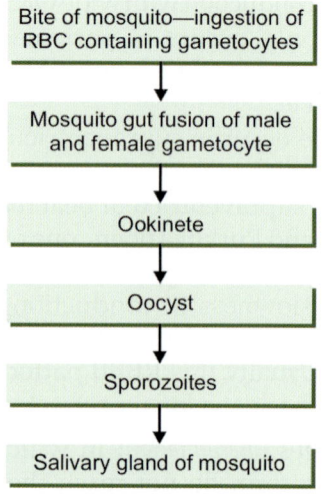

Mosquito cycle:

Bite of mosquito—ingestion of RBC containing gametocytes
↓
Mosquito gut fusion of male and female gametocyte
↓
Ookinete
↓
Oocyst
↓
Sporozoites
↓
Salivary gland of mosquito

Human cycle

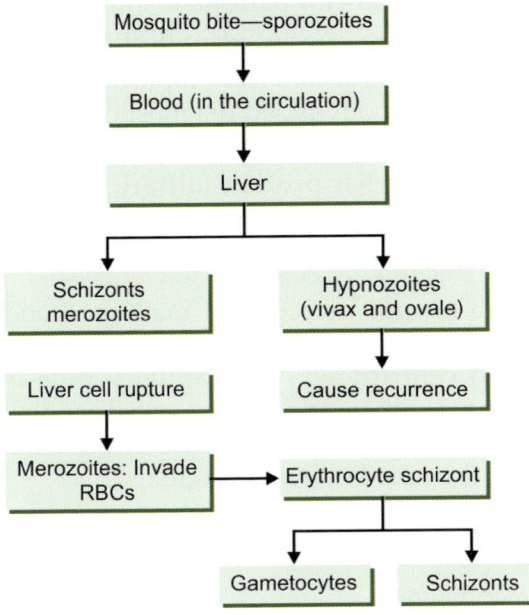

Human cycle:

Mosquito bite—sporozoites
↓
Blood (in the circulation)
↓
Liver
↓
Schizonts merozoites | Hypnozoites (vivax and ovale)
↓ | ↓
Liver cell rupture | Cause recurrence
↓
Merozoites: Invade RBCs → Erythrocyte schizont
↓
Gametocytes | Schizonts

RBC changes caused by the malarial parasite
- Invades RBCs
- Consumes hemoglobin
- Forms malarial pigment called hemozoin from heme.
- Changes in the RBC membranes.
- Changes the antigenic property of RBCs, RBCs alter in their shape.
- Falciparum forms rosetting, agglutination and cyto adherence blocking the micro circulation especially in the brain.

Types of RBCs infected by malarial parasites
- *Plasmodium vivax* and *Plasmodium ovale*: Young RBCs.
- *Plasmodium malariae*—older RBCs
- *Plasmodium falciparum*—all stages of RBCs.

Pathological changes in the host
- Removal of parasite by spleen—splenomegaly.
- Release of proinflammatory cytokines—causes fever.
- Significant immunological response with increase…IgG, IgM.

- Chronic parasitemia without fever in hyperendemic area.

Clinical features: Fever, body ache, headache.

Fever pattern
- Vivax and ovale: Benign tertian—every 3rd day (alternate days)
- Malariae-Quartan—every 4th day.
- Falciparum: Malignant tertian alternate day or irregular or daily (quotidian).
- If the fever is present daily in malaria consider—either Falciparum or mixed infection.
- Paroxysms of fever—coincides with rupture of RBCs.

Characteristics of fever
- Cold phase (30–40 minutes) chills, rigors and sudden onset
- Hot phase: High grade fever 104–106° (hyperpyrexia) with flushing and delirium (4–8 hours).
- Wet phase: Severe sweating and fever decreases.

Signs: Anemia, herpes labialis, jaundice, splenomegaly, hepatomegaly.

Signs which are not present in malaria
- Rash, lymphadenopathy, muscle tenderness, petechiae (rare)
- Neck stiffness.

Falciparum malaria
- Severe anemia
- Thrombocytopenia
- Acute kidney injury
- Malarial hepatitis
- Metabolic acidosis
- Severe hypoglycemia
- ARDS
- Cerebral malaria
- Secondary sepsis.

Severe hypoglycemia
Occurs due to
- Glucose consumption by the host and parasite.
- Decreased production of glucose by the liver.
- Quine therapy stimulating pancreatic insulin secretion.

Cerebral malaria

Presence of

- Convulsions
- Focal neurological deficit
- Coma
- Signs of meningitis is usually absent.

 Note

Certain hemoglobins like Hb E, Hb C, alpha thalassemia, ovalocytosis and sickle cell trait protect against falciparum malaria may be due to impaired growth and multiplication of parasites inside abnormal RBCs.

Black water fever

- Occurs in severe falciparum infection due to severe intravascular hemolysis with hemoglobinuria resulting in renal failure.
- Recurrent malaria occurs with *Pl. vivax* and *ovale* (due to persistent hepatic forms)
- Recurrent malaria does not occur with falciparum.
- Chronic complications of malaria
  - Repeated infection with *Plasmodium malariae* causes nephrotic syndrome.
  - Massive splenomegaly: Tropical spleno-megaly syndrome.
  - May predispose to lymphoproliferative disorders like lymphoma.

Malaria in pregnancy

Can cause

- Abortion
- Low birth weight
- Maternal anemia
- Hypoglycemia and pedal edema
- Premature labor and fetal distress
- Congenital malaria
- Doxycycline and primaquine—contraindi-cated in pregnancy.
- Chloroquine—safe in pregnancy

 Note

Malaria can also be transmitted by blood transfusion, needle sharing with shorter incubation period.

Investigations

Blood smear

- Thick smear—for parasite identification
- Thin smear—species identification.
- Finger prick, or card test—rapid diagnostic tests: Antibody-based diagnostic tests.
- For example, LDH, aldolase antigen and histidine rich protein (all are malaria specific).

QBC (Quantitative buffy coat test for malaria)

- Lab test for detection of malaria. Blood sample is taken in a QBC capillary tube and centrifuged. The capillary tube is coated with fluorescent dye called acridine orange. Parasites with fluorescent dye can be examined under UV light.

PCR: Amplication of nucleic acid of the parasite.

Other findings

- Severe anemia thrombocytopenia, raised blood urea, creatinine.
- Abnormal LFT, prolonged PT and APTT.

CSF: High opening pressure (otherwise normal) in cerebral malaria.

TROPICAL SPLENOMEGALY SYNDROME

Also called hyperactive malarial syndrome.

- Found in endemic area of malaria.
- Occurs due to chronic antigenic stimula-tion.
- There is severe stimulation of lymphoid series (B lymphocytes) with increased production of IgM.

Clinical features

- Patient is from endemic area of malaria.
- Abdominal distention with massive splenomegaly.
- Associated with severe anemia and weight loss.
- Fever is usually not present.
- Mild hepatomegaly and jaundice may be associated.

Diagnostic features

- Massive splenomegaly.
- Raised IGM levels
- Hepatic sinusoidal lymphocytosis.
- Responds to antimalarial treatment
- Peripheral smear for malaria is usually negative.
- PCR indirect immunological tests may be positive for malarial antibodies.

Lichen Planus

- Papulosquamous disorder of skin.
- Lesions are covered by grey lines called Wickham's striae.

Site of involvement

- Skin over the wrist
- Legs and scalp
- Oral mucosa
- It may from whitish lesion in the tongue and oral mucosa and can cause alopecia.
- There can be associated with hepatitis C and may be a predisposing factor for squamous cell carcinoma.
- Local application of steroids is helpful.

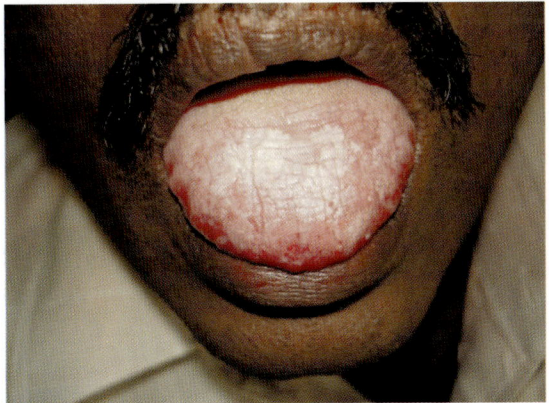

Fig. 10.6: Oral white lesions—lichen planus

Pemphigus Vulgaris

- Blistering form of skin disease.
- Age group involved—usually 4th to 5th decade.
- It is usually the IgA autoantibody mediated.

- Pathology
  - There is separation of epidermis.
  - There is loss of binding between epithelial cells.
  - There is involvement of skin and mucosa.
  - Inflammatory infiltration with leucocytes and eosinophils.
  - IgA antibodies get deposited on keratinocytes.

Features

- Itching
- Pain
- Secondary infection
- Scarring
- Pigmentation

Treatment: Corticosteroids.

Leprosy

Causative organism: *Mycobacterium leprae*: Acid-fast bacillus.

Transmission

- Close contact with infected persons
- Respiratory secretions can contain *M. leprae*.

Clinical features: A form of granulomatous disease.

Incubation period: 5 or more years.

Part affected: Cooler parts of the body—skin, nerves, eye, testes, etc.

Spectrum of disease

- Tuberculoid
- Borderline tuberculoid (BT)
- Borderline borderline
- Borderline lepromatous
- Lepromatous.

Tuberculoid leprosy (Paucibacillary)

- Immunologically more reactive patients
- Less severe disease
- Affects peripheral nerves and skin.

Skin lesions

- Maculoanaesthetic patches
- Few
- Asymmetrical

- Red and raised borders.
- Scaly, dry without sweating with loss of hair.
- Few number of bacillus in the lesion (paucibacillary)
- Enlarged peripheral nerves (ulnar, posterior auricular, lateral popliteal).
- Anesthesia in the distribution of the nerve with muscle involvement.
- Patients produce strong positive lepromin test.

Lepromatous Leprosy (Multibacillary)

- Immunologically less reactive.
- More severe disease.
- Multiple may be symmetrical skin lesions less demarcated with nodules and skin infiltration.
- Can have involvement of eyebrows (madarosis), ear lobes, face (leonine facies).
- Large number of bacilli are present and cause nerve involvement (with symmetrically thickened nerves).
- Systemic involvement can occur except lungs and CNS (are usually spared in leprosy).
- Immunologically less competent and so lepromin skin test is negative.

Lepra reactions: Usually occurs after starting chemotherapy.

Type I reaction

- Can have exacerbation of previous lesions/fresh lesions appear.
- Nerve involvement with nerve damage.
- Systemic steroids are indicated if nerves are involved.
- If occurs after starting the treatment, indicates more immunologically reactive (reversal reaction) and more tendency to become tuberculoid. If occurs before starting the treatment, indicates less immunologically reactive (downgrading) and tendency to become more lepromatous.

Type 2 reactions (ENL: Erythema Nodosum Leprosum)

- Occurs in lepromatous leprosy
- Usually after starting chemotherapy

- Possibly TNF mediated.
- Develop fever, increased number of red popular lesions, nerve involvement and multisystem involvement (eye, testes, kidney, blood, etc.).

Lucio phenomenon

- Found in lepromatous leprosy
- Ulcerative lesions in the lower limb
- Becomes infected secondarily
- Multiple bacilli causing necrosis of epidermis and dermis.

Diagnosis: Skin smear/biopsy of the lesion for AFV.

Complications

Neuropathy

- Painless ulcers
- Polyneuropathy
- Mononeuropathy/mononeuropathy multiplex
- Vth nerve palsy
- Facial palsy
- Wrist drop, foot drop
- Clawhand
- Nerve abscess.

Involves eye, nose, and testes

Eye

- Exposure keratitis
- Loss of corneal sensation
- Uveitis
- Corneal damage.

Nose

- Rhinitis
- Epistaxis
- Saddle nose

Testes: Orchitis, infertility, impotence.

Systemic complications of leprosy

- In lepramatous leprosy
- Glomerulonephritis
- Amyloidosis
- Secondary bacterial infection.

Kala Azar (Black Fever)/Visceral Leishmaniasis

Causative agent: Leishmania donovani.

Clinical features

- Fever with chills and rigors and sweating, weight loss.
- Increased pigmentation of skin (kala azar)
- Massive splenomegaly
- Mid hepatomegaly + lymphadenopathy.
- Pancytopenia.

Investigations

- Skin smear for the parasite
- Skin test for Leishmania is positive
- Bone marrow aspiration for the parasite
- Splenic aspiration for the parasite.

Other methods: Like PCR, monoclonal antibody techniques.

Cysticercosis

Causative agent: Larvae from the eggs of the tapeworm: Tenia solium.

Occurs due to

- Swallowing of eggs of Tenia solium (may be fecal matter)
- Usually from close contact of person who is a tapeworm carrier or vegetables contaminated with eggs.
- Eating meat of pork which is not properly cooked does not result in cysticercosis but can cause intestinal tapeworm infestation.

Parts affected

- Brain—can present with seizures.
- Muscle—can produce subcutaneous swellings.
- Other internal organs including eye.

Diagnosis

- Neuroimaging studies
- Demonstration of antibodies to cysticerci.

Treatment

- Albendazole/Praziquantel
- Anticerebral edema measures
- Antiepileptics, corticosteroids, surgery.

Syphilis

Causative organism: Treponema pallidum (spirochete).

Type of disease

- Infectious disease involving multiple systems.
- Incubation period 4–6 weeks
- Route of spread—usually sexual route.
- Other modes of spread
  - Blood transfusion
  - Fetus from utero
  - Organ transplantation

Clinical manifestations

- Primary syphilis (after 4–6 weeks of contact)
- Characteristic lesion—syphilitic chancre.
- Site—at genitalia
- Homosexuals—anal canal and rectum

Features

- Ulcerative lesion with indurated base with well-defined borders.
- Local lymphadenopathy—usually inguinal firm, painless.
- Primary lesion heal spontaneously within 4–6 weeks.

Secondary syphilis: Occurs after 6 weeks to 8 weeks of healing of primary infection.

Features: Involvement of skin, mucosa, parenchymal lesions and lymph nodes.

General features: Fever body ache and weight loss.

Skin lesions: Maculopapular/coppery brown rash, involving extremities trunk.

Mucosal lesions

- Snail tract ulcers over the mucosa.
- Ulcers with red erythematous margins.

Condyloma lata

- Moist areas—perineum, pink/grey white lesions.
- Can develop generalized lymphadenopathy and alopecia areata.

Other features: Uveitis, hepatitis, nephritis, optic neuritis.

Latent syphilis: Suggested by: No clinical manifestations, positive serological tests for syphilis, normal CSF.

Early latent: 1st year after the infection.

Late latent: After 1st year after the infection.

Tertiary syphilis (late syphilis)

- Usually after 2 years of latent syphilis.
- Can occur after decades of latent stage.
- Involvement of skin, mucosa, CNS and cardiovascular system.

Benign tertiary syphilis

Syphilitic gumma

- Granulomatous lesion
- Central area of necrosis
- Can involve skin, bones
- Can develop ulcers with slough

CNS syphilis

- CNS can be involved in early stages of syphilis
- May be asymptomatic
  - No clinical manifestations
  - CSF +ve for VDRL
  - CSF cell count is increased.

Symptomatic neurosyphilis

- Meningeal meningitis
- Meningovascular can cause endarteritis obliterans and CVA.

Parenchymatous syphilis

- Usually occurs in late syphilis
- For example, general paresis of insane
- Tabes dorsalis.

General paresis of insane

- Usually after 10–40 years of primary infection
- Form of chronic encephalitis
- There will be atrophy of frontal and temporal lobes.

Features

- Memory loss
- Decreasing intelligence
- Cognitive defect

- Speech disturbance
- Exaggerated reflexes
- Argyll Robertson pupil

Tabes dorsalis

- After 20–30 years of primary infection.
- Involvement of posterior root, ganglia and posterior column.

Features

- Severe sensory ataxia
- Posterior column sensory loss
- Joint and position sense loss
- Optic atrophy
- Argyll Robertson pupil
- Charcot's joints.

Congenital syphilis

- Due to transmission of infection from mother to fetus.
- Immunological reaction causing damage to fetal structures.

Early congenital syphilis

- Within 1st 2 years of birth.
- Involves mucosal lesion, skin involvement. Appearance of rash.
- Formation of blebs and condyloma lata.
- Can cause hepatitis, jaundice, heptosplenomegaly, lymphadenopathy.

Late congenital syphilis

After 2 years of birth

- Deafness—8th cranial nerve palsy
- Palatal gumma
- Keratitis.

Can have stigmata of syphilis

- Saddle nose
- Mulberry molars
- Clutton's joints
- Hutchinson's teeth

Diagnosis: 2 types of tests: Treponemal and non-treponemal tests.

Non-treponemal antibody tests

- IgM/IgG type of reactive antibodies against cardiolipin-lecithin and cholesterol antigen. For example, VDRL and RPR tests.

- VDL and RPR can be used as screening tests.
- Confirmation is by FTA-Abs test

Treponemal tests
- Reactive against treponemal antigens. For example, TPHA (treponema pallidum hemagglutination test)
- FTA-Abs (fluorescent treponema antibody absorption test).

CSF test-Gold standard for CNS syphilis: A non-reactive CSF FTA test—rules out neurosyphilis.

False positive serological tests: Occurs in following conditions

SLE	Elderly
TB	Malaria
Leprosy	After vaccination

STEVENS-JOHNSON SYNDROME

It is a type of hypersensitivity reaction of skin and mucosa usually due to drugs.

Pathological Features

- Detachment of mucosa and epidermis
- Epidermal necrosis.
- If there is less than 10% of epidermis is involved, it is Stevens-Johnson syndrome.
- If the involvement is more than 30% of epidermal involvement, it indicates toxic epidermal necrolysis (TEN).

Offending agents
Usually drug induced
- Sulpha drugs
- Cotrimoxazole
- NSAIDs
- Nevirapine.

Features
- Mucosal involvement
- Blister formation over the skin
- Conjunctival involvement
- There can be associated fever
- Secondary infection
- Rarely pulmonary and intestinal involvement.

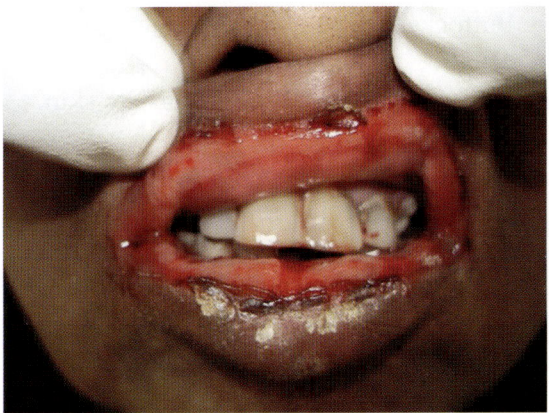

Fig. 10.7: Oral lesions: Drug-induced Stevens-Johnson syndrome

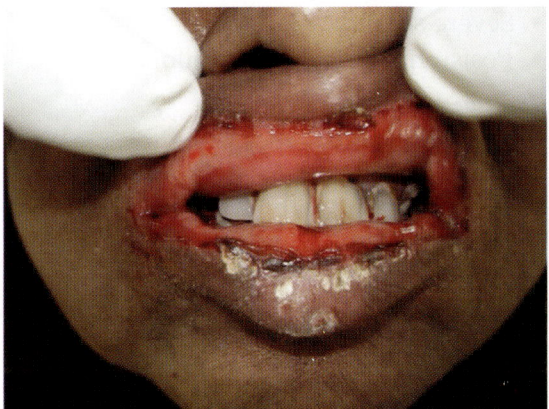

Fig. 10.8: Oral lesions: Drug-induced Stevens-Johnson syndrome

Treatment
- Stop the offending agent
- Corticosteroids.

SCABIES

Causative organism: *Sarcoptes scabiei* (itch mite).

Mode of spread
- Direct skin contact
- From person to person—female mites are transmitted from person to person.

Site involved
- Web spaces of digits
- Genitalia

- Buttocks
- Thigh

Characteristic lesions: Burrows in the skin.

Features
- Severe itching especially nocturnal.
- Hypersensitivity reaction with severe inflammatory lesions.
- Develops secondary streptococcal infection.

Norwegian scabies
- Occurs in immune compromised individuals.
- There will be infection with large numbers of itch mites.

Complications
- Severe secondary infection
- Poststreptococcal glomerulonephritis.

Treatment
- Topical application of pyrethrin cream
- Personal hygiene
- Rx of contacts.

Cutaneous Larva Migrans

Caused by larvae of
- *Ancylostoma braziliense* (cat hookworm)
- *Ancylostoma caninum* (dog hookworm)
- Due to the migration of larvae through the skin.

Features
Site involved
- They form the track with red papules—slowly moving 2–3 cm/day
- Associated with severe itching
- Can become infected/vesiculated. It can progress for a few weeks.
- Systemic features are absent.

Treatment: Thiabendazle/Albendazole/Ivermectin.

Visceral Larva Migrans

Caused by migration of larvae of *Toxocara canis* and *Toxocara catis*. Can spread to other organs through blood stream and can cause organ damage.

Can affect
- Liver
- Myocardium
- CNS causing seizures
- Eye: May mimic retinoblastoma

DIAGNOSIS OF HIV INFECTION

Following laboratory tests are used
1. By direct detection of HIV
2. Detection of components of HIV
3. Detection of antibodies to HIV (appears around 2–3 weeks after the initial infection).

Screening test
- Detects antibody to HIV by ELISA technique.
- Usually lab detects—both HIV-1 and HIV-2 viruses.
- Tests are scored as non-reactive (negative) or highly reactive (positive) or partially reactive (indeterminate).

Tests can be false positive
- After recurrent blood transfusion
- Transplantation
- Liver disease
- Vaccination
- Viral infection.
- Rarely HIV infected individuals can be negative if treated early but can become positive if treatment is discontinued.

Confirmatory tests
- *Western blot*: Detects specific antigens with different molecular weight. Specific antibodies to these antigens can be detected by western blot as bands. Negative western blot—no bands are seen.
- Positive or indeterminate ELISA but negative western blot—test is false positive.
- If antibodies to all 3 major genes—gag, pol and env are present—infection with HIV.
- Positive western blot: If antibodies to 2 of the 3 major HIV proteins—p24, gp 41 and gp120/160 are present.

- If there is absence of p24 band—more likely that test is negative—confirm with RNA-based test-for HIV-1 or follow-up western blot.
- Indeterminate western blot—less immune response individuals/repeat test after 1 month.
- If initial ELISA is negative—test to be repeated if clinically indicated (if exposed within 3 months).
- If ELISA is positive/indeterminate—repeat the test.
- If ELISA is negative or two occasions: Test is negative.
- If repeat test is positive/indeterminate—perform western blot.
- If western blot is positive: Indicative of HIV infection.
- If western blot is negative: Not indicative of HIV infection
- If western blot is indeterminate—repeat after 6 weeks—or perform p24 capture assay, or
  - HIV-1 RNA assay or
  - HIV-1 DNA PCR or
  - Tests for HIV-2
- Rapid diagnostic tests: Gives results in 1 to 60 minutes
- Oral quick rapid HIV-1 antibody test
- Can be done on blood, saliva or plasma.

Direct detection of HIV components
P24-antigen capture assay:
- Present initially before immune response occurs.
- Its level increases as the disease progresses.
- Very useful test in the stage of acute HIV syndrome before antibody detection by ELISA.
- HIV-RNA assay for detecting the level of viremia and response to treatment.
- RT-PCR can also be used for HIV RNA level.

Laboratory monitoring of HIV infection
CD4 count
- Determines the patient's immunological status

- If count is <200 cell/cmm—diagnostic of AIDS
- Increased risk of *Pneumocystis jiroveci* infection.
- If <50 cells/cumm—infection with CMV, *Mycobacterium avium intracellulare* and *Toxoplasma gondii*.
- CD4 count is measured once in 3–6 months.
- Hypersplenism and bone marrow suppressive therapy can interfere with CD4 count.

HIV RNA determination
- For monitoring the therapeutic response.
- Usual technique used: RT PCR
- Indicated at the time of diagnosis and even after 3–6 months
- After starting ART-HIV RNA copy will be less than 50 copies/ml within 6 months of therapy.

HIV resistance testing
- Indicated at the time of diagnosis
- At starting ART
- If there is virological failure.

ACQUIRED IMMUNE DEFICIENCY SYNDROME
Aetiological agent: Retrovirus.
Retrovirus causing disease in humans:
- HIV-1 and HIV-2 viruses
- HTLV-1 and HTLV-2 viruses
- Commonest cause of HV infection: HIV-1 virus.
- HIV-2 virus was initially found in Africa.

Important aspects of HIV virus: It is a RNA virus and with the enzyme reverse transcriptase genomic RNA reverse transcriptases to DNA. Its major envelop proteins are gp120 and gp 41.

Transmission
Sexual
- Heterosexual and homosexual
- Mother to infant: Perinatal and through breast milk.
- Needle sharing/needle prick
- Blood transfusion and blood product transfusion.

Not transmitted by
- Casual contact or through mosquitoes.
- Body secretions—urine, sweat, tears and saliva—do not transmit.

Pathogenesis
- Binds to CD4 receptors
- There will be occurrence of viremia causing clinical HIV infection.
- Characterised by severe immune deficiency of CD4 (T helper) cells.
- Replication of virus occurs in the lymphatic system.

Mechanism of immune deficiency
- Destruction of CD4 lymphocytes
- Death of cell (direct infection of the cells)
- Exhaustion of immune system and cell dysfunction.

Acute HIV infection: Can occur within 2 to 4 weeks after contacting the infection.

Features
- Fever, bodyache, joint pain
- Vomiting and diarrhea
- Lymphadenopathy
- Mucocutaneous rash
- Meningoencephalitis
- Peripheral neuropathy

Asymptomatic stage: Can be up to 8–10 years without significant decline in the CD4 count/increase in the HIV RNA load.

Clinical HIV infection: Occurs after latency with decrease in the CD4 count (<200 cells/L) and increase in the viral load.

Manifestations of HIV infection: Acquired immune deficiency syndrome.

Clinical manifestations
Cardiovascular
- Increased incidence of IHD (presence of procoagulant state)
- Pulmonary hypertension
- Cardiomyopathy
- Pericardial effusion.

Gastrointestinal
- Oral—candidiasis, aphthous ulcers
- Hairy leucoplakia.

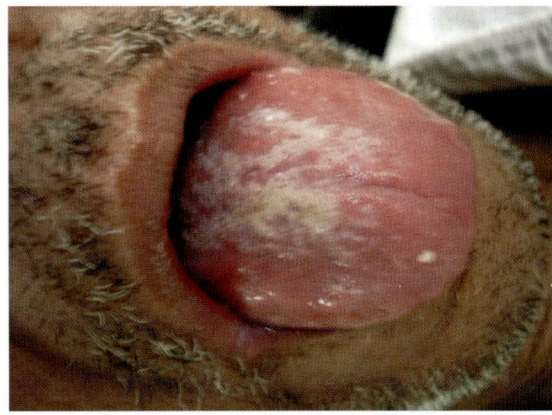

Fig. 10.9: Oral candidiasis

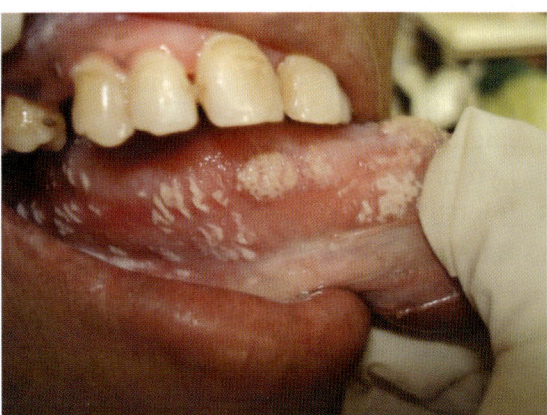

Fig. 10.10: Oral candidiasis

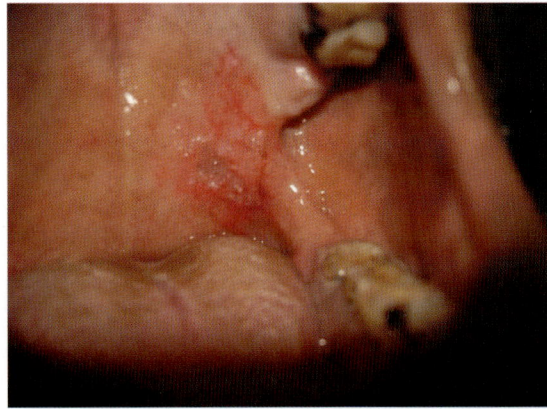

Fig. 10.11: Oral aphthous ulcers

Intestinal
- Gram-negative infection
- Compylobacter infection

- *Isospora belli* infection
- *Salmonella typhimurium*
- Cryptosporidiosis
- Microsporidia infection
- Tuberculosis
- HSV and EBV infection.

Oesophageal
- Candidiasis
- Herpes, simplex/EBV infection
- Kaposis sarcoma

HIV enteropathy, lymphoma
Disseminated strongyloidosis

Respiratory
- Gram positive/Gram-negative pneumonia
- Pulmonary TB/atypical mycobacterial infection
- Pneumocystis/fungal infection
- Lymphoma/Kaposi's sarcoma
- Interstitial pneumonia

Hepatobiliary—including pancreas
- Hepatitis including granulomatous hepatitis
- Co-infection with hepatitis B and C
- Fungal infection
- Pancreatitis

Hematological
- Pancytopenia
- Generalised lymphadenopathy
- Persistant generalized lymphadenopathy
- Lymphoma
- Venous thrombosis.

Renal and urogenital
- HIV nephropathy (collapsing glomerulopathy: FSGS)
- Tenofovir-induced renal failure
- UTI
- Genital infection: Candidial/herpetic

Endocrinal
- Thyroid dysfunction
- Metabolic syndrome mainly due to protease
- Hypogonadism
- SIADH

Rheumatological
- Athralgia
- Polyarthritis: Reactive arthritis
- Septic arthritis

Immunoglogical
- Drug reactions
- Immune reconstitution syndrome.

Nervous system manifestations
CNS infections
- Tuberculosis
- Toxoplasmosis
- Cryptococcosis
- Trypanasomiasis
- CMV infection
- Due to syphilis

CNS: Lymphoma
HIV dementia complex
Progressive multifocal leucoencephalopathy (JC virus infection)
Cerebrovascular accident.

Spinal cord manifestations
- Vascular myelopathy
- Posterior column dysfunction with sensory ataxia.

Peripheral nervous system
- AIDP in acute seroconversion stage
- CIDP
- Distal sensory neuropathy
- Drug induced: Stavudine induced
- Mononeuritis multiplex

Muscular involvement
- Myopathy
- Drug induced: Zudovidine induced.

Causes of convulsions in a patient of HIV infection
- Toxoplasma of brain
- Cryptococcal infection/TB infection
- HIV encephalopathy
- Progressive multifocal leucoencephalopthy.
- Lymphoma

Skin manifestations
- Herpes zoster
- Psoriasis
- Folliculitis

- Molluscum contagiosum
- Herpes simplex infection
- Kaposi's sarcoma
- Drug induced: Stevens-Johnson syndrome
- Pigmentation of nails
  - HIV-induced yellow nails
  - Zudovidine-induced blue nails.

Eye involvement
- Retinopathy: Exudates and hemorrhage
- CMV retinopathy
- Herpes zoster and simplex infection

Miscellaneous manifestations
- Severe emaciation—wasting syndrome
- Leishmaniasis
- Histoplasmosis
- Bartonellosis

Malignant disorders associated with HIV infection
- Kaposis sarcoma
- Lymphoma
  - CNS lymphoma
  - Burkitt's lymphoma
- Castleman's disease—lymphoproliferative disorder
- Cervical/anal dysplasia—associated human papillomavirus.

HERPES ZOSTER

Causative agent: Varicella zoster virus.

Common predisposing conditions
- Immune compromised conditions (diabetes mellitus, on steroids).
- HIV infection
- Age group >60 years.

Occurs due to: Reactivation of the virus which is present in dorsal root ganglia.

Features
- Localised pain in the dermatomal pattern: Unilateral.
- Usual dermatomes involved:
  - T3 to L3 dermatomes.
  - Ophthalmic division of trigeminal nerve.
- Fever
- Maculopapular to vesicular eruption in the distribution of the dermatome with crust formation.

Complications
- Herpes zoster ophthalmicus
- Ramsay Hunt syndrome (due to herpes zoster of geniculate ganglion)
- Rare—meningoencephalitis.
- Transverse myelitis
- Transmission of chickenpox
- Chronic: Postherpetic neuralgia

Multidermatomal herpes zoster
- More than one dermatome is involved
- Common on HIV infection.

Other causes of unilateral distribution of lesions/ rash
- HSV infection
- Coxsackie infection

Index